W9-CNM-332

Pulmonary Disease and Pregnancy

Guest Editor

GHADA BOURJEILY, MD

CLINICS IN CHEST MEDICINE

www.chestmed.theclinics.com

March 2011 • Volume 32 • Number 1

SAUNDERS an imprint of ELSEVIER, Inc.

W.B. SAUNDERS COMPANY
A Division of Elsevier Inc.

1600 John F. Kennedy Boulevard • Suite 1800 • Philadelphia, Pennsylvania 19103

http://www.theclinics.com

CLINICS IN CHEST MEDICINE Volume 32, Number 1
March 2011 ISSN 0272-5231, ISBN-13: 978-1-4557-0429-3

Editor: Sarah E. Barth
Developmental Editor: Jessica Demetriou

© **2011 Elsevier Inc. All rights reserved.**

This journal and the individual contributions contained in it are protected under copyright by Elsevier, and the following terms and conditions apply to their use:

Photocopying
Single photocopies of single articles may be made for personal use as allowed by national copyright laws. Permission of the Publisher and payment of a fee is required for all other photocopying, including multiple or systematic copying, copying for advertising or promotional purposes, resale, and all forms of document delivery. Special rates are available for educational institutions that wish to make photocopies for non-profit educational classroom use. For information on how to seek permission visit www.elsevier.com/permissions or call: (+44) 1865 843830 (UK)/(+1) 215 239 3804 (USA).

Derivative Works
Subscribers may reproduce tables of contents or prepare lists of articles including abstracts for internal circulation within their institutions. Permission of the Publisher is required for resale or distribution outside the institution. Permission of the Publisher is required for all other derivative works, including compilations and translations (please consult www.elsevier.com/permissions).

Electronic Storage or Usage
Permission of the Publisher is required to store or use electronically any material contained in this journal, including any article or part of an article (please consult www.elsevier.com/permissions). Except as outlined above, no part of this publication may be reproduced, stored in a retrieval system or transmitted in any form or by any means, electronic, mechanical, photocopying, recording or otherwise, without prior written permission of the Publisher.

Notice
No responsibility is assumed by the Publisher for any injury and/or damage to persons or property as a matter of products liability, negligence or otherwise, or from any use or operation of any methods, products, instructions or ideas contained in the material herein. Because of rapid advances in the medical sciences, in particular, independent verification of diagnoses and drug dosages should be made.

Although all advertising material is expected to conform to ethical (medical) standards, inclusion in this publication does not constitute a guarantee or endorsement of the quality or value of such product or of the claims made of it by its manufacturer.

Clinics in Chest Medicine (ISSN 0272-5231) is published quarterly by Elsevier Inc., 360 Park Avenue South, New York, NY 10010-1710. Months of issue are March, June, September, and December. Periodicals postage paid at New York, NY and additional mailing offices. Subscription prices are $293.00 per year (domestic individuals), $475.00 per year (domestic institutions), $140.00 per year (domestic students/residents), $321.00 per year (Canadian individuals), $583.00 per year (Canadian institutions), $399.00 per year (international individuals), $583.00 per year (international institutions), and $195.00 per year (international and Canadian students/residents). International air speed delivery is included in all Clinics subscription prices. All prices are subject to change without notice. **POSTMASTER:** Send address changes to Clinics in Chest Medicine, Elsevier Health Sciences Division, Subscription Customer Service, 3251 Riverport Lane, Maryland Heights, MO 63043. **Customer Service: Telephone: 1-800-654-2452** (U.S. and Canada); **1-314-447-8871** (outside U.S. and Canada). **Fax: 1-314-447-8029. E-mail: journalscustomerservice-usa@elsevier.com** (for print support); **journalsonlinesupport-usa@elsevier.com** (for online support).

Reprints. For copies of 100 or more of articles in this publication, please contact the Commercial Reprints Department, Elsevier Inc., 360 Park Avenue South, New York, NY 10010-1710. Tel.: 212-633-3812; Fax: 212-462-1935; E-mail: reprints@elsevier.com.

Clinics in Chest Medicine is covered in *MEDLINE/PubMed (Index Medicus), Current Contents/Clinical Medicine, EMBASE/ Excerpta Medica, Science Citation Index,* and *ISI/BIOMED.*

Printed in the United States of America.

Contributors

GUEST EDITOR

GHADA BOURJEILY, MD
Assistant Professor of Medicine, Pulmonary and Critical Care Medicine, Department of Medicine, Women and Infants Hospital of Rhode Island, The Warren Alpert Medical School of Brown University, Providence, Rhode Island

AUTHORS

GINA ANKNER, RN, MSN
Senior Nurse Coordinator, Department of Medicine, Women and Infants Hospital of Rhode Island, Providence, Rhode Island

VENKATA BANDI, MD
Associate Professor, Pulmonary, Critical Care and Sleep Medicine, Baylor College of Medicine, Houston, Texas

KATHRYN BILELLO, MD
Associate Clinical Professor of Medicine, Department of Medicine, University of California San Francisco-Fresno Program, Fresno, California

GHADA BOURJEILY, MD
Assistant Professor of Medicine, Pulmonary and Critical Care Medicine, Department of Medicine, Women and Infants Hospital of Rhode Island, The Warren Alpert Medical School of Brown University, Providence, Rhode Island

ROBERT BRENT, MD, PhD, DSc (Hon)
Distinguished Professor of Pediatrics, Radiology, Pathology, Anatomy, and Cell Biology; Louis and Bess Stein Professor of Pediatrics; Emeritus Professor of the Department of Pediatrics, Jefferson Medical College, Philadelphia, Pennsylvania; Head, Laboratory of Clinical and Environmental Teratology, Research Department, Alfred I. duPont Hospital for Children, Wilmington, Delaware

VERONICA BRITO, MD
Fellow, Pulmonary and Critical Care Medicine, Winthrop-University Hospital, Mineola, New York

MICHEL CHALHOUB, MD
Associate Clinical Professor of Medicine, Director of Interventional Endoscopy and Fellowship Program, Department of Medicine, Pulmonary and Critical Care Medicine, Staten Island University Hospital, Staten Island, New York

J.F. CORDIER, MD
Department of Respiratory Medicine, Reference Centre for Rare Pulmonary Diseases, Hospices Civils de Lyon, Louis Pradel Hospital, University of Lyon I, Lyon, France

V. COTTIN, MD, PhD
Department of Respiratory Medicine, Reference Centre for Rare Pulmonary Diseases, Hospices Civils de Lyon, Louis Pradel Hospital, University of Lyon I, Lyon, France

ROBERT O. CRAPO, MD
Professor of Medicine, Division of Pulmonary and Critical Care Medicine, LDS Hospital, University of Utah, Utah

ARMIN ERNST, MD, FCCP
Chief, Interventional Pulmonology, Beth Israel Deaconess Medical Center; Associate Professor of Medicine and Surgery, Harvard Medical School, Boston, Massachusetts

N. FREYMOND, MD
Department of Respiratory Medicine,
Reference Centre for Rare Pulmonary
Diseases, Hospices Civils de Lyon,
Louis Pradel Hospital, University of Lyon I,
Lyon, France

PETER G. GIBSON, MBBS (Hons), FRACP
Conjoint Professor, Centre for Asthma and
Respiratory Diseases, University of
Newcastle and Hunter Medical Research
Institute; Department of Respiratory
and Sleep Medicine, John Hunter Hospital,
Newcastle, New South Wales, Australia;
Woolcock Institute of Medical Research,
Sydney, New South Wales, Australia

KALPALATHA K. GUNTUPALLI, MD
Professor of Medicine, Pulmonary, Critical
Care and Sleep Medicine Section, Baylor
College of Medicine, Houston, Texas

MATTHEW J. HEGEWALD, MD
Assistant Professor of Medicine, Division
of Pulmonary and Critical Care Medicine,
Intermountain Medical Center, University of
Utah, Murray; Director, Pulmonary Function
Laboratory, Intermountain Medical Center,
Murray, Utah

COLLEEN GLYDE JULIAN, PhD
Altitude Research Center, Department of
Emergency Medicine, Anschutz Medical
Campus, University of Colorado Denver,
Aurora, Colorado

C. RANDALL LANE, MD
Postdoctoral Fellow, Section of Pulmonary
and Critical Care Medicine, Yale University
School of Medicine, New Haven,
Connecticut

LUCIA LARSON, MD
Assistant Professor of Medicine and
Obstetrics and Gynecology, Division
Director and Fellowship Director,
Division of Obstetric and Consultative
Medicine, Department of Medicine,
Women and Infants Hospital of Rhode
Island, The Warren Alpert Medical
School of Brown University,
Providence, Rhode Island

JOHN R. MCARDLE, MD, FCCP
Associate Professor of Medicine,
Section of Pulmonary and Critical Care
Medicine, Yale University School of
Medicine, New Haven, Connecticut

NIHARIKA MEHTA, MD
Assistant Professor of Medicine,
Division of Obstetric and Consultative
Medicine, Department of Medicine, Women
and Infants Hospital of Rhode Island, The
Warren Alpert Medical School of Brown
University, Providence, Rhode Island

GIACOMO MESCHIA, MD
Professor Emeritus, Departments of
Physiology and Pediatrics, Perinatal
Research Facility, University of Colorado
School of Medicine, Aurora, Colorado

MARGARET A. MILLER, MD
Assistant Professor of Medicine and
Obstetrics and Gynecology, Director of
Ambulatory Services, Division of Obstetric
and Consultative Medicine, Women and
Infants' Hospital of Rhode Island,
The Warren Alpert Medical School of
Brown University, Providence,
Rhode Island

VAHID MOHSENIN, MD
Professor of Medicine, Yale Center for
Sleep Medicine, Division of Pulmonary,
Critical Care and Sleep Medicine, Yale
University School of Medicine,
New Haven, Connecticut

ROSS K. MORGAN, MD, FRCPI, FCCP
Consultant Respiratory Physician, Department
of Respiratory Medicine, Beaumont Hospital,
Dublin, Ireland

UMA MUNNUR, MD
Associate Professor, Department of
Anesthesiology, Baylor College of Medicine,
Houston, Texas

SUSAN MURIN, MD, MSc
Professor of Clinical Medicine, Division
of Pulmonary, Critical Care and Sleep
Medicine, University of California Davis
School of Medicine; Veterans Affairs
Northern California Health System,
Sacramento, California

VANESSA E. MURPHY, BMedChem (Hons), PhD
Postdoctoral Research Fellow, Centre for
Asthma and Respiratory Diseases, University
of Newcastle and Hunter Medical Research
Institute, New Lambton Heights; Department of
Respiratory and Sleep Medicine, John Hunter
Hospital, Newcastle, New South Wales,
Australia

**MICHAEL S. NIEDERMAN, MD, FACP,
FCCP, FCCM**
Chairman, Department of Medicine, Winthrop
University Hospital, Mineola, New York;
Department of Medicine, SUNY at Stony
Brook, New York

ROKHSARA RAFII, MD, MPH
Senior Pulmonary/Critical Care Fellow,
Division of Pulmonary, Critical Care and
Sleep Medicine, University of California
Davis School of Medicine; Veterans Affairs
Northern California Health System,
Sacramento, California

TERENCE K. TROW, MD
Assistant Professor of Medicine, Director, Yale
Pulmonary Hypertension Center, Section of
Pulmonary and Critical Care Medicine, Yale
University School of Medicine, New Haven,
Connecticut

Contents

Preface   xiii

Ghada Bourjeily

Respiratory Physiology in Pregnancy   1

Matthew J. Hegewald and Robert O. Crapo

Pregnancy induces marked changes in the respiratory and cardiovascular systems that are essential for meeting the increased metabolic demands of the mother and fetus. Important respiratory system changes occur in the upper airway, chest wall, static lung volumes, and ventilation and gas exchange. Marked cardiovascular changes also occur during pregnancy including increased plasma volume, increased cardiac output, and reduced vascular resistance. Knowledge of these physiologic adaptations is necessary for the clinician to distinguish the common "physiologic dyspnea" from disease states that occur during pregnancy.

Fetal Oxygenation and Maternal Ventilation   15

Giacomo Meschia

In the past 20 years, measurements of umbilical blood flow and umbilical venous Po_2, oxygen saturation, pH, and oxygen capacity have provided reliable information about the state of oxygenation of normal and growth restricted human fetuses. However, no comparable information is available about the uterine circulation. Therefore, understanding of oxygen transport across the human placenta and the effect of maternal ventilation on fetal oxygenation is tentative, and currently based on a model that is derived from evidence in another species. The main purpose of this model is to illustrate the kind of information that is needed to make further progress in this area.

High Altitude During Pregnancy   21

Colleen Glyde Julian

One of the greatest physiologic challenges during pregnancy is to maintain an adequate supply of oxygenated blood to the uteroplacental circulation for fetal development. This challenge is magnified under conditions of limited oxygen availability. High altitude impairs fetal growth, increases the incidence of preeclampsia, and, as a result, significantly increases the risk of perinatal and/or maternal morbidity and mortality. This review summarizes the clinical consequences and physiologic challenges that emerge when pregnancy and high altitude coincide and highlights the adaptations that serve to protect oxygenation and fetal growth under conditions of chronic hypoxia.

The Pulmonologist's Role in Caring for Pregnant Women with Regard to the Reproductive Risks of Diagnostic Radiological Studies or Radiation Therapy   33

Robert Brent

Radiography of the chest, head, neck, teeth, or extremity exposes the embryo or ovary to insignificant exposures of radiation except when radionuclides are utilized. In some instances, there is no exposure at all. Pulmonologists are fortunate with regard to the specific studies they request to provide clinical care because most of the diagnostic tests do not directly expose the uterus (embryo) or ovary. This article discusses radiation risks and their evaluation and pregnancy-related issues in diagnostic radiological studies.

Pharmacotherapy in Pregnancy and Lactation   43

Niharika Mehta and Lucia Larson

Prescribing for patients who are pregnant and breastfeeding can be a challenge for clinicians facing insufficient information regarding medication safety, overestimation of perceived risk of medication both by patients and care providers, and increasing litigation costs. This article aims to guide the clinician in choosing the safest and most effective strategy when prescribing medications to patients who are pregnant and breastfeeding.

Management Principles of the Critically Ill Obstetric Patient   53

Uma Munnur, Venkata Bandi, and Kalpalatha K. Guntupalli

The goals in management of critically ill obstetric patients involve intensive monitoring and physiologic support for patients with life-threatening but potentially reversible conditions. Management principles of the mother should also take the fetus and gestational age into consideration. The most common reasons for intensive care admissions (ICU) in the United States and United Kingdom are hypertensive disorders, sepsis, and hemorrhage. The critically ill obstetric patient poses several challenges to the clinicians involved in her care, because of the anatomic and physiologic changes that take place during pregnancy.

Interventional Chest Procedures in Pregnancy   61

Ross K. Morgan and Armin Ernst

Interventional pulmonology encompasses diagnostic and therapeutic bronchoscopic procedures, and pleural interventions. In the last 10 years older techniques have been refined and exciting new technologies have extended the reach and application of the instruments used. The main areas within pulmonary medicine for which these interventions have a role are malignant and nonmalignant airway disease, pleural effusion, pneumothorax, and artificial airways. There are no data from well-designed prospective trials to guide recommendations for interventional pulmonary procedures in pregnancy. The recommendations provided in this article are based on critical review of reported case series, opinion from recognized experts, and personal observations.

Smoking and Smoking Cessation in Pregnancy   75

Susan Murin, Rokhsara Rafii, and Kathryn Bilello

Smoking during pregnancy is among the leading preventable causes of adverse maternal and fetal outcomes. Smoking prevalence among young women is the primary determinant of smoking prevalence during pregnancy. Smoking among women of childbearing age is associated with reduced fertility, increased complications of pregnancy, and a variety of adverse fetal outcomes. There is increasing evidence of lasting adverse effects on offspring. Guidelines for smoking cessation during pregnancy have been developed. This article reviews the epidemiology of smoking during pregnancy, the adverse effects of smoking on the mother, fetus, and offspring, and recommended approaches to smoking cessation for pregnant women.

Asthma in Pregnancy   93

Vanessa E. Murphy and Peter G. Gibson

> Worldwide the prevalence of asthma among pregnant women is on the rise, and pregnancy leads to a worsening of asthma for many women. This article examines the changes in asthma that may occur during pregnancy, with particular reference to asthma exacerbations. Asthma affects not only the mother but the baby as well, with potential complications including low birth weight, preterm delivery, perinatal mortality, and preeclampsia. Barriers to effective asthma management and opportunities for optimized care and treatment are discussed, and a summary of the clinical guidelines for the management of asthma during pregnancy is presented.

Pregnancy in Cystic Fibrosis   111

John R. McArdle

> The challenges posed by cystic fibrosis (CF), including poor nutrition and progressive lung function decline, may pose problems for pregnancy for both mother and child. A multidisciplinary team of providers is optimal to help address the variety of issues that might arise in such a pregnancy. Careful attention to maternal weight gain, pulmonary function and exacerbations, and screening for gestational diabetes is necessary. Pregnancies among women with CF are associated with more frequent use of intravenous antibiotics and hospitalization than is seen in nonpregnant CF women. This article reviews maternal and fetal outcomes for CF in pregnancy.

Pneumonia Complicating Pregnancy   121

Veronica Brito and Michael S. Niederman

> Community-acquired pneumonia (CAP) can affect pregnancy, posing risks to mother and fetus. CAP is the most common fatal nonobstetric infectious complication and a common cause of hospital readmission. Risk factors of pneumonia in pregnancy relate to anatomic and physiologic respiratory changes and immune changes. Aspiration can occur during labor, can cause life-threatening disease, and is more common in cesarean deliveries. Influenza pneumonia can cause severe disease, increasing the risk of preterm delivery, abortion, cesarean section, maternal respiratory failure, and death. CAP treatment requires considering antimicrobial appropriateness and safety, choosing therapy in line with guidelines, but considering maternal and fetal risk.

Infiltrative Lung Diseases in Pregnancy   133

N. Freymond, V. Cottin, and J.F. Cordier

> Pregnancy may affect the diagnosis, management, and outcome of infiltrative lung disease (ILD). Conversely, ILD may affect pregnancy. ILD may occur as a result of drugs administered commonly or specifically during pregnancy. Most ILDs predominate in patients older than 40 years and are thus rare in pregnant women. During pregnancy ILD may arise de novo and preexisting ILD may be exacerbated or significantly worsened. Some ILDs generally do not alter the management of pregnancy, labor, or delivery. Preexisting ILD no longer contraindicates pregnancy systematically, but thorough evaluation of ILD before pregnancy is required to identify potential contraindications and adapt monitoring.

Peripartum Pulmonary Embolism   147

Margaret A. Miller, Michel Chalhoub, and Ghada Bourjeily

> Pregnancy is an example of Virchow's triad predisposing to the development of venous thromboembolism (VTE). Specific risk factors for antepartum and postpartum

VTE have been identified. The diagnosis of pulmonary embolism in pregnancy is complicated by the physiologic changes of pregnancy as well as physicians' apprehension about ordering radiologic studies during pregnancy because of concerns with fetal well-being. Therapy for VTE is complicated by pregnancy physiology affecting medication pharmacokinetics and bioavailability, and the unpredictable occurrence of labor during therapeutic anticoagulation.

Pregnancy and Pulmonary Hypertension   **165**

C. Randall Lane and Terence K. Trow

When pulmonary hypertension (PH) occurs in pregnancy, physiologic stress can overwhelm an already strained right ventricle resulting in right ventricular failure and death. Mortality remains unacceptably high (25%–30%). Patients with PH should be counseled to avoid pregnancy. This article discusses the physiologic changes of pregnancy that make it difficult for patients with PH, the pitfalls of transthoracic echocardiography in diagnosing PH in pregnancy, and the historical data regarding mortality. The causes of development of PH during pregnancy are discussed, and the limited data on management of patients with PH who choose to carry their pregnancy to term are reviewed.

Sleep-disordered Breathing in Pregnancy   **175**

Ghada Bourjeily, Gina Ankner, and Vahid Mohsenin

Symptoms of sleep-disordered breathing are more common in pregnant women compared with nonpregnant women. It is likely that physiology of pregnancy predisposes to the development or worsening of sleep-disordered breathing, but some physiologic changes may also be protective against the development of this disease. Clinical presentation may be less predictive of sleep disordered breathing in pregnancy than in the non-pregnant population; nonetheless, snoring is associated with adverse pregnancy outcomes. Treatment strategies are similar to the nonpregnant population, however, pregnancy-specific scenarios may arise and these subtleties are addressed in this review.

Index   **191**

Clinics in Chest Medicine

FORTHCOMING ISSUES

June 2011

Lung Transplantation
Robert M. Kotloff, MD,
Guest Editor

September 2011

Respiratory Infections
Michael S. Niederman, MD,
Guest Editor

December 2011

Lung Cancer
Lynn Tanoue, MD, and
Richard Matthay, MD,
Guest Editors

RECENT ISSUES

December 2010

Venous Thromboembolism
Terence K. Trow, MD, and
C. Gregory Elliott, MD,
Guest Editors

September 2010

Pulmonary Manifestations of Rheumatic Disease
Kristin B. Highland, MD, MSCR,
Guest Editor

June 2010

Sleep
H. Klar Yaggi, MD, MPH,
Teofilo L. Lee Chiong Jr, MD, and
Vahid Mohsenin, MD,
Guest Editors

ISSUES OF RELATED INTEREST

Obstetrics and Gynecology Clinics of North America, Volume 37, Issue 2 (June 2010)
Update on Medical Disorders in Pregnancy
Judith U. Hibbard, MD, *Guest Editor*

THE CLINICS ARE NOW AVAILABLE ONLINE!

Access your subscription at:
www.theclinics.com

Preface

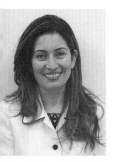

Ghada Bourjeily, MD
Guest Editor

t has been close to two decades since *Clinics in Chest Medicine* has devoted an issue to lung disease in pregnancy. Pregnancy is a unique and special time in a woman's life and most pregnancies are healthy and uneventful. In the twenty-first century, pregnancies are likely more medically complicated than they had ever been. Women in the western world are choosing to conceive later in life. With advances in medical therapy, children with severe hereditary diseases such as cystic fibrosis are now living longer and reaching reproductive years, with many desiring and achieving pregnancy. Assisted reproductive technologies are also helping women with chronic medical illnesses, who would not otherwise have conceived, get pregnant.

With all these cultural and technological changes in the past few decades, many medical practitioners including pulmonologists and intensivists are faced with the multiple challenges of pregnancy. In many circumstances, pregnancy clearly affects disease behavior and, in others, the disease strongly impacts pregnancy outcomes. Fetal harm associated with pharmacotherapy of these diseases and concerns for teratogenicity and oncogenicity associated with radiation exposure complicate the picture even further. Labor and delivery pose a significant hemodynamic challenge and intensify the burden of pregnancy on the respiratory system, leading to a potential for decompensation of many cardiac and respiratory conditions. All these challenges have the potential to lead to adverse outcomes if the clinician is ill-equipped to care for these women.

The purpose of this issue is to arm clinicians with basic knowledge of pregnancy that would help them weigh the risks associated with diagnosis and treatment against the risks of undiagnosed or untreated disease.

This issue dedicates a few articles to discussions of basic principles of pregnancy care. The issue opens with discussions of maternal respiratory and cardiac physiology and the hemodynamic effects of labor and delivery followed by a discussion of fetal oxygenation and ventilation. The article on high altitude in pregnancy is then introduced to highlight the available data linking chronic hypoxia to pregnancy outcomes. Following these reviews, the next articles focus on the use of pharmacotherapy in pregnancy and the effects of radiation exposure in utero. Other articles focusing on the management principles of gravidas include chest interventional procedures and intensive care unit procedures. A variety of airway, vascular, and parenchymal disorders is then followed by a discussion of sleep-disordered breathing in pregnancy. We have opted against a discussion of obstetric disorders in the ICU since a recent article was published in the issue on nonpulmonary critical care in March 2009.

I hope the issue identifies knowledge gaps and promotes pulmonary, critical care, and sleep research in this special population, while discouraging the systematic exclusion of pregnant women from many clinical trials.

I am truly thankful to all of my collaborators and am extremely fortunate to have worked with an

Clin Chest Med 32 (2011) xiii–xiv
doi:10.1016/j.ccm.2010.12.001
0272-5231/11/$ – see front matter © 2011 Elsevier Inc. All rights reserved.

amazing group of scientists, pulmonologists, intensivists, obstetric internists, anesthesiologists, and pediatricians from around the world who have agreed to share their knowledge and expertise in providing these comprehensive reviews. I could not thank the wonderful publisher Sarah Barth and her team enough for making the process so seamless and for everyone's assistance in seeing this product to completion. I would also like to thank my family for their patience and ongoing support.

Ghada Bourjeily, MD
Pulmonary and Critical Care Medicine
Department of Medicine
Women and Infants Hospital of Rhode Island
The Warren Alpert Medical School
of Brown University
100 Dudley Street, Suite 110C
Providence, RI 02905, USA

E-mail address:
GBourjeily@wihri.org

Respiratory Physiology in Pregnancy

Matthew J. Hegewald, MD[a,b,*], Robert O. Crapo, MD[c]

KEYWORDS
- Respiratory physiology • Pregnancy
- Pulmonary function testing

This review discusses respiratory physiologic changes during normal pregnancy. Cardiovascular physiology is also reviewed, given the important interactions between the respiratory and cardiovascular systems in pregnancy. The combination of hormonal changes, mechanical effects of the enlarging uterus, and marked circulatory changes result in significant changes in pulmonary and cardiovascular physiology. These adaptations are necessary to meet the increased metabolic demands of the mother and fetus. It is important for the clinician to be familiar with the normal physiologic changes in pregnancy. Understanding these changes is critical in distinguishing the common dyspnea that occurs during normal pregnancy from pathophysiologic states associated with cardiopulmonary diseases seen in pregnancy,[1] and in anticipating disease worsening in pregnancy and the peripartum period in those women with cardiopulmonary disorders.

UPPER AIRWAY CHANGES IN PREGNANCY

There are significant changes to the mucosa of the nasopharynx and oropharynx during pregnancy. The mucosal changes in the upper airway include hyperemia, edema, leakage of plasma into the stroma, glandular hypersecretion, increased phagocytic activity, and increased mucopolysaccharide content.[2,3] All of these result in nasal congestion often called rhinitis of pregnancy. The clinical definition of rhinitis of pregnancy is "nasal congestion present during the last 6 or more weeks of pregnancy without other signs of respiratory tract infection and with no known allergic cause, disappearing completely within 2 weeks after delivery."[2] The incidence of rhinitis of pregnancy has been reported to be between 18% and 42%.[4–6] Nasal congestion is often noted early in the first trimester, peaks late in pregnancy, and disappears within 48 hours of delivery.[2,4] The etiology of rhinitis of pregnancy is not clear,[2] though increased blood volume and hormonal factors likely play a role. Blood volume changes are discussed later. Hormonal factors include estrogen and placental growth hormone. Nasal mucosal biopsies obtained during pregnancy and from women taking oral contraceptive medications have implicated estrogen as a cause.[3] However, other factors are likely involved, as estrogen levels are not higher in women who have rhinitis of pregnancy than in women who do not.[7] Placental growth hormone may contribute to rhinitis of pregnancy, as levels are significantly higher in patients with the syndrome.[2] Nonhormonal factors implicated in nasal congestion in pregnancy include smoking, nasal allergy, infections, and chronic use of topical vasoconstrictor medication.

Rhinitis of pregnancy has the potential to contribute to maternal-fetal complications. Nasal obstruction contributes to snoring and sleep-disordered breathing, both of which are associated with hypertension and preeclampsia and may

[a] Division of Pulmonary and Critical Care Medicine, Intermountain Medical Center, University of Utah, 5121 South Cottonwood Street, UT 84157, USA
[b] Pulmonary Function Laboratory, Intermountain Medical Center, 5121 South Cottonwood Street, Murray, UT 84157, USA
[c] Division of Pulmonary and Critical Care Medicine, LDS Hospital, University of Utah, 8th Avenue and C Street, Salt Lake City, UT 84103, USA
* Corresponding author. Pulmonary Department, Intermountain Medical Center, PO Box 577000, Murray, UT 84157.
E-mail address: matt.hegewald@imail.org

Clin Chest Med 32 (2011) 1–13
doi:10.1016/j.ccm.2010.11.001
0272-5231/11/$ – see front matter © 2011 Elsevier Inc. All rights reserved.

contribute to intrauterine growth retardation, although the relationship between sleep-disordered breathing and intrauterine growth retardation is controversial.[2,8] Nasal congestion and resultant mouth breathing reduces concentrations of inhaled nitric oxide, primarily produced in the maxillary sinuses.[9] Nitric oxide is a potent mediator of pulmonary vascular tone, and reduced nitric oxide may contribute to the complications associated with snoring. The upper airway congestion and obstruction common in pregnancy may adversely affect the ability of air to pass through nasal and oral tubes.

Mallampati score, a common predictor of airway patency, has been shown to increase during the course of pregnancy.[10] Neck circumference has also been found to be increased with pregnancy,[11,12] and decreases in the postpartum period.[11]

Using acoustic reflectance measurements, oropharyngeal junction size is smaller in the seated position, and mean pharyngeal cross-sectional area is smaller in the supine, lateral, and seated position in pregnant women compared with nonpregnant controls.[11] In addition, there was a much larger drop in the size of the upper airway on laying down in pregnant women in their third trimester compared with nonpregnant controls in one study[13] but not in another.[11] Factors potentially affecting airway collapsibility in these patients include reduced lung volumes—leading to less caudal traction on the upper airway[14]—and fat infiltration of the upper airway. Functional residual capacity is reduced in pregnancy in the upright position with an additional reduction occurring in the supine position. Pregnant women may gain an average of 25 to 35 pounds (11–16 kg) during the course of pregnancy. However, in the study by Iczi and colleagues,[13] the drop in airway size between the seated and the supine position in the pregnant group did not appear to be related to body mass index, suggesting that other factors such as changes in functional residual capacity or changes in the upper airway related to interstitial fluid may play a role. Mean pharyngeal cross-sectional area increases significantly postpartum compared with intrapartum,[11] but it is not clear when or whether these changes return to preconception size. The measurements discussed here may be even more pronounced during sleep, with the loss of upper airway muscle dilation, but this theory needs to be tested further.

CHEST WALL CHANGES IN PREGNANCY

The thorax undergoes significant structural changes in pregnancy: The subcostal angle of the rib cage and the circumference of the lower chest wall increase and the diaphragm moves up.[15–18] These changes are necessary to accommodate the enlarging uterus and increasing maternal weight, but the changes occur early in pregnancy before the uterus is significantly enlarged.[15,18] Hormonal changes rather than the mechanical effects of the enlarging uterus cause relaxation of the ligamentous attachments of the lower ribs. Relaxin, the hormone responsible for relaxation of the pelvic ligaments, likely also causes relaxation of the lower rib-cage ligaments.[19] The subcostal angle progressively widens from 68.5° to 103.5° during pregnancy.[18] The anterior-posterior and transverse diameters of the chest wall each increase by 2 cm, resulting in an increase of 5 to 7 cm in the circumference of the lower rib cage. The anatomic changes of the chest wall peak at week 37. The chest wall configuration normalizes by 24 weeks postpartum but the subcostal angle remains about 20% wider than the baseline value.[15] The enlarging uterus causes the diaphragm to be displaced cephalad 4 cm in late pregnancy, but the increase in chest wall size mitigates any changes in lung volumes caused by the upward displacement of the diaphragm. The anatomic changes of the thorax with pregnancy are illustrated in **Fig. 1**.

RESPIRATORY MUSCLE FUNCTION

There is no significant change in respiratory muscle strength during pregnancy despite the cephalad displacement of the diaphragm and changes in the chest wall configuration. Maximal inspiratory and expiratory mouth pressures and maximum transdiaphragmatic pressure, measured as gastric pressure minus esophageal pressure, in late pregnancy and after delivery show no significant changes.[15,20] Despite the upward displacement of the diaphragm by the gravid uterus, diaphragm excursion actually increases by 2 cm compared with the nonpregnant state.[18,20] Increased diaphragmatic excursion and preserved respiratory muscle strength are important adaptations, given the increase in tidal volume and minute ventilation that accompanies pregnancy. Improved diaphragm mechanics in pregnancy are explained by an increased area of apposition of the diaphragm to the rib cage.[20]

LUNG FUNCTION IN PREGNANCY
Static Lung Function

Static lung function stays the same in pregnancy except for decreases in functional residual capacity (FRC) and its components: expiratory reserve volume (ERV) and residual volume (RV). FRC depends on 2 opposing forces: the elastic recoil of the lungs and the outward and downward

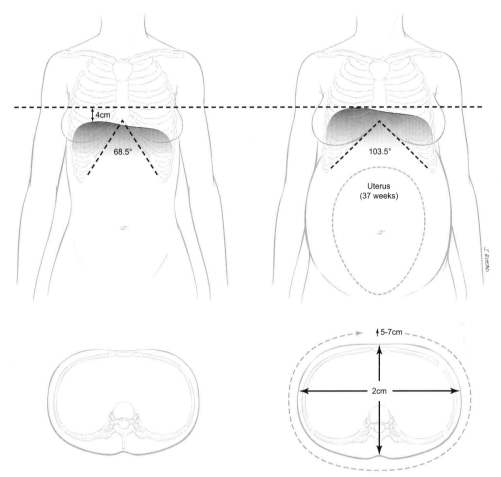

Fig. 1. Chest wall changes that occur during pregnancy. The subcostal angle increases, as does the anterior-posterior and transverse diameters of the chest wall and the chest wall circumference. These changes compensate for the 4-cm elevation of the diaphragm so that total lung capacity is not significantly reduced.

pull of the chest wall and abdominal contents. A reduction in FRC in pregnancy is expected given the 4-cm elevation of the diaphragm, decreased downward pull of the abdomen, and changes in chest wall configuration that decrease outward recoil.[17] As anticipated, chest wall compliance is decreased antepartum compared with postpartum.[21] Lung compliance is unaffected by pregnancy.[21,22]

Several studies have measured serial static lung volumes during pregnancy and after delivery.[23–27] The changes in lung function in pregnancy are illustrated in **Fig. 2**. FRC decreases by approximately 20% to 30% or 400 to 700 mL during pregnancy. FRC is composed of ERV, which decreases 15% to 20% or 200 to 300 mL, and RV, which decreases 20% to 25% or 200 to 400 mL. Significant reductions in FRC are noted at 6 months' gestation with a progressive decline as pregnancy continues.[23,28] At term, there is a further 25%

decrease in FRC in the supine position compared with sitting.[26]

Inspiratory capacity (IC), the maximum volume that can be inhaled from FRC, increases by 5% to 10% or 200 to 350 mL during pregnancy. Total lung capacity (TLC), the combination of FRC and IC, is unchanged or decreases minimally (less than 5%) at term.

Lung volume measurements can be made using inert gas techniques and by body plethysmography.[29] In patients without lung disease the 2 techniques produce similar results.[30] Garcia-Rio and colleagues[27] measured lung volumes by plethysmography and inert gas (helium dilution) techniques during pregnancy and postpartum. At 36 weeks of pregnancy there were significant differences in lung volumes between the 2 techniques. FRC measured by body plethysmography was decreased by 27% compared with postpartum whereas FRC measured by helium dilution

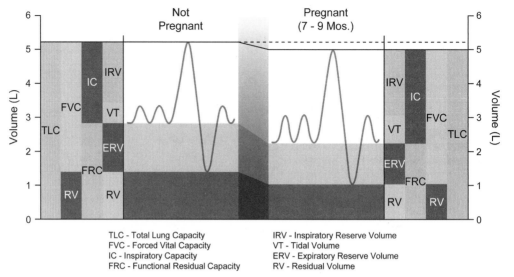

Fig. 2. Changes in lung volumes with pregnancy. The most significant changes are reductions in FRC and its subcomponents ERV and RV, and increases in IC and VT.

was decreased 38% compared with postpartum. FRC was larger by 18% or 350 mL when measured by plethysmography. The underestimation of lung volumes by inert gas technique has been attributed to airway closure during tidal breathing in late pregnancy.[27]

Both pregnancy and obesity are associated with an increase in abdominal mass, resulting in a reduction in FRC. However, significant differences are seen in other lung volumes between the 2 processes. Specifically, RV is decreased in pregnancy and increased in obesity.[31] The increase in RV in obesity is attributed to significant air trapping.[31]

Spirometry

Airflow mechanics during pregnancy have been extensively studied and are well characterized. Beginning with the classic study by Cugell in 1953, several investigators have measured lung function serially during pregnancy and after delivery.[23,25,27,32–36]

Routine spirometric measurements (forced expiratory volume in 1 second [FEV_1] and FEV_1/forced vital capacity [FVC] ratio) are not significantly different compared with nonpregnant values. FVC has been reported to be either minimally increased, decreased, or unchanged during pregnancy compared with the nonpregnant state; on average, there is no significant change.[23,25,27,32–36] The shape of the flow-volume curve and instantaneous flows that reflect larger airway caliber (peak expiratory flow) and smaller airway caliber (forced expiratory flow at 50% and 25% of vital capacity) are also unchanged.[35,37] Maximum breathing capacity,

also referred to as maximum voluntary ventilation, a measure of respiratory muscle strength and airway mechanics, is not significantly changed with pregnancy.[23,33]

The stability of spirometry during pregnancy suggests that there is no significant change in expiratory airflow resistance with pregnancy. Spirometry is also not significantly different in women with twin pregnancy as compared with singleton pregnancy.[38] Clinicians caring for pregnant patients should be alert to these findings: abnormal spirometry in a pregnant patient is likely not related to pregnancy and suggests respiratory disease.

Airway Resistance/Conductance

Several studies have addressed airway resistance and its reciprocal, airway conductance, during pregnancy.[22,32,34,39] Measurements of airway resistance and conductance quantify the ease with which air flows through the tracheobronchial tree for a given driving pressure. These parameters are primarily determined by the caliber of the large and medium-sized bronchi and because of this lung volume is a key factor.[40] Investigators have found either a decrease in total pulmonary resistance[22,32] or no change[34,39] during pregnancy. The reduced or stable airway resistance indicates that there is no change in the caliber of the large and medium-sized airways in pregnancy, despite factors that would be expected to increase airway resistance, including a reduction in FRC, reduced nasopharyngeal caliber due to upper airway congestion, and bronchoconstriction associated with the significant reduction in alveolar

P_{CO_2}. This outcome may be explained by hormonal changes during pregnancy. Specifically, progesterone and relaxin may have bronchodilatory effects that counterbalance the bronchoconstricting elements.[22,34]

Closing Volume

Measurement of closing volume provides a quantitative assessment of small airway closure.[41] Closing volume and closing capacity are often used synonymously, but technically, closing capacity equals closing volume plus RV. Airway closure occurs when pleural pressure exceeds airway pressure (ie, transpulmonary pressure is negative). Airway closure during tidal breathing occurs when the closing volume is greater than end-expiratory lung volume or closing capacity is greater than FRC. The closure of small airways with tidal breathing has important physiologic consequences, including a maldistribution of ventilation in relation to perfusion, and a resultant impairment of gas exchange and small airway injury from cyclic opening and closing of peripheral airways.[41] The single-breath nitrogen test is the most commonly used method for assessing closing volume.[41]

Closing volume has been extensively studied in pregnancy.[24,27,35,42–45] Given the significant reduction in end-expiratory lung volume and FRC and the increase in pleural pressure during pregnancy,[15] airway closure during tidal breathing was seen as an explanation for the mild decrease in oxygenation commonly seen in late pregnancy.[18,46] Studies of closing capacity in pregnancy have given conflicting results. Most studies indicate that closing volume and closing capacity do not change during pregnancy,[35,43,45] but one study that measured closing capacity at 2-month intervals during pregnancy noted a progressive, linear increase in closing capacity beginning in the second trimester.[24]

More important for gas exchange is the relationship between closing capacity and FRC. Here again, the studies are not consistent. Closing capacity has been reported to exceed FRC in up to 60% of patients in late pregnancy, especially in the supine position,[42,45] whereas others have reported this to be a rare finding.[35,43,44] The differences among studies may be explained by the large variability in closing volume measurements[47] or presence of other factors that affect closing volume such as smoking, asthma, obesity, and kyphoscoliosis.[48] Changes in closing capacity relative to FRC in late pregnancy likely cause a decrease in oxygenation, especially in the supine position, but the effect is likely small and not clinically important.[44]

Diffusing Capacity

The diffusing capacity for carbon monoxide (DL_{CO}) provides a quantitative measure of gas transfer in the lungs. The physiologic changes of pregnancy would be expected to have opposing effects on DL_{CO}. The increase in cardiac output and intravascular volume would be expected to recruit capillary surface area and increase DL_{CO} while the known reduction in hemoglobin concentration in pregnancy would be expected to decrease DL_{CO}. The most comprehensive study of DL_{CO} in pregnancy was performed by Milne and colleagues.[49] Diffusing capacity was measured monthly throughout pregnancy beginning in the first trimester and then 3 to 5 months postpartum. After correcting for alveolar volume and hemoglobin, DL_{CO} was highest in the first trimester, decreasing to a nadir at 24 to 27 weeks with no further reduction thereafter.[49] Alveolar volume measured by inert gas techniques was also significantly less after the first trimester.[49] Another study showed a similar reduction in DL_{CO} after the first trimester,[37] but this has not been a consistent finding.[50] When DL_{CO} is partitioned into its membrane and capillary blood volume components, the membrane component is either stable or slightly decreased while the capillary blood volume is unchanged.[37,50] Diffusing capacity increases with exercise in pregnancy just as it does in normal subjects,[51] indicating that pregnancy does not interfere with the ability to recruit pulmonary capillaries with exercise. Diffusing capacity does not increase when measured in the supine position as it does in nonpregnancy,[26] likely as a result of impaired venous return from the mechanical effects of the gravid uterus on the vena cava. Although most studies addressing DL_{CO} in pregnancy have methodological defects, pregnancy does not appear to cause a significant change in DL_{CO}.

VENTILATION AND GAS EXCHANGE

There is a significant increase in resting minute ventilation (V_E) during pregnancy. At term, V_E is increased by 20% to 50% compared with nonpregnant values.[15,23,25,28,52–55] The increase in V_E is associated with a 30% to 50% (from approximately 450 to 650 mL) increase in tidal volume with no change or only a small increase (1–2 breaths per minute) in respiratory rate. While V_E increases in all studies, the time course of the increase is variable. Some studies reveal a progressive increase throughout pregnancy[23,28] but most indicate that V_E rises sharply in the first 12 weeks with a minimal increase thereafter.[15,25,53,55]

The increase in tidal volume occurs without an increase in inspiratory time or the duration of the respiratory cycle, indicating that inspiratory flow is increased.[15,17,55]

The dead space to tidal volume ratio (V_D/V_T) in pregnancy is unchanged at approximately 30%.[17,56,57] Given the significant increase in tidal volume, this indicates that dead space ventilation is also increased. Studies of dead space ventilation in pregnancy have produced conflicting results.[56–58] Dead space ventilation would be expected to decrease in pregnancy because of the increases in cardiac output and perfusion to the lung apices. However, most studies indicate that there is an increase in dead space ventilation.[56,57] Anatomic dead space is unlikely to be altered by pregnancy, so an increase in alveolar dead space is the likely cause. The mechanism for the increase in alveolar dead space is not clear.

Hyperventilation in pregnancy is primarily caused by a progesterone effect augmented by an increased metabolic rate and increased CO_2 production. There is convincing evidence that progesterone is a respiratory stimulant. Increased ventilation occurs during the luteal phase of the menstrual cycle corresponding to increased plasma progesterone levels.[59] Exogenous progesterone administered to males causes increased minute ventilation and CO_2 chemosensitivity.[60,61] The mechanism by which progesterone causes an increase in ventilation is not completely understood, although progesterone decreases the threshold and increases the sensitivity of the central ventilatory chemoreflex response to CO_2.[59,62,63] Independent of its effect on CO_2 sensitivity, there is also evidence that progesterone, either alone or in combination with estradiol, stimulates central neural sites in the medulla oblongata, thalamus, and hypothalamus, involved in controlling ventilation.[59,62] Progesterone also has a direct effect on the carotid body so as to increase the peripheral ventilatory response to hypoxia. This effect is potentiated by estrogen.[64] In summary, progesterone and estradiol act synergistically to increase minute ventilation and reduce $Paco_2$ by multiple mechanisms.

The discordance between increasing progesterone after the first trimester and relative stability of minute ventilation has not been explained. Progesterone increases progressively during pregnancy. Most studies reveal a sharp increase in minute ventilation early in pregnancy and then only a minimal increase during the remainder of pregnancy.[15,25,53,55] There is a direct relationship between respiratory drive, quantified by mouth occlusion pressure ($P_{0.1}$), the pressure measured at the mouth 100 milliseconds following airway occlusion at FRC, and progesterone levels throughout pregnancy.[15] The lack of an association between $P_{0.1}$ and minute ventilation may be explained by increased respiratory impedance secondary to mechanical changes in the chest wall and abdomen.[15]

Dyspnea is a common complaint in healthy pregnant women. "Physiologic dyspnea" occurs in 60% to 70% of normal pregnant women by 30 weeks of gestation.[53,65,66] Women with physiologic dyspnea when compared with asymptomatic pregnant women have a higher $P_{0.1}$ and an increased ventilatory response to both CO_2 and hypoxia.[55] The increased minute ventilation and chemosensitivity are not explained by higher progesterone levels in patients with physiologic dyspnea compared with those without this symptom.[55] Physiologic dyspnea is likely related to an increased awareness of this augmented drive to breathe.[13]

The increased metabolic demands of the fetus, uterus, and maternal organs result in increased oxygen consumption (Vo_2), carbon dioxide production (Vco_2), and basal metabolic rate. Vo_2 and Vco_2 at term are approximately 20% and 35% greater, respectively, than nonpregnant values.[28,52,54,56,67–69] The respiratory exchange ratio (Vco_2/Vo_2) is unchanged or minimally increased with pregnancy.[52,54,56,69] The increase in V_E exceeds the increase in Vco_2 and Vo_2. The disproportionate increase in V_E leads to an increase in alveolar and arterial partial pressures of oxygen (PAo_2 and Pao_2) and a decrease in alveolar and arterial partial pressures of CO_2 ($PAco_2$ and $Paco_2$).

Normal arterial blood values in pregnancy at sea level are listed in **Table 1**. Templeton and Kelman[57] measured serial arterial blood gases in a cohort of healthy women throughout pregnancy and postpartum at sea level. Pao_2 was 106 mm Hg during the first trimester and decreased to 102 mm Hg near term. Pao_2 values during pregnancy were greater than those measured postpartum and in a control group (Pao_2 93–95 mm Hg). There was no change in the PAo_2-Pao_2 difference throughout pregnancy compared with the postpartum period or the control group. Other studies have also documented an increase in Pao_2 during pregnancy.[63,70,71]

The increased oxygen tension during pregnancy is an important adaptation that facilitates oxygen transfer across the placenta. Despite an increased oxygen tension, the combination of increased oxygen consumption and a lower reservoir of oxygen stores due to reduced functional residual capacity decreases maternal oxygen reserves. Pregnant women are more susceptible

Table 1
Arterial blood gas (ABG) changes in pregnancy (sea level)

| ABG Measurement | Nonpregnant State | Pregnant State | |
		First Trimester	Third Trimester
pH	7.40	7.42–7.46	7.43
P_aO_2 (mm Hg)	93	105–106	101–106
P_aco_2 (mm Hg)	37	28–29	26–30
Serum HCO_3 (mEq/L)	23	18	17

Data from Refs.[44,57,63]

to the development of hypoxemia during periods of apnea, such as during endotracheal intubation.[72]

There is a significant reduction in Pa_{O_2} of approximately 10 mm Hg with changing from the sitting to the supine position in late pregnancy. This reduction has been attributed to closure of dependent airways and resultant ventilation/perfusion mismatch.[44,73]

Hyperventilation during pregnancy results in a significant reduction in Pa_{CO_2}. The Pa_{CO_2} decreases from a baseline value of 35 to 40 mm Hg to 27 to 34 mm Hg during pregnancy.[57,63,70,71] The reduction in Pa_{CO_2} is evident in the first trimester. Some studies reveal a progressive reduction in Pa_{CO_2} throughout pregnancy, reaching a nadir late in pregnancy.[28,63,70,71] Others show an initial reduction in Pa_{CO_2} that remains relatively stable throughout the remainder of pregnancy.[57] The persistently low Pa_{CO_2} results in a chronic respiratory alkalosis. Compensatory renal mechanisms

excrete bicarbonate, reaching a nadir bicarbonate level of 18 to 22 mEq/L in late pregnancy.[63,70,71] pH is maintained at 7.42 to 7.46.[57,63,70,71] The chronic alkalosis stimulates 2,3-diphosphoglycerate synthesis causing a rightward shift of the oxyhemoglobin dissociation curve, which aids oxygen transfer across the placenta.[74]

CARDIOVASCULAR CHANGES IN PREGNANCY

Significant cardiovascular changes during the course of pregnancy affect respiratory physiology. These changes include increased plasma volume, increased cardiac output, and reduced vascular resistance. The adaptations begin early in pregnancy, and are critical in meeting the increasing metabolic demands of the mother and fetus and in tolerating the acute blood loss that occurs with childbirth. The cardiovascular changes with pregnancy are listed in **Table 2**.

Table 2
Hemodynamic changes in pregnancy

| Measurement | Change with Pregnancy | |
	% Change	(Absolute Change)
Cardiac output	30%–50% ↑	(2 L/min)
Heart rate	15%–20% ↑	(12 beats/min)
Stroke volume	20%–30% ↑	(18 mL)
Mean arterial pressure	0%–5% ↓	
Central venous pressure	No change	
Systemic vascular resistance	20%–30% ↓	(320 dyne·s/cm^5)
Left ventricular stroke work index	No change	
Mean pulmonary artery pressure	No change	
Pulmonary capillary wedge pressure	No change	
Pulmonary vascular resistance	30% ↓	(40 dyne·s/cm^5)

Data from Refs.[48,52,81,82]

Blood Volume Changes

Total body volume expansion occurs secondary to sodium and water retention during pregnancy. Total body volume expansion accounts for approximately 6 kg of the weight gained during pregnancy, and is distributed among the maternal extracellular and intracellular spaces, amniotic fluid, and the fetus.[17,75] Maternal blood volume increases progressively during pregnancy, peaking at a value approximately 40% greater than baseline by the third trimester. The increase in maternal plasma blood volume is physiologically important. Smaller increases in maternal plasma blood volume are associated with intrauterine growth retardation and poor fetal outcomes.[76]

The increase in plasma blood volume is best explained by the underfill hypothesis. Vasodilation of the maternal circulation and shunt-like effects created by the low-resistance uteroplacental circulation activate the renin-angiotensin system, and stimulate increased renal sodium reabsorption and water retention. Animal models suggest that the nitric oxide system is the main mediator of the primary peripheral vasodilation in pregnancy.[77] Hormonal factors also contribute to volume expansion and activation of the renin-angiotensin system[75,78,79] However, elevated levels of atrial natriuretic peptide early in pregnancy are not consistent with the underfill hypothesis.[80] The exact mechanism for volume homeostasis in normal pregnancy remains unexplained. The 40% increase (1.2 L on average) in maternal plasma blood volume exceeds the 20% to 30% increase in maternal red blood cell mass, resulting in hemodilution and the relative anemia of pregnancy.[76]

Cardiac Output

Cardiac output begins to increase as early as the fifth week of pregnancy and peaks at 30% to 50% (approximately 2 L per minute) above nonpregnant values at 25 to 32 weeks.[81–85] The increase in cardiac output is a result of a 20% increase in heart rate and a 20% to 30% increase in stroke volume. The increase in stroke volume is a consequence of an increase in preload, due to increased plasma volume and a 20% to 30% decrease in systemic vascular resistance with no significant change in ventricular contractility.[82–84,86] Studies that have used repeated echocardiograms during pregnancy have revealed no significant change in left ventricular ejection fraction, with increases in left ventricular mass and wall thickness as well as increases in all cardiac chamber dimensions.[83,84] Cardiac output may decrease slightly in the third trimester, but is highly dependent on body position. In late pregnancy, cardiac output in the supine position decreases by up to 30% compared with the left lateral decubitus position as a result of compression of the inferior vena cava by the gravid uterus and reduced venous return.[87]

Central Hemodynamic and Pulmonary Vascular Changes

In addition to the significant increase in cardiac output and reduction in systemic vascular resistance discussed earlier, right heart catheterization studies in normal pregnant women revealed no changes in central venous pressure and pulmonary capillary wedge pressure compared with nonpregnant values.[81,82] Mean pulmonary artery pressure is also unchanged during pregnancy.[81,82] Pulmonary artery pressures increase minimally with exercise but remain within the normal range.[81] Pulmonary vascular resistance significantly decreases during pregnancy, as would be expected given the stable mean pulmonary artery pressure and pulmonary wedge pressure as well as the increased cardiac output.

EXERCISE PHYSIOLOGY IN PREGNANCY

Moderate aerobic exercise during pregnancy appears to be safe for the mother and fetus, and may improve some pregnancy outcomes such as gestational diabetes and preeclampsia.[88–91] Most studies addressing the physiologic response to exercise in pregnancy used submaximal, constant load exercise protocols to avoid potential risk to the fetus.[52,56,67,69,89,92,93]

At moderate intensity of exercise, pregnant women respond differently to nonpregnant women. The increase in V_{O_2} for a given workload is greater.[68,69,92] However, V_{O_2} varies with the type of exercise. In pregnant subjects weight-bearing exercise, such as treadmill walking, is associated with a significantly higher V_{O_2} than is cycle ergometry compared with the difference between these 2 modes in nonpregnant controls.[52] When non–weight-bearing exercise is performed and V_{O_2} is adjusted for body weight (V_{O_2} expressed in mL O_2/kg/min), the V_{O_2} increases are similar for a given workload in pregnant and nonpregnant subjects.[89,92]

During pregnancy, minute ventilation (V_E) and alveolar ventilation (V_A) are higher at rest and the rate of increase with exercise is more rapid compared with the nongravid state. Both V_E and V_A increase 20% to 25% compared with nonpregnant values at submaximal work rates.[56,69,89,92] The increase in V_E exceeds the increase in V_{O_2}

resulting in an increase in the ventilatory equivalent for oxygen (V_E/V_{O_2}).

Cardiac output is higher for a given exercise level in pregnant subjects compared with nonpregnant subjects. This difference is primarily due to an increase in stroke volume.[67,92] The proportionally greater increase in cardiac output with exercise results in a reduction in the difference between the arterial and mixed venous oxygen content differences (C_{aO_2}–C_{vO_2}) compared with the nonpregnant state, leading to increased oxygen delivery to the fetus during maternal exercise.[67]

Few studies have performed symptom-limited maximal cardiopulmonary exercise tests in late pregnancy.[69,89] Maximal O_2 consumption has been noted to be reduced in sedentary pregnant women, but is associated with lower peak heart rates and may be partly due to effort. Maximal O_2 consumption is preserved in physically fit pregnant women but anaerobic working capacity may be reduced.

The fetus usually responds to submaximal maternal exercise with an increase in fetal heart rate. The fetal heart rate gradually returns to normal after the mother stops exercise.[89] Transient fetal bradycardia may develop with maximal exercise. The significance of fetal bradycardia with intense exercise is unclear. Prolonged submaximal exercise (greater than 30 minutes) in late pregnancy often results in a moderate reduction in maternal blood glucose concentration and may transiently reduce fetal glucose availability. Maternal core body temperature increases with moderate exercise, but generally less than 1.5°C.[89] The clinical significance of these changes is not clear, but moderate exercise does not appear to be associated with adverse effects to the mother or fetus.

RESPIRATORY PHYSIOLOGY IN LABOR, DELIVERY, AND POSTPARTUM

Hyperventilation, beyond the usual pregnancy-mediated increase in minute ventilation, is common during labor and delivery. Several factors interact to influence minute ventilation during labor and delivery. Pain, anxiety, and coached breathing techniques increase minute ventilation whereas narcotic analgesics have the opposite effect. The result is a wide variation in minute ventilation and breathing patterns, as illustrated by a study of 25 patients during labor that found tidal volumes ranging from 330 to 2250 mL and minute ventilation varying from 7 to 90 L per minute.[94] Pain control with narcotic analgesics minimizes labor-induced hyperventilation, suggesting that the main contributing factor for the hyperventilation is painful uterine contractions.[11] Hyperventilation during labor and delivery results in a reduction in alveolar CO_2 levels from 32 mm Hg during early labor to 26 mm Hg during the second stage.[95] The significant hyperventilation during labor and delivery and resultant hypocarbia can cause uterine vessel vasoconstriction and decreased placental perfusion, and may have deleterious effects in patients with marginal placental reserves.[43] Within 72 hours of delivery, the minute ventilation decreases halfway back toward the nonpregnant value and returns to baseline within a few weeks.[49,51]

The static lung volume changes that occur during pregnancy rapidly normalize after delivery with decompression of the diaphragm and lungs. FRC and RV return to baseline values within 48 hours.[20] The chest wall changes that occur during pregnancy normalize by 24 weeks postpartum, but the subcostal angle does not return to its prepregnancy value, remaining about 20% wider than baseline.[15]

CARDIOVASCULAR PHYSIOLOGY IN LABOR, DELIVERY, AND POSTPARTUM

Labor, delivery and the postpartum period are associated with significant cardiovascular changes. Cardiac output increases 10% to 15% above late pregnancy levels during early labor and by 50% during the second stage of labor.[87,96] The increase in cardiac output is caused by an increase in both heart rate and stroke volume. Factors contributing to the hemodynamic changes during labor include pain and anxiety with resultant increases in circulating catecholamines, and uterine contractions with resultant cyclic "autotransfusions" and increases in central blood volume and preload. Narcotic analgesics and regional anesthesia minimize the pain-mediated changes in cardiac output. Immediately postpartum there is a 60% to 80% increase in cardiac output and stroke volume relative to prelabor values, due to increased preload associated with "autotransfusion" of approximately 500 mL of blood that is no longer diverted to the uteroplacental vascular bed, and the relief of aortocaval compression with delivery.[82,91] Systolic and diastolic blood pressure and systemic vascular resistance increase during active labor, although the magnitude depends on the severity of maternal pain, anxiety, and the intensity of uterine contractions. It is important for the clinician to recognize that patients with underlying cardiac or pulmonary vascular disease may not be able to augment their cardiac output in the peripartum period, resulting in decompensated heart failure.

There is conflicting information regarding the time course for the resolution of the cardiovascular physiologic changes after delivery. Most studies reveal a significant reduction in cardiac output and stroke volume by 2 weeks after delivery, with further reductions to near baseline values over 12 to 24 weeks.[77,79,81,97] However, another study indicated that cardiac output and stroke volume remained significantly elevated above prepregnancy values at 12 weeks postpartum.[98] Some of the cardiovascular changes resolve more slowly. Left ventricular wall thickness and mass remain significantly greater than nonpregnant controls at 24 weeks after delivery, suggesting an element of residual hypertrophy.[92]

SUMMARY

Significant anatomic and physiologic adaptations involving the respiratory and cardiac systems occur during pregnancy and are necessary to meet the increased metabolic demands of both the mother and the fetus. The prominent respiratory changes include: mechanical alterations to the chest wall and diaphragm to accommodate the enlarging uterus; a reduction in FRC and its components ERV and RV, with little or no change in TLC; and an increase in minute ventilation, resulting in reduced Pa_{CO_2} and chronic respiratory alkalosis. There is no significant change in spirometry, DL_{CO}, or oxygenation. The major cardiovascular changes include increased plasma blood volume, increased cardiac output, and a reduction in systemic vascular resistance. A basic knowledge of these expected changes will help health providers distinguish the common physiologic dyspnea from breathlessness caused by the various cardiopulmonary diseases that coexist with pregnancy.

REFERENCES

1. Lapinsky SE. Cardiopulmonary complications of pregnancy. Crit Care Med 2005;33(7):1616–22.
2. Ellegard EK. Pregnancy rhinitis. Immunol Allergy Clin North Am 2006;26(1):119–35, vii.
3. Toppozada H, Michaels L, Toppozada M, et al. The human respiratory nasal mucosa in pregnancy. An electron microscopic and histochemical study. J Laryngol Otol 1982;96(7):613–26.
4. Bende M, Gredmark T. Nasal stuffiness during pregnancy. Laryngoscope 1999;109(7 Pt 1):1108–10.
5. Ellegard E. [Nasal congestion among women. At least every fifth pregnant woman suffers–most common among smokers]. Lakartidningen 2000; 97(34):3619–20, 3623 [in Swedish].
6. Mabry RL. Rhinitis of pregnancy. South Med J 1986; 79(8):965–71.
7. Ellegard EK. Clinical and pathogenetic characteristics of pregnancy rhinitis. Clin Rev Allergy Immunol 2004;26(3):149–59.
8. Pien GW, Schwab RJ. Sleep disorders during pregnancy. Sleep 2004;27(7):1405–17.
9. Lundberg JO, Weitzberg E. Nasal nitric oxide in man. Thorax 1999;54(10):947–52.
10. Pilkington S, Carli F, Dakin MJ, et al. Increase in Mallampati score during pregnancy. Br J Anaesth 1995; 74(6):638–42.
11. Izci B, Vennelle M, Liston WA, et al. Sleep-disordered breathing and upper airway size in pregnancy and post-partum. Eur Respir J 2006;27(2):321–7.
12. Pien GW, Fife D, Pack AI, et al. Changes in symptoms of sleep-disordered breathing during pregnancy. Sleep 2005;28(10):1299–305.
13. Izci B, Riha RL, Martin SE, et al. The upper airway in pregnancy and pre-eclampsia. Am J Respir Crit Care Med 2003;167(2):137–40.
14. White DP. Pathogenesis of obstructive and central sleep apnea. Am J Respir Crit Care Med 2005; 172(11):1363–70.
15. Contreras G, Gutierrez M, Beroiza T, et al. Ventilatory drive and respiratory muscle function in pregnancy. Am Rev Respir Dis 1991;144(4):837–41.
16. Elkus R, Popovich J Jr. Respiratory physiology in pregnancy. Clin Chest Med 1992;13(4):555–65.
17. Crapo RO. Normal cardiopulmonary physiology during pregnancy. Clin Obstet Gynecol 1996;39(1): 3–16.
18. Weinberger SE, Weiss ST, Cohen WR, et al. Pregnancy and the lung. Am Rev Respir Dis 1980; 121(3):559–81.
19. Goldsmith LT, Weiss G, Steinetz BG. Relaxin and its role in pregnancy. Endocrinol Metab Clin North Am 1995;24(1):171–86.
20. Gilroy RJ, Mangura BT, Lavietes MH. Rib cage and abdominal volume displacements during breathing in pregnancy. Am Rev Respir Dis 1988;137(3):668–72.
21. Marx GF, Murthy PK, Orkin LR. Static compliance before and after vaginal delivery. Br J Anaesth 1970;42(12):1100–4.
22. Gee JB, Packer BS, Millen JE, et al. Pulmonary mechanics during pregnancy. J Clin Invest 1967; 46(6):945–52.
23. Cugell DW, Frank NR, Gaensler EA, et al. Pulmonary function in pregnancy. I. Serial observations in normal women. Am Rev Tuberc 1953;67(5):568–97.
24. Garrard GS, Littler WA, Redman CW. Closing volume during normal pregnancy. Thorax 1978; 33(4):488–92.
25. Alaily AB, Carrol KB. Pulmonary ventilation in pregnancy. Br J Obstet Gynaecol 1978;85(7):518–24.

26. Norregaard O, Schultz P, Ostergaard A, et al. Lung function and postural changes during pregnancy. Respir Med 1989;83(6):467–70.

27. Garcia-Rio F, Pino-Garcia JM, Serrano S, et al. Comparison of helium dilution and plethysmographic lung volumes in pregnant women. Eur Respir J 1997;10(10):2371–5.

28. Prowse CM, Gaensler EA. Respiratory and acid-base changes during pregnancy. Anesthesiology 1965;26:381–92.

29. Wanger J, Clausen JL, Coates A, et al. Standardisation of the measurement of lung volumes. Eur Respir J 2005;26(3):511–22.

30. Ferris BG. Epidemiology standardization project (American Thoracic Society). Am Rev Respir Dis 1978;118(6 Pt 2):1–120.

31. Unterborn J. Pulmonary function testing in obesity, pregnancy, and extremes of body habitus. Clin Chest Med 2001;22(4):759–67.

32. Goucher D, Rubin A, Russo N. The effect of pregnancy upon pulmonary function in normal women. Am J Obstet Gynecol 1956;72(5):963–9.

33. Ihrman K. A clinical and physiological study of pregnancy in a material from northern Sweden. II. Vital capacity and maximal breathing capacity during and after pregnancy. Acta Soc Med Ups 1960;65:147–54.

34. Milne JA, Mills RJ, Howie AD, et al. Large airways function during normal pregnancy. Br J Obstet Gynaecol 1977;84(6):448–51.

35. Baldwin GR, Moorthi DS, Whelton JA, et al. New lung functions and pregnancy. Am J Obstet Gynecol 1977;127(3):235–9.

36. Puranik BM, Kaore SB, Kurhade GA, et al. A longitudinal study of pulmonary function tests during pregnancy. Indian J Physiol Pharmacol 1994;38(2):129–32.

37. Gazioglu K, Kaltreider NL, Rosen M, et al. Pulmonary function during pregnancy in normal women and in patients with cardiopulmonary disease. Thorax 1970;25(4):445–50.

38. McAuliffe F, Kametas N, Costello J, et al. Respiratory function in singleton and twin pregnancy. BJOG 2002;109(7):765–9.

39. Kerr JH. Bronchopulmonary resistance in pregnancy. Can Anaesth Soc J 1961;8:347–55.

40. Levitzky MG. Pulmonary physiology. 7th edition. New York (NY): McGraw-Hill; 2007.

41. Milic-Emili J, Torchio R, D'Angelo E. Closing volume: a reappraisal (1967–2007). Eur J Appl Physiol 2007; 99(6):567–83.

42. Bevan DR, Holdcroft A, Loh L, et al. Closing volume and pregnancy. Br Med J 1974;1(5896):13–5.

43. Craig DB, Toole MA. Airway closure in pregnancy. Can Anaesth Soc J 1975;22(6):665–72.

44. Awe RJ, Nicotra MB, Newsom TD, et al. Arterial oxygenation and alveolar-arterial gradients in term pregnancy. Obstet Gynecol 1979;53(2):182–6.

45. Russell IF, Chambers WA. Closing volume in normal pregnancy. Br J Anaesth 1981;53(10):1043–7.

46. Fishburne JI. Physiology and disease of the respiratory system in pregnancy. A review. J Reprod Med 1979;22(4):177–89.

47. Burki NK, Barker DB, Nicholson DP. Variability of the closing volume measurement in normal subjects. Am Rev Respir Dis 1975;112(2):209–12.

48. Camann WR, Ostheimer GW. Physiological adaptations during pregnancy. Int Anesthesiol Clin 1990; 28(1):2–10.

49. Milne JA, Mills RJ, Coutts JR, et al. The effect of human pregnancy on the pulmonary transfer factor for carbon monoxide as measured by the single-breath method. Clin Sci Mol Med 1977;53(3):271–6.

50. Krumholz RA, Echt CR, Ross JC. Pulmonary diffusing capacity, capillary blood volume, lung volumes, and mechanics of ventilation in early and late pregnancy. J Lab Clin Med 1964;63:648–55.

51. Bedell GN, Adams RW. Pulmonary diffusing capacity during rest and exercise. a study of normal persons and persons with atrial septal defect, pregnancy, and pulmonary disease. J Clin Invest 1962; 41(10):1908–14.

52. Knuttgen HG, Emerson K Jr. Physiological response to pregnancy at rest and during exercise. J Appl Physiol 1974;36(5):549–53.

53. Milne JA. The respiratory response to pregnancy. Postgrad Med J 1979;55(643):318–24.

54. Rees GB, Broughton Pipkin F, Symonds EM, et al. A longitudinal study of respiratory changes in normal human pregnancy with cross-sectional data on subjects with pregnancy-induced hypertension. Am J Obstet Gynecol 1990;162(3):826–30.

55. Garcia-Rio F, Pino JM, Gomez L, et al. Regulation of breathing and perception of dyspnea in healthy pregnant women. Chest 1996;110(2):446–53.

56. Pernoll ML, Metcalfe J, Kovach PA, et al. Ventilation during rest and exercise in pregnancy and postpartum. Respir Physiol 1975;25(3):295–310.

57. Templeton A, Kelman GR. Maternal blood-gases, (PAo_2-Pao_2), physiological shunt and VD/VT in normal pregnancy. Br J Anaesth 1976;48(10):1001–4.

58. Shankar KB, Moseley H, Vemula V, et al. Physiological dead space during general anaesthesia for Caesarean section. Can J Anaesth 1987;34(4): 373–6.

59. Bayliss DA, Millhorn DE. Central neural mechanisms of progesterone action: application to the respiratory system. J Appl Physiol 1992;73(2):393–404.

60. Zwillich CW, Natalino MR, Sutton FD, et al. Effects of progesterone on chemosensivity in normal men. J Lab Clin Med 1978;92(2):262–9.

61. Schoene RB, Pierson DJ, Lakshminarayan S, et al. Effect of medroxyprogesterone acetate on respiratory drives and occlusion pressure. Bull Eur Physiopathol Respir 1980;16(5):645–53.

62. Jensen D, Wolfe LA, Slatkovska L, et al. Effects of human pregnancy on the ventilatory chemoreflex response to carbon dioxide. Am J Physiol Regul Integr Comp Physiol 2005;288(5):R1369–75.

63. Liberatore SM, Pistelli R, Patalano F, et al. Respiratory function during pregnancy. Respiration 1984; 46(2):145–50.

64. Hannhart B, Pickett CK, Moore LG. Effects of estrogen and progesterone on carotid body neural output responsiveness to hypoxia. J Appl Physiol 1990;68(5):1909–16.

65. Gilbert R, Auchincloss JH Jr. Dyspnea of pregnancy. Clinical and physiological observations. Am J Med Sci 1966;252(3):270–6.

66. Tenholder MF, South-Paul JE. Dyspnea in pregnancy. Chest 1989;96(2):381–8.

67. Ueland K, Novy MJ, Metcalfe J. Cardiorespiratory responses to pregnancy and exercise in normal women and patients with heart disease. Am J Obstet Gynecol 1973;115(1):4–10.

68. Pernoll ML, Metcalfe J, Schlenker TL, et al. Oxygen consumption at rest and during exercise in pregnancy. Respir Physiol 1975;25(3):285–93.

69. Artal R, Wiswell R, Romem Y, et al. Pulmonary responses to exercise in pregnancy. Am J Obstet Gynecol 1986;154(2):378–83.

70. Lucius H, Gahlenbeck H, Kleine HO, et al. Respiratory functions, buffer system, and electrolyte concentrations of blood during human pregnancy. Respir Physiol 1970;9(3):311–7.

71. Dayal P, Murata Y, Takamura H. Antepartum and postpartum acid-base changes in maternal blood in normal and complicated pregnancies. J Obstet Gynaecol Br Commonw 1972;79:612–24.

72. Archer GW Jr, Marx GF. Arterial oxygen tension during apnoea in parturient women. Br J Anaesth 1974;46(5):358–60.

73. Ang CK, Tan TH, Walters WA, et al. Postural influence on maternal capillary oxygen and carbon dioxide tension. Br Med J 1969;4(5677):201–3.

74. Tsai CH, de Leeuw NK. Changes in 2,3-diphosphoglycerate during pregnancy and puerperium in normal women and in beta-thalassemia heterozygous women. Am J Obstet Gynecol 1982;142(5): 520–3.

75. Brown MA, Gallery ED. Volume homeostasis in normal pregnancy and pre-eclampsia: physiology and clinical implications. Baillieres Clin Obstet Gynaecol 1994;8(2):287–310.

76. Hytten F. Blood volume changes in normal pregnancy. Clin Haematol 1985;14(3):601–12.

77. Cadnapaphornchai MA, Ohara M, Morris KG Jr, et al. Chronic NOS inhibition reverses systemic vasodilation and glomerular hyperfiltration in pregnancy. Am J Physiol Renal Physiol 2001;280(4): F592–8.

78. Longo LD. Maternal blood volume and cardiac output during pregnancy: a hypothesis of endocrinologic control. Am J Physiol 1983;245(5 Pt 1) R720–9.

79. Wilson M, Morganti AA, Zervoudakis I, et al. Blood pressure, the renin-aldosterone system and sex steroids throughout normal pregnancy. Am J Med 1980;68(1):97–104.

80. Sala C, Campise M, Ambroso G, et al. Atrial natriuretic peptide and hemodynamic changes during normal human pregnancy. Hypertension 1995 25(4 Pt 1):631–6.

81. Bader RA, Bader ME, Rose DF, et al. Hemodynamics at rest and during exercise in normal pregnancy as studies by cardiac catheterization. J Clin Invest 1955;34(10):1524–36.

82. Clark SL, Cotton DB, Lee W, et al. Central hemodynamic assessment of normal term pregnancy. Am J Obstet Gynecol 1989;161(6 Pt 1):1439–42.

83. Robson SC, Hunter S, Boys RJ, et al. Serial study of factors influencing changes in cardiac output during human pregnancy. Am J Physiol 1989;256(4 Pt 2) H1060–5.

84. Mabie WC, DiSessa TG, Crocker LG, et al A longitudinal study of cardiac output in normal human pregnancy. Am J Obstet Gynecol 1994 170(3):849–56.

85. van Oppen AC, Stigter RH, Bruinse HW. Cardiac output in normal pregnancy: a critical review. Obstet Gynecol 1996;87(2):310–8.

86. Hunter S, Robson SC. Adaptation of the maternal heart in pregnancy. Br Heart J 1992;68(6):540–3.

87. Ueland K, Metcalfe J. Circulatory changes in pregnancy. Clin Obstet Gynecol 1975;18(3):41–50.

88. Kramer MS, McDonald SW. Aerobic exercise for women during pregnancy. Cochrane Database Syst Rev 2006;3:CD000180.

89. Wolfe LA, Weissgerber TL. Clinical physiology of exercise in pregnancy: a literature review. J Obstet Gynaecol Can 2003;25(6):473–83.

90. Bung P, Bung C, Artal R, et al. Therapeutic exercise for insulin-requiring gestational diabetics: effects on the fetus–results of a randomized prospective longitudinal study. J Perinat Med 1993;21(2):125–37.

91. Dempsey JC, Sorensen TK, Williams MA, et al Prospective study of gestational diabetes mellitus risk in relation to maternal recreational physical activity before and during pregnancy. Am J Epidemiol 2004;159(7):663–70.

92. Gorski J. Exercise during pregnancy: maternal and fetal responses. A brief review. Med Sci Sports Exerc 1985;17(4):407–16.

93. Wolfe LA, Walker RM, Bonen A, et al. Effects of pregnancy and chronic exercise on respiratory responses to graded exercise. J Appl Physiol 1994;76(5):1928–36.

94. Cole PV, Nainby-Luxmoore RC. Respiratory volumes in labour. Br Med J 1962;1(5285):1118.
95. Reid DH. Respiratory changes in labour. Lancet 1966;1(7441):784–5.
96. Fujitani S, Baldisseri MR. Hemodynamic assessment in a pregnant and peripartum patient. Crit Care Med 2005;33(Suppl 10):S354–61.
97. Robson SC, Hunter S, Moore M, et al. Haemodynamic changes during the puerperium: a Doppler and M-mode echocardiographic study. Br J Obstet Gynaecol 1987;94(11):1028–39.
98. Capeless EL, Clapp JF. When do cardiovascular parameters return to their preconception values? Am J Obstet Gynecol 1991;165(4 Pt 1):883–6.

Fetal Oxygenation and Maternal Ventilation

Giacomo Meschia, MD

KEYWORDS

- Fetal oxygenation • Maternal ventilation
- Placental oxygen transport
- Placental venous equilibration model

THE P_{O_2} OF FETAL BLOOD

In the last trimester of pregnancy, the blood that carries oxygen to the human fetus via the umbilical vein has a much lower P_{O_2} than maternal arterial blood. **Table 1** shows representative data for a 35-week human fetus. Umbilical venous P_{O_2} is approximately 28 mm Hg. Two compensatory mechanisms, namely the high oxygen affinity and the high oxygen capacity of fetal blood, produce an umbilical venous oxygen content, which is comparable to normal values of adult arterial blood. **Fig. 1** shows how the oxygen carried by umbilical venous blood is distributed to the fetal organs.[1] This figure is a schematic drawing of the circulation in the near term fetal lamb and presents oxygen saturation values at different sites. Some of the umbilical venous blood that flows to the fetus (percent saturation, 80) enters directly into the inferior vena cava (IVC) through the ductus venosus. The remainder perfuses the liver. The left hepatic lobe is perfused almost exclusively by umbilical venous blood, whereas the right lobe is perfused by a mixture of portal (percent saturation, 27) and umbilical venous blood. The hepatic artery contributes less than 10% of liver flow.

Within the thoracic IVC, the inputs from the ductus venosus, hepatic veins, and abdominal IVC mix and flow toward the heart to be routed in two directions. The first is through the foramen ovale and the left atrium into the left ventricle. The second is through the right atrium, where a mix of IVC and superior vena cava (SVC) blood forms the venous return of the right ventricle. Another complexity, which is not presented in **Fig. 1**, is that the mixing of ductus venosus, hepatic, and abdominal IVC flows in the thoracic IVC is incomplete, and the ductal flow streams preferentially through the foramen ovale.[2] Most of the output of the right ventricle bypasses the lungs and flows through the ductus arteriosus into the abdominal aorta where it mixes with blood from the ascending aorta to form the blood that perfuses the lower body and the placenta. The heart and upper body are perfused by blood ejected from the left ventricle.

An interesting result of this pattern of blood flow distribution is that the blood perfusing the upper body has a higher oxygen content than that perfusing the lower body. In sheep, the ascending versus descending aorta oxygen content difference has been shown to be normally 0.45 ± 0.02 mM, which represents an oxygen saturation difference of approximately 7%. Theoretical considerations suggest that this difference may be greater in the human fetus, but its actual value has not been determined. However, the blood in the ascending aorta is bound to have lower P_{O_2} and oxygen saturation values than the umbilical vein, and the blood flowing through the abdominal aorta has the same composition as umbilical arterial blood. Consequently, all fetal organs are perfused by blood that in postnatal life would be considered extremely hypoxic. The most remarkable aspect of this state of oxygenation is that it

Departments of Physiology and Pediatrics, Perinatal Research Facility, University of Colorado School of Medicine, 13243 East 23rd Avenue, Mail Stop F441, Aurora, CO 80045, USA
E-mail address: Barbara.falk@ucdenver.edu

Clin Chest Med 32 (2011) 15–19
doi:10.1016/j.ccm.2010.11.007
0272-5231/11/$ – see front matter © 2011 Elsevier Inc. All rights reserved.

Table 1
Representative data for blood oxygen transport in a 35-week human fetus

Blood oxygen, capacity (mM)	9.4
Umbilical venous oxygen, saturation (%)	70.0
Umbilical venous oxygen, content (mM)	6.6
Umbilical venous Po_2 (mm Hg)	28.0
Umbilical arterial oxygen saturation (%)	40.0
Umbilical arterial oxygen content (mM)	3.8
Umbilical arterial Po_2 (torr Hg)	19.0
Cardiac output (mL/min/kg)	500.0
Umbilical blood flow (mL/min/kg)	120.0

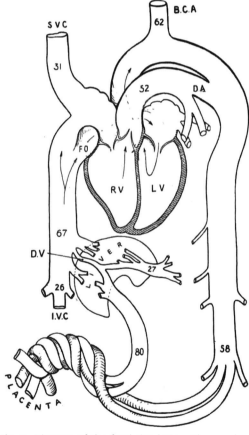

Fig. 1. Diagram of the fetal circulation. The numbers indicate the percentage of oxygen saturation of blood withdrawn simultaneously from various vessels and averaged from determinations on six fetal lambs. BCA, brachiocephalic artery; DA, ductus arteriosus; DV, ductus venosus; FO, foramen ovale; IVC, inferior vena cava; SVC, superior vena cava. (*From* Born GV, Dawes GS, Mott JC, et al. Changes in the heart and lungs at birth. Cold Spring Harb Symp Quant Biol 1954;19:102–7; with permission.)

maintains a rate of fetal oxygen consumption of approximately 300 µM/min per kg body weight (ie, a higher weight-specific oxygen consumption rate than the adult body at rest).

THE VENOUS EQUILIBRATION MODEL OF TRANSPLACENTAL EXCHANGE

The study of transplacental diffusion in sheep has produced a model of placental oxygen transport[3] that may be applicable to the human placenta.[4] According to this model, transplacental diffusion is between maternal and fetal blood streams, which tend to equilibrate the concentration of the diffusing molecules in the uterine and umbilical venous effluents. Several factors prevent equilibration, the most obvious of which is that uterine venous blood is formed through mixing of the maternal placental and myometrial venous outputs. However, in near-term sheep, myometrial flow is approximately 3% of uterine flow and is of negligible importance in determining the large uterine–umbilical venous Po_2 difference present in this species.

Attempts to define the causes of this disequilibrium have produced two interesting results. The first is that the magnitude of the uterine–umbilical venous Po_2 difference (ΔPo_2) is inversely related to placental weight.[5] The second is that experiments aimed at changing fetal oxygenation (ie, maternal inhalation of different gas mixtures,[6] reduction of either uterine[7] or umbilical blood flow)[8] do not appreciably change the ΔPo_2. All of these experimental procedures do change the absolute values of uterine and umbilical venous Po_2, but have virtually no effect on the difference between these variables.

The most important reason for the presence of a large and stable ΔPo_2 is that the placenta has a high rate of oxygen consumption.[9] Oxygen consumption by the placental barrier and the stroma of the placental villi is a hindrance to umbilical oxygen uptake because the placental mitochondria tend to draw oxygen indiscriminately from both the maternal and the fetal circulation. One of the most important functions of the high oxygen affinity and low Po_2 of fetal blood is to reduce the flux of fetal oxygen into placental metabolism.

In ewes with blood having an oxyhemoglobin dissociation curve similar to human adult blood, the normal ΔPo_2 is approximately 14 mm Hg.[10] The ΔPO_2 of the normal human placenta is uncertain; in the only study addressing this question, uterine venous Po_2 was approximately 20 mm Hg higher than umbilical venous Po_2.[4] Current information about near-term human uterine blood flow, umbilical Po_2, and oxygen uptake suggests that the normal ΔPo_2 may be much less than 20 mm Hg.[3] Some of the available evidence about oxygen transport across the human placenta is contradictory and indicates the need for further investigation.

In the third trimester of a normal pregnancy, an exponential increase of umbilical oxygen uptake occurs, which coincides with growth of the placental terminal villi. The structure of these villi indicates that their main function is to increase the rate of transplacental diffusional exchange.[11] In the small placenta of growth-restricted fetuses, the terminal villi are disproportionally reduced compared with the rest of the villous tree.[11] This information may explain why ΔPo_2 is inversely related to placental weight. It suggests that the transplacental venous Po_2 difference is smaller across the terminal villi than across the stem and intermediate villi, so that a reduction in terminal villi would lead to an enlargement of the Po_2 difference between the venous outputs of the maternal and fetal placental blood flows. An enlargement of this difference leads to fetal hypoxia. In a study of 14 cases of human fetal growth restriction, the degree of fetal hypoxia correlated with placental weight. In the 5 most severe cases, umbilical venous Po_2 and oxygen saturation averaged 21.7 ± 1.5 mm Hg and $50.2\% \pm 4.1\%$, respectively.[12]

THE ROLE OF MATERNAL VENTILATION IN FETAL OXYGENATION

Alveolar ventilation increases in pregnancy disproportionally more than the rate of oxidative metabolism. Consequently, at sea level arterial Po_2 increases approximately 10 mm Hg and Pco_2 decreases to approximately 30 mm Hg.[13] Arterial pH also increases o approximately 7.45. At the normal, sea level values of arterial O_2 saturation a 10-mm Hg Po_2 increase has a negligible effect on the oxygen content of maternal blood. The major function of this hyperventilation may be to control fetal Pco_2, because the transplacental excretion of carbon dioxide requires the Pco_2 of umbilical blood to be higher than that in the maternal circulation. In sheep, the Pco_2 of umbilical venous blood is normally approximately 3 mm Hg higher than in the uterine vein, and the Pco_2 of umbilical arterial blood is approximately 13 mm Hg higher than in maternal arterial blood.[10] Fetal pH is regulated to be approximately 7.41 and 7.38 in umbilical venous and arterial blood, respectively. The role of transplacental ion exchange in determining fetal pH has not been defined. Bicarbonate and chloride ions cross the ovine placenta slowly, as shown in tracer studies and from evidence that the infusion of ammonium

chloride in the maternal circulation has been used to create a metabolic acidosis that is limited to the maternal compartment.[6] However, marked differences in placental ion permeability exist among species, suggesting that bicarbonate transport across the human placenta may be faster than in sheep.

Hyperventilation may also be one of the factors that control the redistribution of maternal cardiac output. In pregnancy, cerebral blood flow decreases approximately 20%.[14] At high altitude, the hyperventilation of pregnancy combines with the hypoxic stimulation of breathing to cause a substantial increase in the Po_2 and oxygen saturation of maternal arterial blood. For example, a study of women who were permanent residents of Cerro de Pasco, Peru (altitude 4300 m), showed significantly higher end tidal Po_2 (65.3 vs 57.8 mm Hg) and arterial oxygen saturation (87.4% vs 83.4%) at 36 weeks gestation than at 13 weeks postpartum.[15]

According to evidence in sheep, placental growth and development can compensate for chronic differences in the Po_2 of maternal blood, so that identical levels of fetal oxygenation are possible at two different states of maternal oxygenation.[10] Whether this is true for the human placenta is unclear. Statistical evidence about high altitude human populations has led to the assumption that maternal hypoxia causes fetal growth restriction. However, wide variations in placental development and fetal weight are common in any human population. Because not all the sources of this variability are known, the effect of high-altitude hypoxia on fetal growth remains conjectural.

In pregnant ewes, acute changes in maternal arterial Po_2 have a predictable effect on umbilical venous Po_2, so that this effect can be quantitatively described.[3] This description is based on a knowledge about maternal and fetal oxygen dissociation curves and two boundary conditions. The first condition is that ΔPo_2 remains virtually constant in response to changes in maternal and fetal Po_2. The second is that, within broad physiologic limits, acute changes in maternal arterial Po_2 do not cause a significant change in uterine blood flow.[16]

Whether a similar description is applicable to human pregnancy is debatable, but no credible alternative is currently available. If the sheep descriptive model is applicable, then the steps leading from a change in maternal arterial Po_2 to a change in umbilical vein oxygenation would be like those shown in the numerical example of **Table 2**. Assuming that an acute drop in partial pressure of inspired oxygen causes the changes in maternal arterial Po_2, pH, and oxygen saturation

Table 2
Step-by-step procedure for estimating the change in umbilical venous oxygenation that follows an acute decrease in maternal partial pressure of inspired oxygen

	Steps		Normoxia	Hypoxia
Maternal artery	1	P_{O_2}, mm Hg	102	44
	2	pH	7.45	7.50
	3	Oxygen saturation, %	96	85
Uterine vein	4	Oxygen saturation, %	71	60
	5	pH	7.42	7.47
	6	P_{O_2}, mm Hg	35	27
Umbilical vein	7	P_{O_2}, mm Hg	28	20
	8	pH	7.41	7.46
	9	Oxygen saturation, %	70	55

shown in steps 1, 2, and 3, and with no appreciable changes in uterine blood flow, maternal blood oxygen capacity, and uterine oxygen uptake, the uterine arteriovenous difference of oxygen saturation would remain constant (ie, the decrease in uterine venous saturation would be equal to the decrease in arterial oxygen saturation [step 4]). Of course, if the change in maternal oxygenation is large enough, uterine oxygen uptake would decrease and, consequently, venous saturation would decrease less than arterial saturation. Therefore, step 4 describes the maximum decrease in venous oxygen saturation that may be expected at constant flow and oxygen capacity. The change in uterine venous pH would be approximately equal to the arterial (step 5); whether exactly equal or different by ± 0.01 units is inconsequential.

The next step (step 6) uses the uterine venous saturation and pH data and knowledge of the human maternal oxygen dissociation curve[17] to calculate that uterine venous P_{O_2} changed from 35 to 27 mm Hg. Step 7 applies the notion of a nearly constant ΔP_{O_2} to estimate that an 8–mm Hg decrease in uterine venous P_{O_2} would cause an equal drop of umbilical venous P_{O_2} from the initial 28 to 20 mm Hg. In steps 8 and 9, umbilical venous P_{O_2} and pH are used to calculate umbilical venous oxygen saturation using a human fetal oxygen dissociation curve.[17]

In this example, a 58–mm Hg decrease in maternal arterial P_{O_2} (44 vs 102) results in an 8–mm Hg decrease in umbilical venous P_{O_2} (20 vs 28). This effect may seem small but it causes an important change in fetal oxygenation because it decreases umbilical venous oxygen saturation from 70% to 55%. Given the P_{50} and steep slope of the fetal oxyhemoglobin dissociation curve, a small decrease in P_{O_2} causes a large decrease in oxygen saturation to less than 70%. In the fetal lamb, for normal values of umbilical blood flow and oxygen capacity, the threshold to severe hypoxia and metabolic acidosis

is crossed when umbilical oxygen saturation decreases to less than 50%.[7] An extension of the theoretical exercise shown in **Table 2** would be to show that for an identical decrease in maternal arterial P_{O_2} and oxygen saturation, a variable effect would occur on fetal oxygenation, depending on the initial values of uterine and umbilical oxygen saturation, pH, and P_{O_2}. To be useful, however, this calculation should be based on more accurate data about oxygen transport across the human placenta than are now available.

In conclusion, in the past 20 years, measurements of umbilical blood flow and umbilical venous P_{O_2}, oxygen saturation, pH, and oxygen capacity have provided reliable information about the state of oxygenation of normal and growth restricted human fetuses. However, no comparable information is available about the uterine circulation. Therefore, understanding of oxygen transport across the human placenta and the effect of maternal ventilation on fetal oxygenation is tentative, and currently based on a model that is derived from evidence in another species. The main purpose of this model is to illustrate the kind of information that is needed to make further progress in this area.

REFERENCES

1. Born GV, Dawes GS, Mott JC, et al. Changes in the heart and lungs at birth. Cold Spring Harb Symp Quant Biol 1954;19:102–7.
2. Edelstone DI, Rudolph AM. Preferential streaming of ductus venosus blood to the brain and heart in fetal lambs. Am J Physiol 1979;237:H724–9.
3. Meschia G. Placental respiratory gas exchange and fetal oxygenation. In: Creasy RK, Resnik R, Iams JD, et al, editors. Creasy & Resnik's maternal-fetal medicine: principles and practice. 6th edition. Philadelphia: Saunders Elsevier Inc; 2009. p. 181–91.

4. Pardi G, Cetin I, Marconi AM, et al. Venous drainage of the human uterus: respiratory gas studies in normal and fetal growth retarded pregnancies. Am J Obstet Gynecol 1992;166:699–706.

5. Regnault TR, de Vrijer B, Galan HL, et al. Development and mechanisms of fetal hypoxia in severe fetal growth restriction. Placenta 2007;28(7):714–23.

6. Rankin JH, Meschia G, Makowski EL, et al. Relationship between uterine and umbilical venous PO_2 in sheep. Am J Physiol 1971;220(6):1688–92.

7. Wilkening RB, Meschia G. Fetal oxygen uptake, oxygenation, and acid-base balance as a function of uterine blood flow. Am J Physiol 1983;244:H749–55.

8. Wilkening RB, Meschia G. Effect of umbilical blood flow on transplacental diffusion of ethanol and oxygen. Am J Physiol 1989;256(3 Pt 2):H813–20.

9. Meschia G, Battaglia FC, Hay WW Jr, et al. Utilization of substrates by the ovine placenta in vivo. Fed Proc 1979;39(2):245–99.

10. Wilkening RB, Molina RD, Meschia G. Placental oxygen transport in sheep with different haemoglobin types. Am J Physiol 1988;254:R585–9.

11. Jackson MR, Walsh AJ, Morrow RJ, et al. Reduced placental villous tree elaboration in small-for-gestational-age pregnancies: relationship with umbilical artery Doppler waveforms. Am J Obstet Gynecol 1995;172:518–25.

12. Marconi AM, Paolini CL, Stramare L, et al. Steady state maternal-fetal leucine enrichments in normal and intrauterine growth-restricted pregnancies. Pediatr Res 1999;46:114–9.

13. Templeton A, Kelman GR. Maternal blood-gases, (PAO_2-PaO_2), physiological shunt and V_D/V_T in normal pregnancy. Br J Anaesth 1996;48(10):1001–4.

14. Zeeman GG, Hatab M, Twickler DM. Maternal cerebral blood flow changes in pregnancy. Am J Obstet Gynecol 2003;189(4):968–72.

15. Moore LG, Brodeur P, Chumbe O, et al. Maternal hypoxic ventilatory response, ventilation, and infant birth weight at 4,300 m. J Appl Physiol 1986;60(4):1401–6.

16. Makowski EL, Hertz RH, Meschia G. Effects of acute maternal hypoxia and hyperoxia on the blood flow to the pregnant uterus. Am J Obstet Gynecol 1973;115(5):624–31.

17. Hellegers AE, Schruefer JJ. Nomograms and empirical equations relating oxygen tension, percentage saturation, and pH in maternal and fetal blood. Am J Obstet Gynecol 1961;81(2):377–84.

High Altitude During Pregnancy

Colleen Glyde Julian, PhD

KEYWORDS

- Hypoxia • Pregnancy • Altitude • Fetal growth
- Preeclampsia

Pregnancy initiates a series of dynamic physiologic responses to compensate for the metabolic demands and anatomic load associated with advancing gestation. On the maternal side, one of the greatest physiologic challenges is to maintain an adequate supply of oxygenated blood to the uteroplacental circulation for fetal development. This challenge of oxygen transport is magnified under conditions of limited oxygen availability, such as hypoxia from high-altitude exposure or pathologic states such as pulmonary disease or anemia. However, among healthy women living at high altitude, maternal physiologic adjustments act to counter arterial hypoxemia and to facilitate the hemodynamic adaptations necessary to aid increased uteroplacental blood flow. Despite this partial compensation for environmental hypoxia, high altitude impairs fetal growth, increases the incidence of preeclampsia, and, as a result, significantly increases the risk of perinatal and/or maternal morbidity and mortality. For these reasons, high altitude has been and will continue to be an invaluable model to explore the physiologic and genetic mechanisms that govern beneficial and pathologic responses to chronic hypoxia during pregnancy without the confounding effect of existing hypoxia-related disease (eg, congenital heart disease, anemia, low blood volume). Resolution of this knowledge gap has tremendous potential to contribute to the development of diagnostic, preventative, and/or treatment strategies to minimize the detrimental consequences of chronic hypoxia during pregnancy, irrespective of altitude.

This review summarizes the clinical consequences and physiologic challenges that emerge when pregnancy and high altitude coincide and highlights the adaptations that serve to protect oxygenation and fetal growth under conditions of chronic hypoxia.

THE CHALLENGE OF HIGH-ALTITUDE HYPOXIA

Again on passing the Great Headache Mountain, the little Headache Mountain, the Red Land and the Fever Slope, men's bodies become feverish, they lose color and are attacked with headache and vomiting…[1]
Ch'ien Han Shu text (approximately 32–37 BC)

High-altitude hypoxia poses one of the greatest environmental threats to human survival. Barometric pressure decreases with ascending altitude, decreasing the P_{O_2} and, in turn, oxygen availability in ambient air. This hypobaric hypoxia is the most pervasive physiologic challenge associated with high-altitude exposure, given that the lower humidity, colder temperatures, and increased solar radiation that also accompany higher elevations can largely be ameliorated through behavioral modification. In contrast, aside from supplemental oxygen or descent, there is no such strategy to avert the effects of environmental hypoxia.

High altitude becomes physiologically and clinically relevant at altitudes greater than or equal to 2500 m, corresponding to a Pa_{O_2} of 60 to 70 mm Hg and not so coincidentally, to the point at which arterial oxygen saturation (Sa_{O_2}) begins to decrease exponentially with further Pa_{O_2} decrements. Importantly, the risk of arterial hypoxemia and its associated complications can occur at much lower altitudes in individuals with existing

This work was supported by grant number NIH HLBI-079647 and TW-01188.
Altitude Research Center, Department of Emergency Medicine, Anschutz Medical Campus, University of Colorado Denver, 12469 East 17th Place, Aurora, CO 80045-0508, USA
E-mail address: colleen.julian@ucdenver.edu

Clin Chest Med 32 (2011) 21–31
doi:10.1016/j.ccm.2010.10.008
0272-5231/11/$ – see front matter © 2011 Elsevier Inc. All rights reserved.

conditions that limit oxygen transport (eg, pulmonary or cardiovascular disease).

Physiologic compensations such as alveolar hyperventilation and erythropoiesis facilitate oxygen transport under conditions of hypoxia, although even these responses are, at times, inadequate to achieve sea-level Sa_{O_2} values depending on the altitude, rate of ascent, and other factors that limit oxygen transport (eg, anemia).

INFLUENCE OF HIGH ALTITUDE ON PREGNANCY OUTCOME

The clinical relevance of high-altitude hypoxia for pregnancy outcome is best illustrated by the 3-fold greater incidence of intrauterine growth restriction (IUGR) at high (≥2500 m) altitude relative to low altitude (**Fig. 1**).[2–5] IUGR, defined as birth weight less than the 10th percentile of sea-level values for a given gestational age and sex,[6] is associated with a 4-fold increase in stillbirth and an 8- to 20-fold increase in neonatal mortality depending on the degree of growth restriction.[7] High altitude also reduces birth weight by an average of 120 g per 1000 m elevation gain,[3]

shifting the entire birth weight distribution to the left.[8] Because this altitudinal effect cannot be explained by maternal or socioeconomic traits known to contribute to reduced fetal growth at low altitude (eg, primiparity, small stature, low economic status),[3,9,10] it has, instead, been attributed to an independent effect of chronic hypoxia to slow fetal growth in the third trimester rather than to shorten gestation.[8]

The incidence of preeclampsia, a potentially life-threatening hypertensive disorder of pregnancy, also increases by approximately 3-fold at high altitude.[11] Preeclampsia is defined as newly elevated systolic (>140 mm Hg) and diastolic (>90 mm Hg) blood pressures accompanied by proteinuria (≥1+ or ≥300 mg in 24 hours) that develops after the 20th week of pregnancy. Although preeclampsia is associated with reduced fetal growth, it is only responsible for approximately half of the altitude-associated reduction in birth weight.[3,11]

Preeclampsia occurs in 5% to 8% of all pregnancies in the United States; however, the incidence and severity is markedly higher in developing countries where more than 90% of the most serious outcomes occur.[12,13] Even among developed countries with comparatively low maternal mortality rates, the proportion of maternal deaths attributed to preeclampsia-related complications is high, accounting for up to two-thirds of maternal deaths in the United Kingdom.[14] The likelihood of poor fetal outcome in cases of preeclampsia depends, in part, on the timing of disease onset. The authors' research group recently identified that women at high altitude with early-onset preeclampsia (ie, before 34 weeks' gestation) delivered preterm, and nearly half (43%) of the women delivered stillborn, growth-restricted infants (Vaughn Browne, MD, PhD, Aurora, CO, USA, personal communication, June 2010). In contrast, women with late-onset disease (ie, after 34 weeks' gestation) delivered at term, but they delivered IUGR infants more often than women who remained normotensive during pregnancy. The prevalence and potential severity of preeclampsia highlights the utility of high altitude as a research model for this disease.

High altitude also increases the risk of several other pregnancy complications (eg, bleeding in the first trimester, premature rupture of membranes, preterm labor, oligohydramnios or polyhydramnios, placental abruption or previa), perinatal morbidity (eg, fetal and neonatal respiratory distress, nuchal cord, congenital abnormalities, early arterial desaturation, perinatal respiratory infections, increased pulmonary vascular resistance, and pulmonary hypertension), and mortality.[10,15–17]

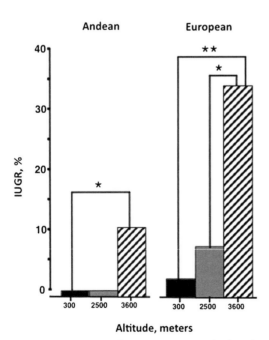

Fig. 1. The incidence of IUGR increases with altitude. At high altitude, IUGR frequency is 5-fold greater in Europeans compared with Andeans after accounting for the effects of other factors that influence fetal growth (unadjusted values shown). Significant differences between altitudes are denoted by * $P<.05$ or ** $P<.01$.

To summarize, chronic hypoxia of high altitude markedly decreases birth weight and increases the incidence of numerous pregnancy complications, including IUGR and preeclampsia. In the following section, unique physiologic responses to pregnancy at high altitude and their potential effects on pregnancy outcome are described.

UNIQUE PHYSIOLOGIC COMPENSATIONS DURING HIGH-ALTITUDE PREGNANCY

Successful pregnancy outcome at high altitude depends on maternal and, ultimately, fetal physiologic compensations for diminished oxygen availability and its secondary effects (eg, hypoxia-regulated gene expression). Failure to maintain maternal arterial oxygenation, impaired maternal vascular adaptation to pregnancy, and/or altered placental/fetal nutrient transport or consumption seem to be important factors for compromised fetal growth at high altitude.[18–22]

Determinants of Maternal Arterial Oxygenation

Maternal arterial oxygenation is an important determinant of infant birth weight at high altitude,[18,19,23–25] and depends on numerous factors (eg, ambient oxygen availability, ventilatory sensitivity, respiratory function, diffusion capacity, oxygen-carrying capacity).

Ventilation

Alveolar ventilation and tidal volume increase with pregnancy (**Table 1**), largely because of the stimulatory effect of progesterone on the medullary respiratory centers,[26] increased carotid body sensitivity to hypoxia, and greater central nervous system translation of carotid body signals that are mediated by estrogen.[27] The 2-fold increase in hypoxic ventilatory response (HVR) with pregnancy is also thought to be regulated by the hormonal stimulation of progesterone and estrogen.[27–30] Pregnancy-induced hyperventilation under normal sea-level conditions raises maternal Pao_2 but has a negligible effect on Sao_2 because these values are already near their physiologic limits (see **Table 1**). In contrast, hyperventilation during pregnancy at high altitude increases both maternal Pao_2 and Sao_2, thereby maintaining oxygen content near the values in nonpregnant women.[24,25,29,31] Women with higher ventilation and higher blood oxygen levels deliver heavier infants, highlighting the importance of maternal arterial oxygenation for the preservation of fetal growth at high altitude.[24,25,32] However, given that pregnancy-induced hyperventilation preserves maternal arterial oxygen content, ventilation does not seem to be central to altitude-associated decrements in birth weight.

Hematologic considerations

The hemodilutional effect of pregnancy, caused by an increase in plasma volume across gestation that is not matched by an equivalent increase in red cell mass, is independent of altitude.[21] As a result, maternal hemoglobin concentration is generally reduced by a similar proportion at low and high altitudes during pregnancy. However, because chronic hypoxia provides a constant erythropoietic stimulus, women at high altitude begin pregnancy with elevated hemoglobin relative to their low-altitude counterparts, and this difference remains across gestation (see **Table 1**).[21]

Diffusion capacity

Pulmonary diffusing capacity of lung for carbon monoxide corrected for hemoglobin concentrations ($DLco_c$) is not influenced by pregnancy at low altitude.[33] Increased pulmonary blood volume and cardiac output during pregnancy should increase capillary surface area for gas exchange; however, the reduced hemoglobin concentrations characteristic of pregnancy effectively equalizes $DLco_c$ of pregnant women with that of nonpregnant women. In contrast, $DLco_c$ is lower during the third trimester compared with nonpregnant women at high altitude, an observation that may be explained by greater ventilation-perfusion mismatch during the later portion of gestation.[34] Comparing altitudes, $DLco_c$ is greater at high than at low altitude during pregnancy as well as in the nonpregnant state, possibly because of greater hemoglobin, ventilation, and pulmonary blood volume during high-altitude pregnancy.[34,35]

Respiratory function

Similar to sea-level conditions, pregnancy does not alter forced expiratory volume in the first second of expiration (FEV_1), forced vital capacity (FVC), or the ratio of FEV_1 to FVC (FEV_1/FVC) among women residing at high altitude in Colorado (3100 m) (**Table 2**).[32,36,37] In contrast, one study reported that FEV_1 declined across pregnancy at 4300 m (Cerro de Pasco, Peru).[38] In this study, McAuliffe and colleagues[38] suggested that increased pulmonary blood volume associated with pregnancy may reduce FEV_1 by increasing interstitial edema and, in turn, raising airway resistance. Functional residual capacity (FRC) decreases with pregnancy at low and high altitudes as a result of the increasing uterus size, increased abdominal pressure, reduced chest wall compliance, and greater subcostal angle associated with advancing gestation.[33,39] Reduced FRC during pregnancy is associated with small airway

Table 1
Determinants of uteroplacental oxygen delivery

Variable	North America, Rocky Mountains				South America, Andes				Asia, Himalayas	
	United States				Bolivia		Peru		Tibet	
	Low Altitude, 1600 m		High Altitude, 3100 m		High Altitude, 3600 m		High Altitude, 4300 m		High Altitude, 3658 m	
	Nonpregnant	Pregnant	Nonpregnant	Pregnant	Nonpregnant	Pregnant	Nonpregnant	Pregnant	Nonpregnant	Pregnant
V_E, L BTPS/min	7.1 ± 0.4	9.6 ± 0.4	8.8 ± 0.3	11.4 ± 0.3	8.5 ± 0.4	8.9 ± 0.4	9.5 ± 0.4	12.0 ± 0.7	10.1 ± 0.5	11.7 ± 0.3
V_{O_2}, ml STPD/min/kg	3.1 ± 0.1	3.5 ± 0.2	3.1 ± 0.8	3.3 ± 0.1	...	...	...	...	5.2 ± 0.2	4.7 ± 0.1
Sa_{O_2}, %	94.6 ± 0.5	95.4 ± 0.4	90.9 ± 0.2	92.2 ± 0.2	92.3 ± 0.3	94.0 ± 0.3	82.9 ± 1.2	87.4 ± 0.4	89.0 ± 0.5	89.9 ± 0.3
Hgb, g/100 mL blood	13.9	12.6	15.1 ± 0.2	13.8 ± 0.2	14.3 ± 0.2	13.2 ± 0.2	14.0 ± 0.4	13.1 ± 0.3	14.9 ± 0.2	12.6 ± 0.3
Ca_{O_2}, mL O_2/100 mL blood	17.5	14.5	18.7 ± 0.2	17.3 ± 0.2	17.9 ± 0.2	17.1 ± 0.2	15.9 ± 0.4	15.6 ± 0.4	18.1 ± 0.3	15.5 ± 0.3
Blood volume, mL/kg	66.6	79.7	58.3 ± 1.2	69.9 ± 1.9	75.8 ± 2.3	85.5 ± 1.7	...	...		
CO, L/min	5.3	6.5	...	...	...	...	5.2 ± 0.5	5.8 ± 0.1	...	...
MAP, mm Hg	84	85	87 ± 1	85 ± 1	78.3 ± 1.3	79.8 ± 1.2	NA	NA	76 ± 2	85 ± 2
HR, bpm	74	84	81 ± 1	93 ± 2	75 ± 1	81 ± 2	77 ± 2	79 ± 2	76 ± 2	81 ± 2
UA flow, mL/min	6 ± 2	312 ± 22	8 ± 2	203 ± 48	66.1 ± 15.6	735.3 ± 88.7	...	...	...	...

Mean ± SEM for percentages with 95% confidence interval. Nonpregnant (at least 3 months postpartum) and pregnant (36 weeks' gestation) values for United States, Bolivian, and Peruvian women are longitudinal, whereas Tibetan data are cross-sectional.

Abbreviations: bpm, beats per minute; BTPS, body temperature and pressure, saturated; Ca_{O_2}, arterial oxygen content; CO, cardiac output; Hgb, hemoglobin; HR, heart rate; MAP, mean arterial blood pressure; STPD, standard temperature and pressure, dry; UA flow, uterine artery blood flow; V_E, expired volume per unit time; V_{O_2}, oxygen consumption.

Data from Niermeyer S, Zamudio S, Moore LG. The people. In: Hornbein TF, Schoene RB, editors. High Altitude: an exploration of human adaptation, vol. 161. In Lung Biology In Health and Disease, Lenfant C (series editor). New York: Marcel Dekker; 2001. p. 43–100.

Table 2
Respiratory characteristics at low and high altitude in the nonpregnant and pregnant states

Variable	Low Altitude			High Altitude			References
	Nonpreg	Preg	Altitude	Nonpreg	Preg	Altitude	
FEV$_1$, L	3.0 ± 0.5	2.9 ± 0.4	Sea level	3.2 ± 0.5	3.3 ± 0.4	4300 m	McAuliffe and colleagues,[38] 2004
	3.1	3.0	Sea level				Milne,[37] 1979
FVC, L	...	...	...	3.8 ± 0.1	3.8 ± 0.1	3100 m	Moore and colleagues,[32] 1982
	3.4 ± 0.5	3.3 ± 0.5	Sea level	3.6 ± 0.5	3.8 ± 0.5	4300 m	McAuliffe and colleagues,[38] 2004
FEV$_1$/FVC, %	...	...	...	94 ± 1	94 ± 1	3100 m	Moore and colleagues,[32] 1982
	90 ± 5	88 ± 5	Sea level	87 ± 4	87 ± 6	4300 m	McAuliffe and colleagues,[38] 2004
	84	81.8	Sea level				Milne,[37] 1979
FRC, L	1.9 ± 0.4	2.0 ± 0.4	Sea level	2.6 ± 0.4	2.06 ± 0.5	4300 m	McAuliffe and colleagues,[38] 2004
F$_R$, breaths/min	...	...	...	15.7 ± 0.6	15.6 ± 0.8	3100 m	Moore and colleagues,[32] 1982
	...	...	...	17.4 ± 0.9	17.4 ± 0.8	3600 m	Vargas and colleagues,[24] 2007
	14 ± 1	15 ± 1	1600 m				Moore and colleagues,[30] 1987
V$_T$ L/min BTPS	...	...	...	0.6 ± 0.0	0.8 ± 0.0	3100 m	Moore and colleagues,[25] 1982
	...	...	...	0.7 ± 0.1	0.8 ± 0.1	3600 m	Vargas and colleagues,[24] 2007
	0.5 ± 0.0	0.7 ± 0.1	1600 m				Moore and colleagues,[30] 1987
TLC, L	4.2 ± 0.6	4.5 ± 0.6	Sea level	5.2 ± 0.5	5.3 ± 0.7	4300 m	McAuliffe and colleagues,[38] 2004
RV, L	0.9 ± 0.3	1.1 ± 0.3	Sea level	1.2 ± 0.4	1.2 ± 0.5	4300 m	McAuliffe and colleagues,[38] 2004
HVR, A value	...	...	...	42.7 ± 6.3	112.4 ± 3.0	3600 m	Vargas and colleagues,[24] 2007
	124 ± 13	237 ± 26	1600 m				Moore and colleagues,[30] 1987
D$_{LCO_C}$ mmol/min/kPa	8[a]	7.5[a]	Sea level	24.5[a]	22[a]	4300 m	McAuliffe and colleagues,[33] 2002

Abbreviations: BTPS, body temperature pressure saturated; F$_R$, respiratory frequency; FRC, functional residual capacity; Nonpreg, nonpregnant (ie, postpartum or nulliparous); Preg, third trimester of pregnancy; RV, residual volume; TLC, total lung capacity; V$_T$, tidal volume.

[a] Estimated from the figure presented in McAuliffe,[33] 2002.

closure during normal breathing and, consequently, an increase in alveolar-arterial oxygen gradient in late gestation. In combination with the existing challenges to maternal arterial oxygenation at high altitude, reduced FRC may be of particular consequence at high altitude, given the potential to further increase the risk of maternal hypoxemia. Comparing altitudes, total lung capacity, inspiratory capacity, FRC, expiratory residual volume, residual volume, FVC, and FEV_1 are greater but mean FEV_1/FVC is lower during pregnancy at high altitude than at low altitude.[38]

Oxygen Transport

Sufficient oxygen availability for fetal development depends not only on oxygen content but also on effective transportation of oxygenated blood to the uteroplacental circulation. High altitude decreases the pregnancy-induced increase in cardiac output, likely due to a failure to decrease peripheral vascular resistance and/or the effect of lower absolute blood volume to reduce cardiac filling (ie, preload) and, in turn, stroke volume.[40–42] Expansion of intravascular space is also impaired with pregnancy at high altitude, as evidenced by a lesser gestational augmentation of maternal left atrial diameter (12% vs 25%), end-diastolic diameter (1% vs 5%), and cardiac output (17% vs 41%).[40] The significance of this impairment is that in combination with reduced vascular tone, increased arterial compliance and the expansion of intravascular space compensate for the total increased circulating blood volume that accompanies pregnancy.

Uteroplacental impedance parameters, frequently used to assess placental insufficiency and risk for adverse pregnancy outcome including IUGR or preeclampsia, are reduced at high than at low altitude.[43–45] This reduction suggests that regulation (or diminution) of uteroplacental blood flow at high altitude is likely driven primarily by maternal rather than by placental factors. Therefore, the authors research group has focused primarily on the maternal side of the uteroplacental circulation.

Direct measurements of uteroplacental blood flow in humans are limited by ethical constraints. However, because the bilateral uterine arteries supply two-thirds of the uteroplacental circulation (the ovarian arteries are responsible for the remainder), uterine artery blood flow is often used as an approximation for total uteroplacental blood flow. For orientation, volumetric uterine artery blood flow measurements are calculated using the vessel cross-sectional area (πr^2) and time-averaged mean flow velocity (TAM) [$60 \times (\pi r^2) \times$ TAM].

Permanent high-altitude residence interferes with maternal vascular adjustment to pregnancy, attenuating the normal increase of uterine artery diameter and blood flow.[46] For example, the pregnancy-associated increase in uterine artery diameter among women living at high altitude in Colorado (Leadville, 3100 m) was half that of their healthy counterparts at lower altitudes (1600 m, Denver).[18,46] In parallel, high altitude reduced uterine artery blood flow by one-fifth near term, an effect that was attributed to smaller vessel diameter because blood flow velocities were equivalent between altitudes. Complementing the Colorado studies, the author's recent work in Bolivia (3600 m) demonstrated a positive association between uterine artery blood flow and/or oxygen delivery and fetal growth by week 20 of pregnancy.[21] Zamudio and colleagues[47] also report positive associations between bilateral uterine artery blood flow or oxygen delivery and birth weight at high altitude.

High altitude also alters patterns of blood flow redistribution that accompany pregnancy at low altitude, an effect that likely contributes to the altitudinal reduction in uteroplacental blood flow. Specifically, the proportion of common iliac blood flow distributed to the uterine versus the external iliac artery increases during pregnancy at low altitude, effectively giving precedence to the uteroplacental circulation; this effect of pregnancy is less pronounced at high than at low altitude.[18,19]

Hypoxia regulates the production of numerous circulating factors known to influence vascular function during pregnancy and/or to be associated with pregnancy complications that are accompanied by uteroplacental ischemia (eg, IUGR or preeclampsia). Given the pronounced reduction of uterine artery expansion at high altitude, the author considers it likely that such factors, including vasoactive substances, angiogenic or inflammatory mediators, and reactive oxygen species, contribute to impaired maternal vascular adaptation at high altitude.[48–54] The author's finding that circulating levels of the potent vasoconstrictor endothelin-1 relative to nitric oxide metabolites (NO_x) were greater in pregnant women at high than in those at low altitude in Colorado supports this general hypothesis.[46] However, extensive evaluations are clearly needed to determine the role of these and other related processes in pregnancy complications associated with high-altitude residence.

HIGHLAND ANCESTRY PROTECTS FETAL GROWTH AT HIGH ALTITUDE

A unique dimension of high-altitude models to examine the effect of chronic hypoxia during human pregnancy is that the magnitude by which fetal growth declines with increasing elevation depends, in part, on the population ancestry.[2,21,55–57] Such ancestry-related effects are informative not only for identifying physiologic traits that increase or decrease susceptibility to poor pregnancy outcome but also for determining the potential role of genetics in the modification of biologic processes underlying these effects. For this reason, the authors and others have sought to evaluate and compare the effect of high altitude on maternal and fetal characteristics during pregnancy in populations of lowland and highland ancestry. Most work in this area has been generated from comparative studies conducted in Asia (ie, Tibet) or South America (eg, Bolivia) because large genetically distinguishable populations of lowland or highland ancestry live across a wide range of altitudes in these regions.

Specifically, the effect of high altitude in reducing birth weight is less in populations of highland origin (eg, Tibetan or Andean) compared with that in lowland origin groups (eg, Han Chinese or European).[2,56,58] As a result, the proportion of IUGR infants is greater at high altitude in lowland than in highland origin groups (see **Fig. 1**).[2,56] The magnitude of this ancestry effect is clearly demonstrated by the author's recent finding that the risk of IUGR at 3600 m in Bolivia was 5-fold higher in European than Andean infants.[2] Contrary to numerous large-scale reports including both medical record reviews and physiologic studies, one investigative group recently questioned the protective effect of Andean ancestry for birth weight at high altitude based on their observation that Andean infants weighed more than European infants, irrespective of the altitude.[47] It is possible that their exclusive inclusion of women undergoing scheduled Cesarean delivery, who tend to be of higher socioeconomic status, accounts for the greater Andean birth weights compared with other reports. With the exception of their report, an extensive literature strongly supports that highland ancestry protects against decrements in birth weight associated with high-altitude residence.[2,21,56,57]

In two separate but complementary reports, the author considered the possibility that Andean women had higher levels of arterial oxygenation and/or greater uteroplacental blood flow during pregnancy at high altitude than Europeans and that one or both of these factors contributed to the protection of birth weight, apparent in the Andeans.[19,24] At high altitude, pregnancy increased maternal ventilation, diminished end-tidal P_{CO_2}, and increased both Sa_{O_2} and HVR in Andean and European women.[24] Despite reduced hemoglobin concentrations in both ancestry groups, arterial oxygen content remained close to that

of nonpregnant women because the pregnancy-associated increase in Sa_{O_2} offset the hemoglobin decrease. Past reports support the author's findings in that no differences in HVR or resting ventilation were identified between Tibetans (highland origin) and Han Chinese (lowland origin) women during pregnancy at high altitude.[31] Maternal oxygenation and ventilation were important for fetal growth in that Andeans who had more ventilation (ie, lower end-tidal P_{CO_2} and/or higher expired volume per unit time) delivered larger infants, but given that HVR, resting ventilation, Sa_{O_2}, total blood volume, and plasma volume increased with pregnancy to a similar extent in Andean and European women residing at high altitude, the author concluded that oxygen content was not responsible for ancestry-associated differences in birth weight at high altitude.[24]

Extensive investigations support an alternative explanation. The author's recent prospective studies in Bolivia revealed profound differences between ancestry groups in terms of maternal vascular adjustments to pregnancy at high altitude and that these differences were not only responsible for increasing uterine artery oxygen delivery but also positively associated with birth weight.[19,21] Specifically, at high altitude, pregnancy increased uterine artery diameter and TAM but lowered uterine artery vascular resistance in both groups. Andean compared with European women had similar uterine artery blood flow in the nonpregnant state, but the values were markedly greater at both weeks 20 and 36 of pregnancy (68% and 56%, respectively) because of larger uterine artery diameter. Moreover, in the study, uterine artery oxygen delivery was nearly 2-fold greater in the Andean than in the European women at week 36 at high altitude as the result of greater uterine artery blood flow, not Sa_{O_2} or hemoglobin concentration (**Fig. 2**). Suggesting an etiologic role of these factors for protected birth weight in Andeans, uterine artery blood flow, oxygen delivery, and fetal biometry were distinct between ancestry groups by week 20 in the study.

In contrast, Zamudio and colleagues[47] have reported equivalent reductions in uterine artery blood flow and O_2 delivery in Andeans compared with Europeans at 38 weeks of pregnancy. As discussed briefly later, the cross-sectional study design used by Zamudio and colleagues significantly limits the ability to identify the presence or absence of a causal relationship between uteroplacental blood flow and oxygen delivery for reduced fetal growth. Recently, Postigo and colleagues[59] reported that despite reduced fetal blood flow at high altitude, fetal oxygen consumption was equivalent between altitudes because of

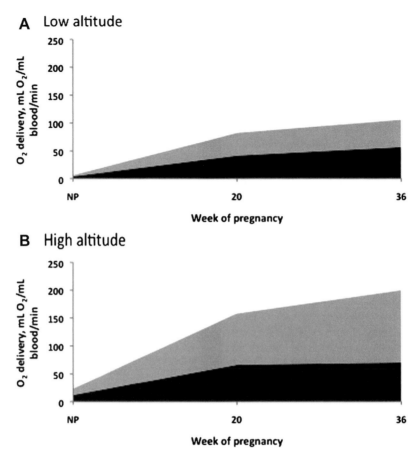

A Low altitude

B High altitude

Fig. 2. At low altitude, the pregnancy-associated increase in uteroplacental oxygen delivery was equivalent in Andean (*black*) and European (*gray*) women (*A*). In contrast, at high altitude, uteroplacental oxygen delivery was more than 2-fold greater in Andean than in European women at 36 weeks' gestation (*B*). NP, nonpregnant.

a greater fetal oxygen extraction at high compared with low altitude. Based on these findings, this research group suggests that diminished fetal glucose availability rather than oxygen delivery is likely responsible for the reduced birth weights seen at altitude. Interpretation of their findings should consider that these studies were designed to explore the role of placental factors for the altitude-associated decline in birth weight, and as such, the measurements were taken 4 days before delivery. Although this sampling strategy is ideal for the intended study, it limits the ability to determine the causal relationship between oxygen delivery and fetal size because fetal growth and, likely, oxygen requirements already begin to slow late in the third trimester. This near-term sampling interval coupled with the investigators' finding that impaired uteroplacental oxygen delivery does contribute to reduced birth weight at high altitude leads to the consideration that the conclusions drawn by the investigators are somewhat premature.

More if not most importantly, the contribution of uteroplacental oxygen delivery to the protection against reduced fetal growth at high altitude does not exclude the involvement of other factors such as variations in glucose availability, glucose transport, placental oxygen consumption or diffusing capacity, or fetal substrate use. The reverse is also true. Evidence does suggest that both fetal and maternal glucose levels are lower at high than at low altitude,[22,60] possibly because of differences in glucose use (placental or maternal), insulin sensitivity, or glucose transport.[22,61] In order to be beneficial for fetal growth and development, increased uteroplacental blood flow must be paralleled by adequate transport mechanisms and use strategies.

SUMMARY

Chronic hypoxia of high-altitude residence significantly increases the risk of poor pregnancy outcome, despite profound physiologic compensations that fully or partially preserve maternal arterial oxygenation and blood flow to the developing fetus. High-altitude research models are invaluable to explore not only the detrimental aspects of chronic hypoxia during pregnancy but also the resolution of these effects. In particular, the protection against hypoxia-associated reductions in fetal growth afforded by highland ancestry provides the unique opportunity to identify physiologic and genetic processes that modify the negative effects of chronic hypoxia for pregnancy outcome. This dimension of the high-altitude research model is particularly intriguing in that improvements in the ability to predict, identify, prevent, and treat complications associated with chronic hypoxia during pregnancy will require an integrated exploration of genetic variants, gene and protein expressions, physiologic characteristics, as well as factors that modify these components (eg, epigenetics, gene-environment interaction). The author considers likely candidates to include alterations in HIF-1α regulated or regulatory genes and their expression, factors that govern vascular growth and remodeling, including angiogenic and/or immunologic substances. Such studies have the potential to improve health outcomes for the more than 140 million high-altitude residents of the world as well as individuals affected by hypoxia-related complications during pregnancy at low altitude.

REFERENCES

1. Ashcroft F. Life at the extremes: the science of survival. Berkeley (CA): University of California Press; 2002. p. 347.
2. Julian CG, Vargas E, Armaza JF, et al. High-altitude ancestry protects against hypoxia-associated reductions in fetal growth. Arch Dis Child Fetal Neonatal Ed 2007;92(5):F372–7.
3. Jensen GM, Moore LG. The effect of high altitude and other risk factors on birthweight: independent or interactive effects? Am J Public Health 1997;87: 1003–7.
4. Unger C, Weiser JK, McCullough RE, et al. Altitude, low birth weight, and infant mortality in Colorado. JAMA 1988;259:3427–32.
5. Krampl E, et al. Fetal biometry at 4300 m compared to sea level in Peru. Ultrasound Obstet Gynecol 2000;16(1):9–18.
6. Williams RL, Creasy RK, Cunningham GC, et al. Fetal growth and perinatal viability in California. Obstet Gynecol 1982;59:624–32.
7. Gilbert WM. Pregnancy outcomes associated with intrauterine growth restriction. Am J Obstet Gynecol 2003;188(6):1596–9.
8. Lichty JL, Ting RY, Bruns PD, et al. Studies of babies born at high altitude. AMA J Dis Child 1957;93:666–9.

9. Giussani DA, Phillips PS, Anstee S, et al. Effects of altitude versus economic status on birth weight and body shape at birth. Pediatr Res 2001;49:490–4.
10. Keyes LE, Armaza JF, Niermeyer S, et al. Intrauterine growth restriction, preeclampsia and intrauterine mortality at high altitude in Bolivia. Pediatr Res 2003;54(1):20–5.
11. Palmer SK, Moore LG, Young D, et al. Altered blood pressure course during normal pregnancy and increased preeclampsia at high altitude (3100 meters) in Colorado. Am J Obstet Gynecol 1999; 180(5):1161–8.
12. Villar K. Eclampsia and pre-eclampsia: a health problem for 2000 years. In: Critchley H, MacLean A, Poston L, editors. London: RCOG Press; 2003. p. 189–207.
13. Lopez-Jaramillo P, Garcia RG, Lopez M. Preventing pregnancy-induced hypertension: are there regional differences for this global problem? J Hypertens 2005;23(6):1121–9.
14. Walker JJ. Pre-eclampsia. Lancet 2000;356(9237): 1260–5.
15. Abman SH, Shanley PF, Accurso FJ. Failure of postnatal adaptation of the pulmonary circulation after chronic intrauterine pulmonary hypertension in fetal lambs. J Clin Invest 1989;83(6):1849–58.
16. Niermeyer S, Shaffer EM, Thilo E, et al. Arterial oxygenation and pulmonary arterial pressure in healthy neonates and infants at high altitude. J Pediatr 1993;123:767–72.
17. Niermeyer S. Cardiopulmonary transition in the high altitude infant. High Alt Med Biol 2003;4(2):225–39.
18. Zamudio S, Palmer SK, Droma T, et al. Effect of altitude on uterine artery blood flow during normal pregnancy. J Appl Physiol 1995;79:7–14.
19. Wilson MJ, Lopez M, Vargas M, et al. Greater uterine artery blood flow during pregnancy in multigenerational (Andean) than shorter-term (European) high-altitude residents. Am J Physiol Regul Integr Comp Physiol 2007;293(3):R1313–24.
20. Zamudio S, Baumann M, Illsley N. Effects of chronic hypoxia in vivo on the expression of human placental glucose transporters. Placenta 2006;27(1):49–55.
21. Julian CG, Wilson MJ, Lopez M, et al. Augmented uterine artery blood flow and oxygen delivery protect andeans from altitude-associated reductions in fetal growth. Am J Physiol Regul Integr Comp Physiol 2009;296(5):R1564–75.
22. Zamudio S, Torricos T, Fik E, et al. Hypoglycemia and the origin of hypoxia-induced reduction in human fetal growth. PLoS One 2010;5(1):e8551.
23. Zamudio S, Palmer SK, Dahms TE, et al. Alterations in uteroplacental blood flow precede hypertension in preeclampsia at high altitude. J Appl Physiol 1995; 79:15–22.
24. Vargas M, Vargas E, Julian CG, et al. Determinants of blood oxygenation during pregnancy in Andean and

European residents of high altitude. Am J Physiol Regul Integr Comp Physiol 2007;293(3):R1303–12.

25. Moore LG, Rounds SS, Jahnigen D, et al. Infant birth weight is related to maternal arterial oxygenation at high altitude. Respiratory, Environmental and Exercise Physiology. J Appl Physiol 1982;52:695–9.

26. Lucius H, Gahlenbeck H, Kleine HO, et al. Respiratory functions, buffer systems, and electrolyte concentrations of blood during human pregnancy. Respir Physiol 1970;9(3):311–7.

27. Hannhart B, Pickett CK, Moore LG. Effects of estrogen and progesterone on carotid body neural output responsiveness to hypoxia. J Appl Physiol 1990;68:1909–16.

28. Hannhart B, Pickett CK, Weil JV, et al. Influence of pregnancy on ventilatory and carotid body neural output responsiveness to hypoxia in cats. J Appl Physiol 1989;67:797–803.

29. Moore LG, Brodeur P, Chumbe O, et al. Maternal hypoxic ventilatory response, ventilation, and infant birth weight at 4,300 m. J Appl Physiol 1986;60:1401–6.

30. Moore LG, McCullough RE, Weil JV. Increased HVR in pregnancy: relationship to hormonal and metabolic changes. J Appl Physiol 1987;62:158–63.

31. Moore LG, Zamudio S, Zhuang J, et al. Oxygen transport in Tibetan women during pregnancy at 3658 m. Am J Phys Anthropol 2001;114:42–53.

32. Moore LG, Jahnigen D, Rounds SS, et al. Maternal hyperventilation helps preserve arterial oxygenation during high-altitude pregnancy. Respiratory, Environmental and Exercise Physiology. J Appl Physiol 1982;52:690–4.

33. McAuliffe F, Kametas N, Costello J, et al. Respiratory function in singleton and twin pregnancy. BJOG 2002;109(7):765–9.

34. McAuliffe F, Kametas N, Rafferty GF, et al. Pulmonary diffusing capacity in pregnancy at sea level and at high altitude. Respir Physiol Neurobiol 2003;134(2):85–92.

35. McAuliffe F, Kametas N, Krampl E, et al. Blood gases in pregnancy at sea level and at high altitude. Br J Obstet Gynaecol 2001;108:980–5.

36. Milne JA, Mills RJ, Howie AD, et al. Large airways function during normal pregnancy. Br J Obstet Gynaecol 1977;84(6):448–51.

37. Milne JA. The respiratory response to pregnancy. Postgrad Med J 1979;55(643):318–24.

38. McAuliffe F, Kametas N, Espinoza J, et al. Respiratory function in pregnancy at sea level and at high altitude. BJOG 2004;111(4):311–5.

39. Alaily AB, Carrol KB. Pulmonary ventilation in pregnancy. Br J Obstet Gynaecol 1978;85(7):518–24.

40. Kametas NA, et al. Maternal cardiac function during pregnancy at high altitude. BJOG 2004;111(10):1051–8.

41. Harrison GL, Moore LG. Systemic vascular reactivity during high-altitude pregnancy. J Appl Physiol 1990;69:201–6.

42. Zamudio S, Palmer SK, Dahms TE, et al. Blood volume expansion, preeclampsia, and infant birth weight at high altitude. J Appl Physiol 1993;75:1566–73.

43. Papageorghiou AT, Yu CK, Erasmus IE, et al. Assessment of risk for the development of preeclampsia by maternal characteristics and uterine artery Doppler. BJOG 2005;112(6):703–9.

44. Bower S, Bewley S, Campbell S. Improved prediction of preecalmpsia by two-stage screening of uterine arteries using the early diastolic notch and color Doppler imaging. Obstet Gynecol 1993;82:78–83.

45. Krampl E, Espinoza-Dorado J, Lees CC, et al. Maternal uterine artery Doppler studies at high altitude and sea level. Ultrasound Obstet Gynecol 2001;18:578–82.

46. Julian CG, Galan HL, Wilson MJ, et al. Lower uterine artery blood flow and higher endothelin relative to nitric oxide metabolite levels are associated with reductions in birth weight at high altitude. Am J Physiol Regul Integr Comp Physiol 2008;295(3):R906–15.

47. Zamudio S, Postigo L, Illsley NP, et al. Maternal oxygen delivery is not related to altitude- and ancestry-associated differences in human fetal growth. J Physiol 2007;582:883–95.

48. Ahmed A, Dunk C, Ahmad S, et al. Regulation of placental vascular endothelial growth factor (VEGF) and placenta growth factor (PlGF) and soluble Flt-1 by oxygen–a review. Placenta 2000;21 (Suppl A):S16–24.

49. Lash GE, Taylor CM, Trew AJ, et al. Vascular endothelial growth factor and placental growth factor release in cultured trophoblast cells under different oxygen tensions. Growth Factors 2002;20(4):189–96.

50. Levine RJ, Maynard SE, Qian C, et al. Circulating angiogenic factors and the risk of preeclampsia. N Engl J Med 2004;350(7):672–83.

51. Nagamatsu T, Fujii T, Kusumi M, et al. Cytotrophoblasts up-regulate soluble fms-like tyrosine kinase-1 expression under reduced oxygen: an implication for the placental vascular development and the pathophysiology of preeclampsia. Endocrinology 2004; 145(11):4838–45.

52. Smith GC, Crossley JA, Aitken DA, et al. Circulating angiogenic factors in early pregnancy and the risk of preeclampsia, intrauterine growth restriction, spontaneous preterm birth, and stillbirth. Obstet Gynecol 2007;109(6):1316–24.

53. Ishihara O, Hayashi M, Osawa H, et al. Isoprostanes, prostaglandins and tocopherols in pre-eclampsia, normal pregnancy and non-pregnancy. Free Radic Res 2004;38(9):913–8.

54. Poston L. Oxidative stress, preeclampsia and anti-oxidants. Reproductive Vascular Medicine 2001;1:106–13.

55. Moore LG, Shriver M, Bemis L, et al. Maternal adaptation to high-altitude pregnancy: an experiment of nature. Placenta 2004;25(Suppl A):S60–71.

56. Moore LG, Young D, McCullough RE, et al. Tibetan protection from intrauterine growth restriction (IUGR) and reproductive loss at high altitude. Am J Hum Biol 2001;13:635–44.

57. Zamudio S, Droma T, Norkyel KY, et al. Protection from intrauterine growth retardation in Tibetans at high altitude. Am J Phys Anthropol 1993;91:215–24.

58. Haas JD, Frongillo EA Jr, Stepick CD, et al. Altitude, ethnic and sex differences in birth weight and length in Bolivia. Hum Biol 1980;52:459–77.

59. Postigo L, Heredia G, Illsley NP, et al. Where the O2 goes to: preservation of human fetal oxygen delivery and consumption at high altitude. J Physiol 2009;587(Pt 3):693–708.

60. Krampl E, Kametas NA, Cacho Zegarra AM, et al. Maternal plasma glucose at high altitude. Br J Obstet Gynaecol 2001;108:254–7.

61. Krampl E, Kametas NA, Nowotny P, et al. Glucose metabolism in pregnancy at high altitude. Diabetes Care 2001;24:817–22.

The Pulmonologist's role in Caring for Pregnant Women with Regard to the Reproductive Risks of Diagnostic Radiological Studies or Radiation Therapy

Robert Brent, MD, PhD, DSc[a,b,*]

KEYWORDS

• Pulmonologist • Exposure • Pregnant • Radiological studies

Almost every practicing physician is aware that the use of diagnostic radiological techniques and radiation therapy using ionizing radiation has increased substantially over the past 30 years.[1] In 1980, the US population received 20% of their exposure to ionizing radiation from medical care. The National Council on Radiation Protection and Measurements (NCRP) No. 160 (2009) reported that almost 50% of the population's radiation exposure came from medical care. Unfortunately, this increased exposure has been presented in the newspapers, television, and Internet, and in many instances, the risks of birth defects, miscarriage, and cancer have been exaggerated and the benefits ignored. It is important for physicians to become as knowledgeable about the risks of ionizing radiation as they are about its benefits. Although pulmonologists do not concentrate their practice on pregnant women or women of reproductive age, these patients are a part of their practice. An important concern is that many women visit their physician, without knowing that they are pregnant or worse, they become pregnant between the time of the office visit and the appointment for the radiological examination. These situations can be concerning for the patient and the physician. In order for the physician to interpret the various forms of exposure measurement, **Table 1** lists the various nomenclatures for radiation exposures, so that the reader will be able to understand radiation exposures in the terms with which they may be familiar.

Pulmonologists are fortunate with regard to the specific studies they request to provide clinical care because most of the diagnostic tests do not directly expose the uterus (embryo) or ovary. Radiography of the chest, head, neck, teeth, or extremity exposes the embryo or ovary to miniscule (insignificant) exposures of radiation. In some instances, there is no exposure at all.

The pulmonologists may infrequently order diagnostic studies that exposes the abdomen or

^a Departments of Pediatrics, Radiology, Pathology, Anatomy and Cell Biology, Thomas Jefferson University, 1025 Walnut Street, Philadelphia, PA 19107, USA
^b Clinical and Environmental Teratology Laboratory, Research Department, Alfred I. duPont Hospital for Children, PO Box 269, Wilmington, DE 19899, USA
* Clinical and Environmental Teratology Laboratory, Research Department, Alfred I. duPont Hospital for Children, PO Box 269, Wilmington, DE 19899.
E-mail address: rbrent@nemours.org

Clin Chest Med 32 (2011) 33–42
doi:10.1016/j.ccm.2010.10.002
0272-5231/11/$ – see front matter © 2011 Elsevier Inc. All rights reserved.

Table 1
Ionizing radiation exposure terminology

Rad/Rem	Millirad/Millirem	Gray (Gy), Milligray (mGy)	Sievert (Sv), Millisievert (mSv)
0.001	1	0.01 mGy	0.01 mSv
0.01	10	0.1 mGy	0.1 mSv
0.1	100	1 mGy	1 mSv
1	1000	0.01 Gy	0.01 Sv
10	10,000	0.1 Gy	0.1 Sv
100	100,000	1 Gy	1 Sv

The units of rad and rem and the gray and sievert are identical for exposures of low energy transfer radiation, such as x-rays, γ-rays, β-rays, and protons. These forms of radiation have a relative biological effectiveness (RBE) rated at one. Exposures to α-rays and neutrons have a biologic effectiveness greater than one. The rem and the sievert take into consideration the RBE of the radiation. For clinicians, the RBE is infrequently relevant because most radiological procedures use radiation with an RBE of 1 so the gray and sievert exposures will be identical.

pelvis to radiation but they should be aware of other studies that could have been ordered by other providers. The vast majority of diagnostic studies exposing the abdomen or pelvis to radiation also expose the embryo or ovary to less than 10 rad (0.1 Gy).

THE REPRODUCTIVE AND DEVELOPMENTAL RISKS OF EXPOSURES OF IONIZING RADIATION TO PREGNANT OR POTENTIALLY PREGNANT WOMEN

The reproductive and developmental risks of in utero exposures to ionizing radiation are listed below (**Tables 2** and **3**).

1. Birth defects, mental retardation, other neurobehavioral effects, growth retardation, and embryonic death (miscarriage) are deterministic effects (threshold effects). These effects have a no observed adverse effect level (NOAEL). Almost all diagnostic radiological procedures provide exposures that are below the NOAEL for these developmental effects. Diagnostic radiological studies rarely exceed 10-rad (0.1 Gy) exposure, whereas the threshold for congenital malformations or miscarriage is more than 20 rad (0.2 Gy) (see **Table 2**).
2. In order for the embryo to be deleteriously affected by ionizing radiation when the mother is exposed to a diagnostic study, the embryo has to be exposed above the NOAEL to increase the risk of deterministic effects. This scenario rarely happens when pregnant women undergo radiographic studies of the head, neck, chest, or extremities.
3. During the preimplantation and preorganogenesis stages of embryonic development, the embryo is least likely to be malformed by the effects of ionizing radiation because the cells of the very young embryo are omnipotent and

can replace adjacent cells that have been deleteriously affected. This early period of development has been designated as "the all or none period."
4. Protraction and fractionation of exposures of ionizing radiation to the embryo decrease the magnitude of the deleterious effects of deterministic effects. The more protracted or fractionated the radiation, the lower the risk because the threshold increases.
5. The increased risk of cancer following high level of exposures to ionizing radiation in adult populations has been demonstrated in the survivors of atomic bomb. Radiation-induced carcinogenesis is assumed to be a stochastic effect (nonthreshold effect), so that there is theoretically a risk at low-level exposures. While there is no question that high-level exposures of ionizing radiation can increase the risk of cancer, the magnitude of cancer risk from embryonic exposures following diagnostic radiological procedures is controversial. Recent publications and analyses indicate that the risk is lower for the irradiated embryo than the irradiated child, which surprised many scientists interested in this subject (**Tables 4–6**).[2]

EVALUATING THE RISKS OF RADIATION EXPOSURE TO THE DEVELOPING EMBRYO

When evaluating the risks of ionizing radiation, the physician is faced with several different clinical situations:

Situation 1

The pulmonologists are fortunate because the radiological tests that would be ordered for their patients do not expose the embryo directly, and therefore, the embryo does not receive an exposure that would increase the risk for birth defects,

Table 2
Radiation effects at different stages of gestation

Stage, Gestation Weeks	Effect
First and second week after last menstrual period (before conception)	First 2 wk after the first day of the last menstrual period. This is preconception radiation. Mother has not yet ovulated
Third and fourth week of gestation (first 2 wk postconception)	Minimum acute lethal dose in humans (from animal studies). Approximately 0.15–0.20 Gy. Most sensitive period for the induction of embryonic death. No increase in risk of malformations in surviving fetuses. All or none stage
Fourth to eighth week of gestation (second to sixth week postconception)	Minimum lethal dose (from animal studies). At 18 d postconception, 0.25 Gy (25 rad). After 50 days postconception, >0.50 Gy (50 rad) Embryo is vulnerable to the induction of major malformations. Threshold for malformations is >0.2–0.5 Gy, depending on the malformation Minimum dose for growth retardation. At 18–36 d, 0.20–0.50 Gy (20–50 rad). At 36–110 d, 0.25–0.50 Gy (25–50 rad) But the induced growth retardation during this period is not as severe as during midgestation (8–15 wk) from similar exposures and is more recuperable[19]
Eighth to fifteenth week of gestation	Most sensitive period for irreversible whole body growth retardation, microcephaly, and severe mental retardation. Threshold for severe metal retardation is 0.35–0.50 Gy (35–50 rad). Miller[20] believes the threshold is >0.5 Gy. Decrease in IQ can occur at lower exposures
Sixteenth week to term of gestation	Higher exposures can produce growth retardation and decreased brain size and intellect, although the effects are not as severe as those from similar exposures during midgestation. There is no documented risk for major anatomic malformations. Minimum lethal dose threshold for mental retardation (from animal studies) is from 15 wk to term >1.5 Gy (150 rad), but decrease in IQ can occur at lower exposures

There is no evidence that radiation exposure in the diagnostic ranges (<0.10 Gy, <10 rad) is associated with measurably increased incidence of congenital malformation, stillbirth, miscarriage, growth retardation, or mental retardation.

miscarriage, growth retardation, mental retardation, or neural behavioral effects (**Table 7**). **Table 7** lists the frequently used diagnostic radiological and radionuclide tests. None of the tests exceed exposures of 10 rad (0.1 Gy or 100 mGy) except for radiation therapy or extensive fluoroscopy to the abdomen or pelvis.

Although most diagnostic radiological studies of the abdomen or pelvis do not expose the embryo to more than 10 rad (0.10 Gy), the family is upset because they are aware that the embryo was directly exposed. Under these circumstances it may be necessary to request the health physicist to calculate the actual exposure to allay the family's concern.

Situation 2

The pregnant patient presents with clinical symptoms that need to be evaluated. What is the appropriate use of diagnostic radiological procedures that may expose the embryo or fetus to ionizing radiation?

A pregnant or possibly pregnant woman complaining of chest symptoms that cannot be attributed to pregnancy deserves the appropriate studies to diagnose and treat the clinical problems, including radiological studies. Furthermore, these studies should not be relegated to one portion of the menstrual cycle if the patient has not yet missed her period. The studies should be performed at the time they are clinically indicated whether or not the patient is in the first or second half of the menstrual cycle. During the second half of the menstrual cycle the pregnancy test result may be negative even though the patient is pregnant. This situation should be explained to the patient and the family.

Table 3
Reproductive risks per million recognized pregnancies

Reproductive Risks	Frequency
Immunologically and clinically diagnosed spontaneous abortions per million conceptions (<20% has lethal malformations or chromosomal abnormalities that cause abortion before the first month of gestation)	350,000
Clinically recognized spontaneous abortions per million clinically recognized pregnancies. Spontaneous abortion after the first missed menstrual period	150,000
Genetic diseases per million births	110,000
Multifactorial or polygenic genetic environmental interactions)	90,000
Dominantly inherited disease	10,000
Autosomal and sex-linked genetic disease	1200
Cytogenetic (chromosomal abnormalities)	5000
New mutations in the developing ova or sperm before conception	3000
Major malformations (genetic, unknown, environmental)	30,000
Prematurity (Ireland 55,000; United States 124,000)	69,000
Fetal growth retardation	30,000
Stillbirths (>20 wk)	4000–20,900
Infertility	7% of couples

Data from Brent RL. Utilization of developmental basic science principles in the evaluation of reproductive risks from pre- and postconception environmental radiation exposures. Teratology 1999;59:182–204.

Situation 3

A patient has completed a diagnostic procedure that has exposed her uterus to ionizing radiation. Her pregnancy test result was negative. She believes she was pregnant at the time of the procedure. What is your response to this situation?

Explain that you would have proceeded with the necessary radiological diagnostic test whether the patient was pregnant or not because diagnostic studies that are indicated in the patient have to take priority over the possible risk to her embryo; however, almost 100% of diagnostic studies do not increase the risks to the embryo (see **Table 1**). Second, she must have been very early in her pregnancy because her pregnancy test result was negative. At this time, obtain the calculated dose to the embryo and determine her stage of pregnancy. If the dose is less than 10 rad (0.1 Gy; 0.1 Sv), you can inform the patient that her

Table 4
Risk of 10-rad (0.1 Gy) exposure to the embryo

Risks	Background Incidence (per 10^6 pregnancies)	Additional Risk of 10-rad (0.1 Gy) Exposure
Very early pregnancy loss, before the first missed period	350,000	0
Spontaneous abortion in a known pregnant women	150,000	0
Major congenital malformations	30,000	0
Severe mental retardation	5000	0
Childhood leukemia per year	40	Very low increased risk, and possibly no measurably identifiable increased risk
Early- or late-onset genetic disease	100,000	Very low risk in next generation
Prematurity	69,000	0
Growth retardation	30,000	0
Stillbirth	20–2000	0
Infertility	7% of couples	0

Table 5
Follow-up of adults with solid cancers in Hiroshima and Nagasaki, who were in utero at the time of detonation of the atomic bombs in 1945

Dose in Sv (rad)	No. of Patients	No. of Cancers	Person-Years	Percentage with Solid Cancers
<0.005 (<0.5)	1547	54	49,326	3.5
0.005−<0.1 (0.5−10.0)	435	16	14,005	3.7
0.1−<0.2 (10−<20)	168	6	5041	3.6
0.2−<0.5 (20−<50)	172	8	5496	4.6
0.5−<1.0 (50−<100)	92	7	2771	7.6
>1	48	3	1404	6.2
Total	2452	94	94	3.5

Data from Preston DL, Cullings H, Suyama A, et al. Solid cancer incidence in atomic bomb survivors exposed in utero or as young children. J Natl Cancer Inst 2008;100:428−36.

risks for birth defects and miscarriage have not been increased. In fact, the threshold for these effects is 20 rad (0.2 Gy) at the most sensitive stage of embryonic development (see **Table 2**). Of course, you are obligated to tell the patient that every healthy woman is at risk for the background incidence of birth defects and miscarriage, which is 3% for birth defects and 15% for miscarriage (see **Table 3**).

Situation 4

A woman delivers a baby with serious birth defects. On her first postpartum visit, she recalls that she had a diagnostic radiological study early in her pregnancy. What is your response when she asks you whether the baby's malformation could be caused by the radiation exposure?

In most instances, the nature of the clinical malformations can rule out radiation teratogenesis (microcephaly, mental retardation, and fetal growth retardation). In such a case, a clinical teratologist or radiation embryologist could be of assistance. On the other hand, if the exposure is less than 10 rad (0.1 Gy), it would not be scientifically supportable to indicate that the radiation exposure was the cause of the malformation. The threshold for malformations is 20 rad (0.2 Gy) (see **Table 2**). The dose, timing, and nature of the malformation are considered in this analysis.

To appropriately and more completely respond to these questions, the physician should rely on the extensive amount of available information on the effects of radiation on embryos. In fact, there is no environmental hazard that has been more extensively studied or on which more information is available (see **Tables 2** and **4**).[3−12]

RADIATION RISKS TO THE EMBRYO

An acute exposure to ionizing radiation more than 50 rad represents a significant risk to the embryo, regardless of the stage of gestation.[6−9,12,13] The

Table 6
Follow-up of adults with solid cancers in Hiroshima and Nagasaki, who were children at the time of detonation of the atomic bombs in 1945

Dose in Sv (rad)	No. of Patients	No. of Cancers	Person-Years	Percentage of Cancers
<0.005 (<0.5)	8549	318	247,744	3.7
0.005−<0.1 (0.5−10)	4528	173	134,621	3.8
0.1−<0.2 (10−<20)	853	38	25,802	4.4
0.2−<0.5 (20−<50)	859	51	25,722	5.9
0.5−<1.0 (50−<100)	325	21	9522	6.5
>1	274	48	7620	17.5
Total	15,388	649	451,031	4.2

Data from Preston DL, Cullings H, Suyama A, et al. Solid cancer incidence in atomic bomb survivors exposed in utero or as young children. J Natl Cancer Inst 2008;100:428−36.

Table 7
Typical doses for selected medical procedures

Type	Description	Embryo/Fetal Dose Range (mGy)	Gonadal Dose (Ovaries, Testes) (mGy)
Radiography	Skull	<0.01	<0.01, <0.01
Radiography	Chest	<0.01	<0.01, <0.01
Radiography	Thoracic spine	<0.01	<0.01, <0.01
Radiography	Mammography	<0.01	<0.01, <0.01
Radiography	Barium meal	0.1−1.1	
Radiography	Pelvis	0.1−1.1	1.2, 4.6
Radiography	Lumbar spine	1−2	4.3, 0.6
Radiography	Abdomen	1−3	2.2, 0.4
Radiography	Barium enema	7−8	16, 3.4
CT	Chest/CTPA	0.1−1	0.08, <0.01
CT	Abdomen	4−16	8.0, 0.7
CT	Pelvis	10−32	23, 1.7
Chest Fluoroscopy	Chest	<0.1 mGy/min	
IR fluoroscopy	Abdominal fluoroscopy	6 mGy/min	
Nuclear Medicine	Lung ventilation	0.1-0.3	0.13−0.5, 0.13−0.5
Nuclear Medicine	Lung perfusion	0.1−0.4	0.06−0.27, 0.04−0.16
Nuclear Medicine	White cell scan	0.7−1.4	
Nuclear Medicine	Renal scan	3−7	1.0−2.0, 0.7−1.4
Nuclear Medicine	Bone scan	4.5−7.0	2.7−4.0, 1.8−2.7
Nuclear Medicine	Cerebral blood flow	5−10	3.7−7.3, 1.3−2.7
Nuclear Medicine	PET	8−16	5.6−11.1, 4.4−8.8
Nuclear Medicine	Myocardial perfusion	16.7−22.2	9.3−12.4, 2.7−3.6
Nuclear Medicine	Therapy	>50	31, 19

Abbreviations: CT, computed tomography; CTPA, CT pulmonary angiography; PET, positron emission tomography.

threshold dose for low energy transfer ionizing radiation that results in an increase in malformations is approximately 20 rad (0.2 Gy) (see **Table 2**). Although congenital malformations are unlikely to be produced by radiation during the first 14 days of human development, there would be a substantial risk of embryonic loss if the dose is high. From approximately the 18th day to the 40th day postconception, the embryo would be at risk for an increased frequency of anatomic malformations if the radiation exposure exceeds 20 to 25 rad (0.20−0.25 Gy). Until about the 15th week, the embryo has an increased susceptibility to central nervous system (CNS) effects, major CNS malformations early in gestation, and mental retardation in midgestation. Of course, with very high doses, in the hundreds of rads, mental retardation can occur in the later part of gestation. Although it is true that the embryo is vulnerable to the deleterious effects of these midrange exposures of ionizing radiation, the measurable effects fall off rapidly as the exposure approaches the usual levels that the embryo receives from diagnostic radiological procedures (<10 rad [0.1 Gy]). The threshold of 20 rad (0.2 Gy) at the most vulnerable stage of development (20−25 days postconception) is increased by protraction of the radiation exposure. If a pregnant woman had a series of radiographic analyses over a period of 3 to 4 days with a total exposure of 15 rad (0.15 Gy), there would be no increased risk for any of the developmental threshold (deterministic) effects.[6,12,13] The recommendations of most radiation embryologists indicate that exposures in the diagnostic range do not increase the risk of birth defects or miscarriage.[6,8,9,12] **Table 4** compares the spontaneous risks facing an embryo at conception and the risks from a low-level exposure of ionizing radiation (10 rad; 100 mGy; 10,000 mrad).

Therefore, the hazards of exposures in the range of diagnostic radiological studies (20−10,000 mrad [0.2 mGy−0.1 Gy]) present an extremely low risk to the embryo when compared with the spontaneous mishaps that can befall human embryos (see **Tables 3** and **4**). Approximately

30% to 40% of human embryos abort spontaneously (many abort before the first missed menstrual period) (see **Table 3**). Human infants have a 3% major malformation rate at term that increases to approximately 6% to 8% once all minor malformations are recorded. Although doses from 1 to 3 rad (0.01−0.03 Gy) can produce cellular effects and diagnostic radiation exposure during pregnancy has been associated with malignancy in childhood, the maximum theoretic risk to human embryos exposed to doses of 10 rad (0.1 Gy) or less is extremely small. When the data and risks are explained to the patient, the family with a wanted pregnancy invariably continues with the pregnancy.

A frequent difficulty is that the risks from diagnostic radiation exposure are evaluated outside the context of the significant normal risks of pregnancy. Furthermore, many physicians approach the evaluation of diagnostic radiation exposure with either of the 2 extremes: a cavalier attitude or panic. The usual procedures in clinical medicine are ignored, and an opinion based on meager information is given to the patient. Frequently, this attitude reflects the physician's bias about radiation effects or his or her ignorance of radiation biology. We have patient records in our files of scores of patients who were not properly evaluated but were advised to have an abortion following radiation exposure. The following case history is an example.

CASE REPORT

A 33-year-old woman was diagnosed with breast cancer and radiation therapy for the breast was initiated. Four weeks into her therapy, it was discovered that she was 11 weeks pregnant. The oncologist, radiation therapist, and surgeon encouraged the patient and her family to abort the pregnancy. She already had received 3800 rad (3.8 Gy) to the breast. The family asked for another opinion, and our counseling service was contacted. The health physicist at the consultee institution had calculated that the fetus had received 50 rad (0.5 Gy) over a period of almost 4 weeks. On each day of therapy the fetus had received 0.9 rad (0.009 Gy). Each week the fetus had 2 days without being exposed. The patient's physicians still suggested a therapeutic abortion but with less certainty. They asked me what I would tell her. I said, "I would not tell her anything. I wanted to talk with her."

When we were able to talk, she immediately asked what should she do. I responded, "Do you have any questions?" She asked, "Could my baby be malformed?" I told her that 3% of babies are malformed and this is the background incidence. But in her case, the fetus's risks for major birth defects were not increased for 2 reasons: (1) the radiation therapy was initiated in the seventh week after all the organs had formed and (2) more important, the dose each day was too low to produce malformations at any stage of pregnancy. Then she asked whether her baby could be severely mentally retarded. I answered her in the negative. But I also had to tell her that 1 in 200 children is born mentally retarded. She then asked whether the baby could be growth retarded. I responded that 4% of newborns are growth retarded but that the radiation exposure would not cause significant growth retardation. Finally, she asked, "Could my baby be normal?" I said, "Yes."

The mother decided against abortion and delivered a 3-kg baby boy who was physically normal and has been developing, according to the mother, very normally.

EVALUATING THE PATIENT

Case histories are transmitted to our laboratory frequently. In 2008, we had 2,200,000 hits on our pregnancy Web site of the Health Physics Society, "Ask the Expert." There were 760,000 downloads and 1646 direct consultations. In most instances, the dose to the embryo is less than 10 rad (0.1 Gy) and is frequently more than 1 rad (0.01 Gy). Our experience has taught us that there are many variables involved in radiation exposure to a pregnant or potentially pregnant woman. Therefore, there is no routine or predetermined advice that can be given in this situation. However, if the physician takes a systematic approach for the evaluation of the possible effects of radiation exposure, he or she can help the patient make an informed decision about continuing the pregnancy. This systematic evaluation can begin only when the following information has been obtained:

- Stage of pregnancy at the time of exposure
- Menstrual history
- Previous pregnancy history
- Family history of congenital malformations and miscarriages
- Other potentially harmful environmental factors during the pregnancy
- Ages of the mother and father
- Type of radiation study and dates and number of studies performed
- Calculation of the embryonic exposure by a medical physicist or competent radiologist
- Status of the pregnancy, wanted or unwanted.

The evaluation should be concluded, with both patient and counselor arriving at a decision. The physician should provide a summary in the medical record, stating that the patient has been informed that every pregnancy has a significant risk of problems and that the decision to continue the pregnancy does not mean that the counselor is guaranteeing the outcome of the pregnancy. The use of amniocentesis and ultrasonography to evaluate the fetus is an individual decision to be made in each pregnancy.

Each consultation should include the following statement. "If you are healthy, young (under 35) and have no personal or family history of reproductive or fetal developmental problems, then you began this pregnancy with a risk of 3% for birth defects and 15% for miscarriage. These are background risks faced by all pregnant women. Good luck with this pregnancy and keep in touch."

THE CARCINOGENIC EFFECTS OF RADIATION

The carcinogenic risks of in utero radiation is an important topic that cannot be addressed adequately in this article. In 1956, Stewart and colleagues[13] published the results of their case-control studies indicating the diagnostic radiation from pelvimetry was associated with a 50% increased risk of childhood leukemia (see **Table 4**). The risk of childhood leukemia could thus increase from 40 cases per million to 60 cases per million in the population of radiation-exposed fetuses. This issue has been a very controversial subject.[12–17] Preston and colleagues[2] presented data from the in utero population of the atomic bomb survivors, and the data indicated that the embryo was less vulnerable to the oncogenic effects of ionizing radiation than a child. It seems that the embryo is much less vulnerable to the oncogenic effects of radiation than previous investigators have believed. Patients can be told that the fetal risk is extremely small to be measured and also because a large exposed population would be necessary (see **Tables 3–5**). Even if one accepts the controversy that the embryo is more vulnerable to the carcinogenic effects of radiation than a child, the risk at these low-level exposures is extremely smaller than spontaneous risks.[1] Furthermore, other studies indicate that Stewart and colleagues'[13] estimate of the risk involved is exaggerated.[10,11,15–17]

DIAGNOSTIC OR THERAPEUTIC ABDOMINAL RADIATION IN WOMEN OF REPRODUCTIVE AGE

In women of reproductive age, it is important for the patient and the physician to be aware of the pregnancy status of the patient before performing any type of radiological procedure in which the ovaries or uterus is exposed. If the embryonic exposure is 10 rad (0.1 Gy) or less, the radiation risk to the embryo are very small when compared with the spontaneous risks (see **Tables 2–5**). Even if the exposure is 10 rad (0.1 Gy), this exposure is far from the threshold or no-effect dose of 20 rad (0.2 Gy). The patient will accept this information if it is offered as part of the preparation for the radiological studies at a time when both the physician and patient are aware that a pregnancy exists or may exist. The pregnancy status of the patient should be determined and noted.

Because the risks of 10-rad (0.1 Gy) fetal irradiation are so small, the immediate medical care of the mother should take priority over the risks of diagnostic radiation exposure to the embryo. Radiological studies that are essential for optimal medical care of the mother and evaluation of medical problems that need to be diagnosed or treated should not be postponed. Elective procedures such as employment examinations or follow-up examinations, once a diagnosis has been made, need not be performed on a pregnant woman even though the risk to the embryo is very small. If other procedures (eg, magnetic resonance imaging or ultrasonography) can provide adequate information without exposing the embryo to ionizing radiation, then they should be used. Naturally, there is a period when the patient is pregnant but the pregnancy test result is negative and the menstrual history is of little use. However, the risks of exposure to 10 rad (0.1 Gy) or less are extremely small during this period of gestation (all or none period,[4] first 2 weeks). The patient will benefit from knowing that the diagnostic study was indicated and should be performed even though she may be pregnant.

SCHEDULING THE EXAMINATION

When elective radiological studies need to be scheduled, it is difficult to know whether to schedule them during the first half of the menstrual cycle just before ovulation or during the second half of the menstrual cycle, when most women are not pregnant. The genetic risk of diagnostic exposures to the oocyte or the embryopathic effects on the preimplanted embryo are extremely small, and there are no data available to compare the relative risk of 10 rad (0.1 Gy) to the oocyte or the preimplanted embryo. If the diagnostic study is performed in the first 14 days of the menstrual cycle, the patient should be advised to defer conception for several months based on the assumption that the deleterious effect of radiation to the ovaries decreases with increasing time between radiation exposure and a subsequent ovulation? The physician is in a quandary because he may be warning the patient about a very-low-risk phenomenon. On the other hand, avoiding conception for several months is not an insurmountable hardship. This potential genetic hazard is quite speculative for man, as indicated by the NCRP and Biological Effects of Ionizing Radiation committee report dealing with preconception radiation[1,6]:

"It is not known whether the interval between irradiation of the gonads and conception has a marked effect on the frequency of genetic changes in human offspring, as has been demonstrated in the female mouse. Nevertheless, it may be advised for patients receiving high doses to the gonads (>25 rads) to wait for several months after such exposures before conceiving additional offspring."[3]

Because the patients exposed during diagnostic radiological procedures absorb considerably less than 25 rad (0.25 Gy), these recommendations may be unnecessary but they involve no hardship to the patient. Because both the NCRP and International Commission on Radiological Protection have previously recommended that elective radiological examinations of the abdomen and pelvis be performed during the first part of the menstrual cycle (10-day rule, 14-day cycle) to protect the zygote from possible but largely conjectural hazards, the recommendation to avoid fertilization of recently irradiated ova perhaps merits equal attention.

IMPORTANCE OF DETERMINING PREGNANCY STATUS OF PATIENTS

If exposures less than 10 rad (0.1 Gy) do not measurably affect the exposed embryos and if it is recommended that diagnostic procedures should be performed at any time during the menstrual cycle, if necessary, for the medical care of the patient, then the question of expending energy to determine the pregnancy status of the patient arises.

There are several reasons why the physician and patient should share the burden of determining the pregnancy status before performing a radiological or nuclear medicine procedure that exposes the uterus:

1. If the physician is forced to include the possibility of pregnancy in the differential diagnosis, a small percentage of diagnostic studies may no longer be considered necessary. Early symptoms of pregnancy may mimic certain types of gastrointestinal or genitourinary disease.

2. If the physician and patient are both aware that pregnancy is a possibility and the procedure is still performed, it is much less likely that the patient will be upset if she subsequently proves to be pregnant.

3. The careful evaluation of the reproductive status of women undergoing diagnostic procedures prevents many unnecessary lawsuits. Many lawsuits are stimulated by the factor of surprise. In some instances, the jury is not concerned with cause and effect but with the fact that something was not done properly by the physicians.[18,19] In this day and age, failure to communicate adequately can be interpreted as less-than-adequate medical care. Both these factors are eliminated if the patient's pregnancy status has been evaluated properly and the situation discussed adequately with the patient. Physicians should learn that practicing good technical medicine may not be good enough in a litigation-prone society. Even more important, the patient will have more confidence if the decision to continue the pregnancy is made before the radiological procedure is performed, because the necessity of performing the procedure would have been determined with the knowledge that the patient was pregnant. In every consultation dealing with the exposure of the embryo to diagnostic studies involving ionizing radiation (radiography, computed tomography, use of radionuclides) in which the reproductive risks or developmental risks for a fetus have not been increased by the radiation exposure, the patient should be informed that every healthy woman with a negative personal and genetic family reproductive history has background reproductive risks, which are 3% for birth defects and 15% for miscarriage. These background risks cannot be changed.

REFERENCES

1. National Council on Radiation Protection and Measurements. Ionizing radiation exposure of the population of the United States. Report No. 160. Washington, DC: NCRP; 2009.

2. Preston DL, Cullings H, Suyama A, et al. Solid cancer incidence in atomic bomb survivors exposed in utero or as young children. J Natl Cancer Inst 2008;100:428–36.

3. Committee on the Biological Effects of Ionizing Radiation. BEIR VII report: the effects on populations of exposure to low levels of ionizing radiation. Washington, DC: National Academy of Science Press; 2005. p. 1–524.

4. National Council on Radiation Protection and Measurements. Basic radiation criteria, report No. 39. Washington, DC: NCRP; 1971.

5. Brent RL. Radiations and other physical agents. In: Wilson JG, Fraser FC, editors, In: Handbook of teratology, vol. 1. New York: Plenum Press; 1977. p. 153—223.

6. Brent RL. Utilization of developmental basic science principles in the evaluation of reproductive risks from pre- and postconception environmental radiation exposures. Teratology 1999;59:182—204.

7. Brent RL. The effects of embryonic and fetal exposure to x-rays and isotopes. In: Barron WM, Lindheimer MD, editors. Medical disorders during pregnancy. 3rd edition. St Louis (MO): Mosby-Yearbook, Inc; 2000. p. 586—610.

8. National Council on Radiation Protection and Measurements. Medical radiation exposure of pregnant and potentially pregnant women, report no. 54. Washington, DC: NCRP; 1977. p. 1—32.

9. Mettler FA, Jr, Brent RL, Streffer C, et al. Pregnancy and medical radiation. In: Valentin J, editor. Annals of the International Commission on Radiological Protection (ICRP), vol. 30. Publication 84, Tarrytown (NY): Elsevier Science Inc; 2000. p. 1—43.

10. Court Brown WM, Doll R, Hill AB. Incidence of leukemia after exposure to diagnostic radiation in utero. Br Med J 1960;2:1539—45.

11. Brent RL, Lauriston S. Taylor lecture: fifty years of scientific research: the importance of scholarship and the influence of politics and controversy. Health Phys 2007;93(5):348—79.

12. Brent RL. Saving lives and changing family histories: appropriate counseling of pregnant women and men and women of reproductive age, concerning the risk of radiation exposures during and before pregnancy. Am J Obstet Gynecol 2009;200(1): 4—24.

13. Stewart A, Webb D, Giles D, et al. Malignant disease in childhood and diagnostic irradiation in utero. Lancet 1956;2:447.

14. McMahon B, Hutchinson GB. Prenatal X-ray and childhood: a review. Acta Unio Int Contra Cancrum 1964;20:1172.

15. Boice JD Jr, Miller RW. Childhood and adult cancer after intrauterine exposure to ionizing radiation. Teratology 1999;59(4):227—33.

16. Wakeford R, Little MP. Risk coefficients for childhood cancer after intrauterine irradiation: a review. Int J Radiat Biol 2003;79:203—9.

17. Brent RL. The effect of embryonic and fetal exposure to X-ray, microwaves, and ultrasound: counseling the pregnant and non-pregnant patient about these risks. Semin Oncol 1989;16: 347—69.

18. Brent RL. Litigation-produced pain, disease and suffering: an experience with congenital malformation lawsuits. Teratology 1977;16:1—14.

19. Rugh R. Low levels of x-irradiation and he early mammalian embryo. Am J Roentgenol 1962;87: 559—66.

20. Miller RW. Discussion: severe mental retardation and cancer among atomic bomb survivors exposed in utero. Teratology 1999;59:234—5.

Pharmacotherapy in Pregnancy and Lactation

Niharika Mehta, MD*, Lucia Larson, MD

KEYWORDS

- Pharmacotherapy • Pregnancy • Lactation • Teratogenicity

Prescription medication use in pregnancy is frequent, with an estimated prevalence of more than 50%.[1] As we grow increasingly dependent on pharmacotherapy for disease management, medication exposure in pregnancy is inevitable. Although some medications, such as thalidomide and isotretinoin, have clearly been shown to be teratogenic, data about fetal effects of most medications is unsatisfactory.

Prescribing for patients who are pregnant and breastfeeding can be a challenge for clinicians facing insufficient information regarding medication safety, overestimation of perceived risk of medication both by patients and care providers, and increasing litigation costs. This article aims to guide the clinician in choosing the safest and most effective strategy when prescribing medications to patients who are pregnant and breastfeeding.

KEY PRINCIPLES

It is important to consider the following key concepts when prescribing for patients who are pregnant:

1. The placental barrier (or the nonexistence thereof): Any drug or chemical substance given to the mother is able to cross the placenta to some degree. Fetal exposure may be affected by metabolism of the drug in the maternal environment, molecular size, ionization and lipid solubility of the drug, and the ability of the fetal organs to process the chemical substance. In general, lipophilic drugs, drugs of a low molecular weight, and drugs that are nonionized at physiologic pH cross the placenta more efficiently than others. Among commonly prescribed medications, notable exceptions to placental crossing include heparins and insulin.

2. The safe period (or the absence thereof): Although it is true that the fetus is most at risk for anatomic malformations related to drug exposure in the first trimester, fetal neurologic and behavioral development, fetal survival, or function of specific organs can be affected even after the first trimester. For most medications, it is unknown if a safe period truly exists. It is useful to divide fetal development in 3 phases when considering in utero drug exposure: (1) The first 14 days after conception (generally the period before patients are aware of pregnancy): This phase is often referred to as the all-or-none period because exposures of the pluripotential cluster of cells that exist at this point are generally thought to either cause a miscarriage or no effect at all. (2) Days 14 to 60 after conception (the period immediately following the first missed period or the earliest positive home pregnancy test): This phase is a period of cell differentiation and organogenesis. Exposures during this time probably have specific window periods during which the embryo is susceptible to particular toxicities. Thalidomide effects were seen only if the drug was taken between days 21 to 36. Valproic acid effects on the neural tube occur between days 14 to 27. (3) From day 60 until

Division of Obstetric and Consultative Medicine, Department of Medicine, Women and Infants Hospital of Rhode Island, The Warren Alpert Medical School of Brown University, 101 Dudley Street, Providence, RI 02905, USA
* Corresponding author.
E-mail address: NMehta@wihri.org

Clin Chest Med 32 (2011) 43–52
doi:10.1016/j.ccm.2010.11.002
0272-5231/11/$ – see front matter
© 2011 Elsevier Inc. All rights reserved.

delivery: This phase is the period of fetal development when the effects of medication exposure may be less obvious than an anatomic malformation, but would qualify as teratogenic nonetheless. A glaring example would be exposure to angiotensin converting enzyme inhibitors in the second or third trimester resulting in fetal oligohydramnios or neonatal anuria, pulmonary hypoplasia, intrauterine growth restriction, and fetal death. Other exposures may result in subtle and delayed effects, such as learning and behavioral problems resulting from chronic prenatal exposure to certain older antiepileptic agents.

3. Pharmacokinetics in pregnancy: Physiologic changes of pregnancy, such as increased plasma volume, increased glomerular filtration rate, and dilutional hypoalbuminemia, can affect pharmacokinetics of many medications. Absorption of oral agents may also be affected by the slowing of gastric motility in pregnancy. Although these physiologic alterations do not routinely warrant a change in drug dosing, they may be important considerations when choosing an appropriate agent. For example, medications with multiple doses per day are more likely to have sustained effect rather than once-daily medications that would be rapidly cleared in patients who are pregnant.

4. Drug safety data in pregnancy: Definitive pregnancy safety data from large, long-term prospective trials exists for few drugs. Most data pertaining to safety of a medication in pregnancy comes from animal studies, case reports/series, case-control studies, or pregnancy registries. There are significant limitations with each of these data sources. There is no information suggesting that data from animal models of teratogenicity can be reliably applied to humans. Case reports/series can overestimate the risk associated with a particular medication. Case control studies in which infants with adverse outcomes, such as a birth defect, are compared with normal infants with respect to in utero exposure may be helpful in identifying a particular toxicity and producing reassuring data for commonly used medications. However, they often cannot separate the effects of medication exposure from the effects of underlying disease. Pregnancy registries are useful in identifying broad margins of risk, but the information obtained depends on the quality of data collection and the follow-up of patients.

5. The US Food and Drug Administration (FDA) pregnancy categories: In an effort to communicate evidence-based pregnancy safety information to the prescriber, the FDA first published specific pregnancy labeling in 1979.[2] The FDA pregnancy categories are listed in **Box 1**. However, there are several shortcomings with such classification: (1) The categories are often seen as a grading system where the risk increases from the lowest in category A to highest in category X and the safety information in the accompanying narrative is not always appreciated by prescribers. (2) Clinicians incorrectly assume that drugs in a particular category carry a similar risk. However, 65% to 70% of all medications are in category C. This category includes medications with adverse animal data or no animal data at all. In addition, adverse animal data may vary in severity from decreased fetal weights to major structural malformation and fetal loss, indicating difference in expected risk. (3) The categories do not distinguish between supporting data from animals and humans. A category B drug may have animal studies that show no risk but have no adequate human studies or have animal studies showing risk but human studies that do not. So, although the FDA pregnancy risk classification is useful as a quick reference with regards to available safety data, it is inadequate when used as the only source. Besides, it is unable to address the potential harm from withholding a medication in pregnancy (see **Box 1**).

Several other useful resources exist in addition to the FDA classification that may assist the clinician in the therapeutic decision-making process. These resources are listed in **Table 1**.

Choosing the Appropriate Agent

Thankfully for pulmonary physicians, most commonly prescribed respiratory agents can be readily used in pregnancy without significant concern about fetal safety. **Table 2** lists some of the most commonly used medications for treating respiratory disease. When prescribing a medication, it is useful to consider whether available data suggest its use for this indication in pregnancy is 'justifiable in most circumstances' or is 'almost never justified.' Some medications may fall in a middle category where there is a paucity of published pregnancy data rather than presence of known fetal ill effects. Such agents may be used in pregnancy but caution suggests that until more human data becomes available, their use should be reserved for patients in whom medications from the first column have failed or are contraindicated because of intolerance or allergy. It is best to make all decisions about medication use in

Box 1
FDA pregnancy categories

US Food and Drug Administration Pregnancy Risk Classification

Category A: Controlled studies show no risk

> Controlled studies in women fail to demonstrate a risk to the fetus in the first trimester, there is no evidence of a risk in later trimesters and therefore the possibility of fetal harm appears remote.

Category B: No evidence of risk in humans

> Either animal reproduction studies have not demonstrated a fetal risk but there are no controlled studies in pregnant women, or animal-reproduction studies have shown an adverse effect (other than a decrease in fertility) that was not confirmed in controlled studies in women in the first trimester (and there is no evidence of a risk in later trimesters).

Category C: Risk cannot be ruled out

> Either studies in animals have revealed adverse effect on the fetus (teratogenic) or appropriate animal data is not available. Drugs should be given only if the potential benefit justifies the potential risk to the fetus.

Category D: Positive evidence of risk

> There is positive evidence of human fetal risk, but the benefits from use in pregnant women may be acceptable despite the risk (eg, if the drug is needed in a life-threatening situation or for a serious disease for which safer drugs cannot be used or are ineffective). There will be an appropriate statement in the warnings section of the labeling.

Category X: Contraindicated in pregnancy

> Studies in animals or human beings have demonstrated fetal abnormalities or there is evidence of fetal risk based on human experience, or both, and the risk of the use of the drug in pregnant women clearly outweighs any possible benefit. The drug is contraindicated in women who are or may be pregnant.

pregnancy on an individual basis, after careful consideration of both the potential risks and benefits and in conjunction with patients, while bearing in mind that fetal wellbeing is dependant on maternal health.

Medication Use in Lactating Mothers

Breastfeeding is associated with significant long-term and short-term benefits for both the infant and the mother. Besides providing the perfect source of nutrition for the infant, breast milk enhances the maturity of the neonate's gastrointestinal (GI) tract and is associated with a lower risk of necrotizing enterocolitis.[3,4] Breastfeeding is also associated with a decreased risk of acute infections, such as GI and respiratory tract infections.[5–8] This benefit persists long after breastfeeding has been completed. Other long-term benefits for the breastfeeding infant include a lower risk for the development of obesity,[9–11] childhood cancers as well as leukemia and lymphoma,[12,13] diabetes mellitus,[14] adult

cardiovascular risk factors,[15,16] allergic disorders, and there may also be improved neurodevelopment outcome in breastfed infants.[17,18] Benefits for the breastfeeding mother include lower risks of breast[19–21] and ovarian cancer[22] as well as decreased cardiovascular risk.[23–25] The additional economic benefit of not needing to buy formula and decreased costs associated with fewer illnesses in both the offspring and the mother result in a significant economic savings in both the short term and the long term. It has been estimated that the Women, Infants, and Children Program, which supports low-income families, saved more than $950 million in 1997 for infants who were exclusively breastfed for the first 6 months of life.[26] Certainly the economic benefit would only be significantly greater if more infants were breastfed and if the cost savings of fewer short-term and long-term medical illnesses were considered. Given the unequivocal health benefits of breastfeeding, the American Academy of Pediatrics (AAP) recommends exclusive breastfeeding of the infant for the first 6 months of life and then

Table 1
Resources to assess pregnancy and lactation safety data on individual drugs

Publication	Source and Brief Description
Medications in Pregnancy and Lactation Briggs GS, Freeman R, Yaffe S	Lippincott Williams & Wilkins Publishers, ISBN-13: 978-07817-7876-3, 8th edition (2008) Hardcover reference text
Shepard's Catalog of Teratogenic Agents Shepard TH, Lemire RJ	Johns Hopkins University Press, ISBN: 0,801,879,531, 11th edition (August 2004) Hardcover listing of 2393 agents, lactation not included
Teratogenic Effects of Drugs Friedman JM and Polifka JE	Johns Hopkins University Press, ISBN: 0,801,863,872, 2nd edition (July 15, 2000) Hardcover and more extensive version of text previously listed
Drugs for Pregnant and Lactating Women Weiner CP and Buhimshi C	Churchill Livingstone, 1st edition (2004) Easy to use, reader friendly hardcover text that summarizes pregnancy and lactation data for 725 generic and 2200 brand name drugs
Medication safety in pregnancy and breastfeeding: An evidence based A-Z clinician's pocket guide Koren G	The McGraw-Hill companies (2007) Easy to use, comprehensive pocket reference
Medications & Mothers' Milk: A Manual of Lactational Pharmacology Thomas Hale	Hale Publishing, ISBN-13: 978-09823-3799-8, 14th edition (2010) Easy to use and comprehensive handbook.
http://neonatal.ama.ttuhsc.edu/lact/index.html	Useful online clinical forum and a helpful adjunct to Dr Hale's reference book
Reprotox	www.REPROTOX.org; distributed in Micromedix, Inc TOMES Reprorisk module Online subscription or diskette. PDA version available
TERIS	http://depts.washington.edu/~terisweb/teris/ also distributed in Micromedix, Inc TOMES Reprorisk module Online subscription or diskette
Motherisk	www.motherisk.org provides teratogenic information and updates on continuing reproductive risk research
Some other useful online sources	www.aap.org/advocacy/archives/septdrugs.htm www.rxlist.com www.otispregnancy.org www.perinatology.com

From Mehta N, Newstead-Angel J, Powrie R. Prescribing in pregnancy and lactation. In: Pulmonary problems in pregnancy. Bourjeily G, Rosene-Montella K, editors. 1st edition. New York (NY): Humana Press; 2009. p. 71–88; with permission from Springer Science and Business Media.

continued for the first year[3] and the World Health Organization recommends breastfeeding up to 2 years or beyond.[27]

KEY PRINCIPLES

Most breastfeeding women who require medications to treat medical conditions and their infants can continue to safely breastfeed and enjoy its benefits if the following key principles are considered:

1. In general, a drug that has no oral absorption is unlikely to cause systemic effects in the infant even if it enters the breast milk. For instance, drugs, such as the aminoglycosides, vancomycin,

and some third-generation cephalosporins, are unlikely to have significant adverse effects on the breastfeeding infant given their poor bioavailability (although it is possible there could be potential allergic reactions or GI side effects if a significant amount of a medications remains in the infant's gut).

2. Drugs enter the breast milk mainly by diffusion so that maternal drug levels are directly proportional to that in the breast milk. Ideally, breastfeeding just as the next dose of medication is due to be administered will result in lower amounts of drug in the breast milk, but this is often impractical given the multiple factors that contribute to the timing of an individual infant's feeds. Choosing drugs with shorter half-lives helps to decrease infant exposure so that drugs requiring dosing several times a day are preferable over once-daily dosed drugs.

3. Two important characteristics of drugs that favor entry into the breast milk are high lipid solubility and less protein binding. Therefore, when choosing between drugs, the drug with the highest protein binding and lowest lipid solubility would be preferable for the breastfeeding woman. Drugs with lower molecular weights (<300 daltons), those that are more ionized, and those that have a high pH are also drugs that are more likely to enter the breast milk.

4. The ability of a drug to cross into the breast milk is also dependent on how well established breast milk production is. In early milk production, there is more space between the alveolar cells for even large molecules, such as immunoglobulins or white blood cells, to pass through. As breastfeeding becomes established there is less space between cells and drugs with higher molecular weights cannot pass as easily. Therefore, the first 4 to 10 days of life is a more sensitive time period for the use of drugs in lactation. In addition, individual neonates may have specific issues, such as prematurity, that may impact on their ability to tolerate even small amounts of drugs that would be easily tolerated by an older infant without any medical issues. If a question regarding this arises, it would be prudent to consult the infant's pediatrician.

5. It does not necessarily follow that drugs that can be safely used in pregnancy can also be safely used in breastfeeding because the infant must be able to independently metabolize ingested medications; whereas, the pregnant mother metabolizes medications for her fetus. Drugs that may accumulate in individual breastfeeding infants include the barbiturates, benzodiazepines, fluoxetine, and meperidine.[28] In contrast, some drugs that are not recommended for use in pregnancy can be safely used in the lactating mother. An example is the angiotensin converting enzyme inhibitors, captopril and lisinopril, which are considered acceptable for use in breastfeeding by the American Academy of Pediatricians but are not recommended for use in pregnancy.

6. The use of medication to treat self-limited mild conditions, such as viral upper respiratory tract infections, should probably be discouraged in lactating women because the benefit of treatment is not significant and unlikely to outweigh any potential risks.

7. Obtaining drug levels in the blood of the breastfed infant is a way to determine if there is significant exposure to medication through the breast milk in cases where there may be concern about possible drug effects in the infant. Indirect measures, such as obtaining the prothrombin time/international normalized ratio of infants whose mothers take warfarin, may also be helpful in such circumstances where there is concern.

8. Iodinated contrast material and gadolinium used in radiographic procedures are associated with little, if any, exposure in breastfed infants and are considered safe to use in lactating women without requiring any interruption of breastfeeding.[29]

It should be remembered that although there is justified concern about the use of medication in lactating mothers, most of these woman can be treated with appropriate medication when needed and still be able to safely breastfeed without interruption **Table 1** lists resources that can be used to guide the pulmonologist in choosing appropriate medications for breastfeeding mothers. Of particular interest is the American Academy of Pediatrics, which comments on the acceptability of several medications for lactation though it should be noted that a significant number of medications on the market are not included. In addition, the book *Medication and Mother's Milk* by Dr Thomas Hale is an excellent source of information for the clinician; whereas, the Motherrisk Web site is also a valuable resource for patients and clinicians. **Box 2** lists some of the drugs more commonly used by the pulmonologist and provides information about breastfeeding safety. Armed with the information in this article it is hoped that the clinician can confidently counsel women regarding the use of medication during lactation so that they and their babies will be

Table 2
Commonly used pulmonary medications in pregnancy

Medication Type	Medication Acceptable for use in Pregnancy	Medications Contraindicated in Pregnancy	Comments
Short-acting inhaled beta 2 adrenergic agonists	Albuterol c Bitolterol c Pirbuterol c Metaproterenol c Terbutaline c	—	—
Long-acting inhaled beta 2 adrenergic agonists	Salmeterol c Formoterol c	—	Of the few studies that have examined pregnancy outcomes with prenatal exposure to long-acting beta2 agonists, no adverse events were found. However, because of small numbers in the studies, and because animal models have shown delayed ossification, use of this agent should be reserved for patients who have failed low-potency inhaled steroids alone.
Xanthines	Theophylline c Aminophylline c	—	The clearance of aminophylline and theophylline is increased in pregnancy but may be variable. There is no evidence of teratogenicity.
Inhaled corticosteroids	Low potency: Beclomethasone dipropionate c Medium potency: Triamcinolone acetonide c High potency: Fluticasone propionate c Budesonide B Flunisolide B	—	Beclomethasone and budesonide are the most widely studied of the inhaled corticosteroids in pregnancy and should be considered the preferred inhaled steroids in pregnancy. Although fluticasone has not been studied in pregnancy, its minimal absorption and the safety of other drugs in this category make its use in pregnancy generally justifiable.
Systemic steroids	Prednisone c Methylprednisolone c Dexamethasone c Hydrocortisone c	—	Several case-control studies have found a significant association with first-trimester steroid use and oral clefts; however, this was not seen in cohort studies. But it is important to note that even if this association is real, the risk is still small. For every 1000 embryos exposed during the susceptible days of first trimester, probably no more than 3 will develop an oral cleft. The background risk in the general population is 1 per 1000. Therefore, the benefits of controlling a life-threatening disease makes steroid use, when indicated in the first trimester, still generally justifiable.
Mast cell stabilizers	Cromolyn sodium B Nedocromil B	—	—
Inhaled anticholinergics	Ipratropium B	—	—

Leukotriene inhibitors	Montelukast B Zafirlukast B	Zileuton B	Although these agents have reassuring animal data and are widely used in pregnancy because of the FDA category B rating, published safety data in human pregnancy is limited at this point. Their use should be limited in pregnancy to those cases where significant improvement in asthma control occurred with these medications before becoming pregnant and was not obtainable through other methods. Zileuton is different than other agents in this class because animal studies have revealed evidence of fetotoxicity using doses equivalent to the maximum recommended daily human dose.
Antihistamines	Diphenhydramine B (but avoid in first trimester) Chlorpheniramine Dimenhydrinate B Second-line agents: Cetirizine B Fexofenadine C Loratadine B	—	Although the newest generation antihistaminic agents are widely used in pregnancy and have not had any concerning animal data associated with them, we still consider them to be second-line agents in pregnancy because of the lack of published human pregnancy safety data about them.
Cough	Guaifenesin C Dextromethorphan C Albuterol C Codeine C	—	
Nasal congestion	Pseudoephedrine C Oxymetazoline C Nasal steroids: Beconase C Rhinocort C Flonase C Nasacort C Nasal cromolyn B Nasal ipratropium B	—	
Antibiotics	Erythromycin B base, ethyl succinate or stearate (not estolate) Penicillins B Cephalosporins B Azithromycin B Vancomycin B Nitrofurantoin B Aminoglycosides D Metronidazole B	Tetracycline D Doxycycline D Clarithromycin C Fluoroquinolones C Erythromycin estolate B	Despite concerning animal data, increasing human data suggests fluoroquinolones might warrant their placement in the use may be justified in rare circumstances category. With sulfonamides, there is concern for kernicterus in the newborn with exposure closer to delivery, and these agents should be avoided near term. Because trimethoprim is a folate antagonist, caution has been advocated with its use in pregnancy. Although maternal treatment with aminoglycosides may theoretically be associated with an increased risk for auditory nerve and renal damage in the fetus, these effects have not been demonstrated in humans.

(continued on next page)

Table 2
(continued)

Medication Type	Medication Acceptable for use in Pregnancy	Medications Contraindicated in Pregnancy	Comments
Antifungals	Amphotericin B Nystatin B Clotrimazole B Terbinafine B	Ketoconazole C	—
Anti-TB medications	Isoniazid C Rifampicin C Pyrazinamide C Ethambutol C Rifabutin B	Ethionamide D Kanamycin D Capreomycin C Fluoroquinolones Streptomycin D	Isoniazid warrants monthly monitoring of liver function tests in pregnancy because of a possible increased incidence of hepatotoxicity in pregnancy.
Antiretroviral medications	Lamivudine C Zidovudine C Didanosine B Stavudine C Nevirapine C Nelfinavir B Saquinavir B Ritonavir B	Tenofovir B Zalcitabine C Delavirdine C Efavirenz D Atazanavir B Fosamprenavir C Tipranavir C Emtricitabine B	Although human pregnancy safety data is lacking for most of the newer HIV medications, use of the majority of the older antiretroviral agents is readily justifiable, efavirenz being the notable exception. Pregnancies exposed to antiretroviral therapy should be registered with the Antiretroviral Pregnancy Registry as early in pregnancy as possible to provide data on the risk of birth defects after exposure.
Antivirals	Acyclovir B Ganciclovir C	Amantidine C Zanamivir C Oseltamivir C Peginterferon C Ribavirin X	—
Vasopressors	Ephedrine C	—	Ephedrine is thought to be the vasopressor of choice during pregnancy because it causes less reduction in uterine blood flow; however, based upon recent reviews either phenylephrine or ephedrine may be justified for use in pregnancy. Given that vasopressors are usually used to treat diseases with high morbidity and mortality, the agent with the most expected benefit should be used while monitoring fetal wellbeing.

Subscripts after each agent represents the FDA pregnancy risk classification.
From Mehta N, Newstead-Angel J, Powrie R. Prescribing in pregnancy and lactation. In: Pulmonary problems in pregnancy. Bourjeily G, Rosene-Montella K, editors. 1st edition. New York (NY): Humana Press; 2009. p. 71–88.

Box 2
Breastfeeding safety for commonly used pulmonary medications

Breastfeeding safety categories: L1, safest; L2, safer; L3, moderately safe; L4, possibly hazardous; L5, contraindicated.[28]

Asthma medications: Most inhaled asthma medications are considered safe for breast feeding, including inhaled steroids and long-acting beta antagonists.

Albuterol: L1

Pirbuterol: L2

Terbutaline: L2

Salmeterol: L2

Formoterol: L3

Beclomethasone: L2

Triamcinolone: L3

Budesonide: L3

Fluticasone: L3

Theophylline: L3

Prednisone: L2; L4 for chronic high dose because of the risk of epiphyseal bone growth inhibition, gastric ulceration, and glaucoma in the infant.

Dexamethasone: L3

Cromolyn sodium: L1

Ipratropium: L2

Zafirlukast: L3

Montelukast: L3

Zileuton: L4 because of the potential for tumorigenicity in animal models.

Antihistamines: most antihistaminic agents can be safely used in pregnancy.

Diphenhydramine: L2

Chlorpheniramine: L3

Cetirizine: L2

Fexofenadine: L3

Loratadine: L2

Cough medicines:

Guaifenesin: L2

Dextromethorphan: L1

Codeine: L3

Decongestants:

Pseudoephedrine: L3 to L4 (Studies suggest significant reduction in milk production and prolactin levels following exposure to pseudoephedrine.)

Phenylephrine: L3

Antifungal agents:

Fluconazole, ketoconazole: L2, AAP approved for use in breastfeeding

Nystatin: L1

Amphotericin B: L3

Tuberculosis (TB) medications:

The American Academy of Pediatrics considers use of isoniazid, rifampin, ethambutol, streptomycin (first-line agents), kanamycin, and cycloserine (second-line agents) compatible with breastfeeding.

HIV medications:

Mothers who are HIV-infected in the United States are advised against breastfeeding because of the risk of transmission of HIV to infants through breast milk.

Antiviral agents:

acyclovir: L2

valacyclovir: L1

Cytomegalovirus transfer into breast milk is known but of low risk to infants born of mothers who are cytomegalovirus-positive.

Vasopressors:

Epinephrine: L1

Ephedrine: L4

Data from Mehta N, Newstead-Angel J, Powrie R. Prescribing in Pregnancy and Lactation. In: Pulmonary Problems in Pregnancy. Bourjeily G, Rosene-Montella K, editors. 1st edition. New York (NY): Humana Press; 2009. p. 71–88.

able to reap the significant short-term and long-term benefits of breastfeeding.

REFERENCES

1. Andrade SE, Gurwitz JH, Davis RL, et al. Prescription drug use in pregnancy. Am J Obstet Gynecol 2004;191:398.

2. Feibus KB. FDA's proposed rule for pregnancy and lactation labeling: improving maternal child health through well-informed medicine use. J Med Toxicol 2008;4(4):284–8.

3. Gartner LM, Morton J, Lawrence RA, et al. Breastfeeding and the use of human milk. Pediatrics 2005;115:496.

4. Claud EC, Walker WA. Hypothesis:inappropriate colonization of the premature intestine can cause

neonatal necrotizing enterocolitis. FASEB J 2001;15: 1398.

5. Leon-Cava N, Lutter C, Ross J, et al. Quantifying the benefits of breastfeeding: a summary of evidence. Food and nutrition program. Washington, DC: Pan American Health Organization; 2001.

6. Glass RI, Stoll BJ. The protective effect of human milk against diarrhea. A review of studies from Bangladesh. Acta Paediatr Scand Suppl 1989;351:131.

7. Paricio Talayero JM, Lizan-Garcia M, et al. Full breastfeeding and hospitalization as a result of infections in the first year of life. Pediatrics 2006; 118:e92.

8. Chantry CJ, Howard CR, Auinger P. Full beast feeding duration and associated decrease in respi-ratory tract infection in US children. Pediatrics 2006;117:425.

9. Gillman MW, Rifas-Shiman SL, Camargo CA Jr, et al. Risk of overweight among adolescents who were breastfed as infants. JAMA 2001;285:2461.

10. Armstrong J, Reilly JJ. Breastfeeding and lowering the risk of childhood obesity. Lancet 2002;359:2003.

11. Von Dries R, Koletzko B, Sauerwald T, et al. Breast feeding and obesity: cross sectional study. BMJ 1999;319:147.

12. Breastfeeding and childhood cancer. Br J Cancer 2001;85:1685.

13. Kwan ML, Buffler PA, Abrams B, et al. Breastfeeding and the risk of childhood leukemia: a meta-analysis. Public Health Rep 2004;119:521.

14. Owen CG, Martin RM, Whincup PH, et al. Does breastfeeding influence risk of type 2 diabetes later in life? a quantitative analysis of published evidence. Am J Clin Nutr 2006;84:1043.

15. Owen CG, Whincup PH, Kaye SJ, et al. Does initial breastfeeding lead to lower blood cholesterol in adult life? a quantitative review of the evidence. Am J Clin Nutr 2008;88:305.

16. Owen CG, Whincup PH, Odoki K, et al. Infant feeding and blood cholesterol: a study in adolescents and a systematic review. Pediatrics 2002;110:597.

17. Mortensen EL, Michaelsen KF, Sanders SA, et al. The association between duration of breastfeeding and adult intelligence. JAMA 2002;287:2365.

18. Sacker A, Quigley MA, Kelly YJ. Breastfeeding ar developmental delay: findings from the millenniu cohort study. Pediatrics 2006;118:e682.

19. Collaborative Group on Hormonal Factors in Brea Cancer. Breast cancer and breast feeding: a collab orative reanalysis of individual data from 47 epide miological studies in 30 countries including 503C women with breast cancer and 96973 wome without the disease. Lancet 2002;360:187.

20. Stuebe AM, Willett WC, Xue F, et al. Lactation an incidence of premenopausal breast cancer: a long tudinal study. Arch Intern Med 2009;169:1364.

21. Martini RM, Middleton N, Gunnell D, et al. Breas feeding and cancer: the Boyd Orr cohort an a systematic review with meta-analysis. J Na Cancer Inst 2005;97:1446.

22. Ness RB, Grisso JA, Cottreau C, et al. Facto related to inflammation of the ovarian epitheliur and risk of ovarian cancer. Epidemiology 200C 11(2):111.

23. Schwarz EB, McClure CK, Tepper PG, et al. Lacta tion and maternal measures of subclinical cardic vascular disease. Obstet Gynecol 2010;115:41.

24. Stuebe AM, Michels KB, Willett WC, et al. Duration c lactation and incidence of myocardial infarction . middle to late adulthood. Am J Obstet Gynec 2009;200:138.

25. Schwarz EB, Ray RM, Stuebe AM, et al. Duration c lactation and risk factors for maternal cardiovascula disease. Obstet Gynecol 2009;113:974.

26. Montgomery DL, Splett PL. Economic benefit c breast-feeding infants enrolled in WIC. J Am Diet As soc 1997;97:379.

27. World Health Organization. Global strategy for infar and young child feeding. Geneva (Switzerland World Health Organization; 2002.

28. Hale T. Medications and mothers' milk: a manual c lactational pharmacology. 13th edition. Amarill (TX): Pharmasoft Publishing; 2008.

29. ACR Committee on Drugs and Contrast Medi Administration of contrast medium to breastfeedin mothers. ACR Bulletin Web based document; 2001 Available at: www.acr.org. Accessed November 4 2010.

Management Principles of the Critically Ill Obstetric Patient

Uma Munnur, MD[a],*, Venkata Bandi, MD[b],
Kalpalatha K. Guntupalli, MD[b]

KEYWORDS

- Critical illness • Pregnancy • Peripartum cardiomyopathy
- Cardiopulmonary resuscitation • Hypertensive crisis
- Massive transfusion protocol

The goals in management of critically ill obstetric patients involve intensive monitoring and physiologic support for patients with life-threatening but potentially reversible conditions. Management principles of the mother should also take the fetus and gestational age into consideration. The most common reasons for intensive care admissions (ICU) in the United States and United Kingdom are hypertensive disorders, sepsis, and hemorrhage. The critically ill obstetric patient poses several challenges to the clinicians involved in her care, because of the anatomic and physiologic changes that take place during pregnancy.

CRITICAL ILLNESS IN PREGNANCY
Prevalence

The estimated prevalence of obstetric patients requiring ICU admission is 0.9% both in the United States and the United Kingdom. Mortality of critically ill obstetric patients ranges from 12% to 20%.[1] The most common cause of maternal death in the ICU is acute respiratory distress syndrome (ARDS).[2]

Prognosis

Patients with primary obstetric disorders tend to have a better overall prognosis as delivery of the fetus usually reverses the illness and resuscitation is more effective. Preterm babies also have a chance of survival in hospitals with established neonatal intensive care units. Several retrospective studies have analyzed the racial differences with regard to ICU admissions and the outcome of parturients. Ethnic minorities, recent immigrants, and low socioeconomic status have been associated with poor outcome.[3] Obstetric patients admitted to the ICU have a better prognosis and mortality is lower than for general medical ICU patients. Nonobstetric critical illness in pregnant women significantly affects fetal and neonatal outcomes. Maternal shock, blood product transfusion, and lower gestational age are associated with an increased risk of fetal loss.[4]

The Confidential Enquiry into Maternal and Child Health in the United Kingdom made a few recommendations aimed at improving child health and reducing maternal mortality.[5] These recommendations highlighted the importance of early recognition and management of severely ill pregnant women, and routine use of early warning scoring systems to be used for obstetric patients.[6] Early recognition of critical illness is essential for a favorable outcome for mother and baby. Prognostic criteria such as APACHE scoring may not predict mortality as accurately in pregnancy as they do

[a] Department of Anesthesiology, Baylor College of Medicine, 1709 Dryden Road, Suite 1700, Houston, TX 77030, USA
[b] Pulmonary, Critical Care and Sleep Medicine, Baylor College of Medicine, 1709 Dryden Road, 9th Floor, Houston, TX 77030, USA
* Corresponding author.
E-mail address: umunnur@bcm.edu

Clin Chest Med 32 (2011) 53–60
doi:10.1016/j.ccm.2010.10.003
0272-5231/11/$ – see front matter © 2011 Elsevier Inc. All rights reserved.

chestmed.theclinics.com

outside of pregnancy. One of the reasons for this difference is the physiologic changes of pregnancy such as an increase in heart rate, change in white cell count, or even a drop in normal values for creatinine that can affect the score. In many cases, delivery results in a drastic improvement in the disease course and a lower mortality, even when initial indicators suggest a high mortality.

Obstetric Versus Nonobstetric Disorders

Primary obstetric disorders account for 50% to 80% of ICU admissions during pregnancy and the puerperium in all parts of the world.[3,7] More than 80% of these admissions are because of preeclampsia and its complications, hemorrhage, and sepsis. Nonobstetric disorders in pregnancy show large geographic variations. In developed countries, asthma, pneumonia, drug abuse, complicated urinary infections, preexisting autoimmune disorders, chronic pulmonary disease, endocrine disorders, trauma, and pulmonary thromboembolism are common.[8,9] Medical disorders commonly seen in developing countries include severe malaria, viral hepatitis, cerebral venous sinus thrombosis, tetanus, tuberculosis, rheumatic valvular heart disease, and anemia.[7] Some of the common obstetric and nonobstetric causes are listed in **Box 1**.

ICUs in developed countries are increasingly challenged with a unique subgroup of pregnant women. Advances in health care have resulted in survival to child-bearing age of women with disorders such as surgically corrected complex congenital heart disease and organ transplant, and chronic disorders such as cystic fibrosis. Pregnant women with these conditions have increased morbidity and tend to require intensive medical care.[10,11]

MANAGEMENT PRINCIPLES OF A CRITICALLY ILL PARTURIENT

Some of the common indications for transfer of patients to the ICU are listed in **Table 1**. As in a nonpregnant critically ill patient, the initial assessment of a parturient is focused on airway, breathing, and circulation.

Airway

Airway evaluation and management remains the first priority as in a nonpregnant patient. Supplemental oxygen may be required in some patients depending on their oxygen saturation. Tracheal intubation is needed in the setting of persistent hypoxemia, airway obstruction, impaired laryngeal reflexes, or altered consciousness. Because

pregnant women are at a high risk for aspiration of gastric contents, endotracheal intubation should be performed sooner rather than later to protect the airway. If the airway examination indicates that tracheal intubation is likely to be difficult, awake intubation should be performed with

---

Box 1
Causes for critical illness in pregnancy

Obstetric causes

  Obstetric hemorrhage

  Placental abruption

  Preeclampsia/eclampsia

  HELLP syndrome (HELLP is an abbreviation of the main findings: hemolytic anemia; elevated liver enzymes and low platelet count)

  Acute fatty liver of pregnancy

  Chorioamnionitis

  Amniotic fluid embolism

  Puerperal sepsis

  Pelvic septic thrombophlebitis

  Peripartum cardiomyopathy

Nonobstetric causes

  Respiratory failure

  ARDS

  Acute renal failure

  Urinary tract infection

  Diabetic ketoacidosis

  Drug abuse

Table 1
Causes of shock in obstetric patients

Hypovolemic shock	Hyperemesis gravidarum, ruptured ectopic pregnancy, placental abruption, placenta previa, postpartum hemorrhage, uterine rupture, trauma
Septic shock	Chorioamnionitis, puerperal sepsis, septic abortion, pneumonia, pyelonephritis
Cardiogenic shock	Valvular heart disease, peripartum cardiomyopathy, acute myocardial infarction, myocarditis

good topical anesthesia. Rapid sequence induction with cricoid pressure and orotracheal intubation is recommended in the obtunded or unconscious parturient without a potentially difficult airway. Difficult airway equipment for airway management must always be available in the ICU and intensivists should be familiar with use of at least a few alternative airway devices.

Breathing

Adequacy of respiration must be established rapidly. Supplemental oxygen and bag/mask ventilation may be required initially. If respiratory effort is inadequate, tracheal intubation is performed and mechanical ventilation initiated without any further delay.

Circulation

Hypotension and shock should be treated promptly to maintain uteroplacental perfusion. After 20 weeks of gestation, pressure of the gravid uterus on the inferior vena cava and abdominal aorta in the supine position can cause supine hypotension syndrome and decrease cardiac output by up to 30%. For chest compressions to be more effective during the second half of pregnancy, studies have confirmed that applying a partial left lateral tilt to the patient relieves the aortocaval compression.[12] Rees and Willis[13] concluded that the best compromise for cardiopulmonary resuscitation is achieved by wedging the patient at 27°.

Two large-bore intravenous cannulae (14G or 16G) should be placed to administer fluids and a Foley catheter should be placed to monitor urine output. Central venous access may be needed for volume resuscitation, bolus drug administration, infusion of vasopressors and central venous oxygen saturation monitoring. Femoral vein catheterization should be avoided if possible because of the risk of thromboembolism and infection. The jugular route is preferred over the subclavian route in patients with coagulopathy, as the subclavian site cannot be compressed in case of excessive bleeding or accidental arterial puncture. Hypotension is treated by aggressive volume resuscitation. If hemorrhage is life threatening, blood group O Rh-negative packed red blood cells are transfused until type specific or cross-matched blood is available. It is preferable to place an arterial line at the earliest to measure the blood pressure continuously. Severe maternal hypotension may require treatment with vasopressors.

If the parturient has pulseless ventricular tachycardia (VT) or ventricular fibrillation (VF), defibrillation is the treatment of choice and is not contraindicated in pregnancy. However, if defibrillation is required, it is important to remember to remove any internal fetal monitoring equipment that might conduct the electricity to the fetus.[14]

The next step during resuscitation of a patient with pulseless VT or VF is to administer appropriate medications that improve cardiac response to defibrillation. Vasopressin has been added to the Advanced Cardiac Life Support (ACLS) guidelines as an alternative to epinephrine. However, in middle to late pregnancy, there is a 4-fold increase in vasopressinase, a cystine aminopeptidase produced by placental trophoblasts, that enhances the clearance of vasopressin. The effect of vasopressors on uteroplacental perfusion in a cardiac arrest situation is unknown; however, the ACLS guidelines must be followed and the use of these vasopressors must not be withheld.[15] The use of epinephrine can enhance placental blood flow and improve fetal outcome.[16] Circulate the medication with 60 to 90 seconds of cardiopulmonary resuscitation (CPR), then defibrillate at 360 J.

Maternal and Fetal Evaluation

After stability of the airway, breathing, and circulation, a thorough evaluation with a detailed history and physical examination is performed. Routine ICU monitoring includes electrocardiogram, pulse oximetry, and noninvasive blood pressure monitoring. As well as blood grouping and cross-matching, blood should be sent for analysis of arterial pH and blood gases, hemoglobin concentration, electrolytes, glucose, renal and liver function. Platelet count, prothrombin time (PT), partial thromboplastin time (PTT), and serum fibrinogen and fibrin degradation product levels are obtained if disseminated intravascular coagulopathy is suspected. Thromboelastography is an alternative test that measures the viscoelastic properties of clot formation, to diagnose thrombocytopenia, platelet dysfunction, and coagulation factor abnormalities. The Kleihauer-Betke analysis should be obtained to detect the presence and percentage of fetal red blood cells in the maternal circulation. Commercially available anti-D immunoglobulin should be administered in the situation of an Rh-positive fetus carried by an Rh-negative mother. Ultrasonography is performed to evaluate the fetus and uteroplacenta.

Fetal well-being is closely monitored in the critically ill parturient. The biophysical profile has gained popularity as a test of fetal well-being. This includes fetal breathing, tone, movement, amniotic fluid volume, and the results of a nonstress test. Each parameter is assigned a score of 2 when present and 0 when absent. Scores of

8 and 10 imply fetal well-being, 6 is equivocal and 4 or less indicates the need to deliver, provided that delivery does not pose a serious risk to the mother. If preterm delivery is anticipated and there is no medical contraindication, betamethasone (2 intramuscular doses of 12 mg, 24 hours apart) may be given to enhance fetal lung maturity. The fetus should be monitored either intermittently or continuously by a trained obstetric nurse in the ICU according to the fetal status.

CARDIOVASCULAR DYSFUNCTION
Shock

Causes of shock in obstetric patients are listed in **Table 1**. Shock presents as tachycardia, tachypnea, hypotension, oliguria, altered mental status, and lactic acidosis.[17–19] Orthostatic hypotension can be the only manifestation of early hemorrhagic shock; the diagnosis may be missed in the supine patient. Signs of external or internal hemorrhage may be present. Rales on auscultation are found in left ventricular failure or ARDS, a third heart sound in peripartum cardiomyopathy and pulmonary thromboembolism, and cardiac murmurs in valvular heart disease.

Patients with shock require invasive monitoring of arterial and central venous pressures. Pulmonary artery catheterization (PAC) is used to monitor pulmonary artery wedge pressure (left ventricular filling pressure), pulmonary arterial pressure, and cardiac output. The role of PAC is controversial. Recent studies in nonpregnant patients show that it does not increase mortality, but failed to show any benefit.[20–22] Echocardiography may therefore be preferred in coagulopathic patients or those requiring only a single hemodynamic evaluation to classify their disease, but PAC remains the mainstay of management of complex problems in critically ill obstetric patients similar to nonobstetric patients.

The parturient should be placed in the left lateral position to relieve aortocaval compression. Cardiac filling should be optimized with rapid intravenous infusion of crystalloids such as normal saline or lactated Ringer's solution. Approximately 3 L of crystalloids are required to replenish 1 L of lost blood (3:1 ratio). Colloids such as hetastarch or albumin remain in the circulation longer than crystalloids. However, in a large multicenter, randomized, double-blind study, Finfer and colleagues[23] found that fluid replacement with normal saline was as effective as human albumin and a lot cheaper. Low central venous pressure (CVP) or pulmonary arterial wedge pressure (PAWP) indicates decreased cardiac preload requiring fluid replacement. However, a normal CVP or PAWP does not rule out hypovolemia and should be treated by repeated fluid challenges with 200 to 500 mL of crystalloids infused over 10 to 15 minutes until the CVP or PAWP increases by 3 mm Hg or more and stays persistently increased.

If the mean arterial pressure (MAP) remains less than 60 mm Hg after fluid replacement, vasopressor therapy is started with infusion of dopamine (2–20 μg/kg/min) or norepinephrine (0.5–20 μg/min) through the central line. Vasopressin (0.01–0.04 units/min) infusion may work if hypotension does not respond to norepinephrine or dopamine. In cardiogenic shock, inotropic agents such as dobutamine (intravenous infusion at 2–20 μg/kg/min) can be started when the MAP is less than 60 mm Hg once intravascular volume status is optimized. Most vasopressors are known to negatively affect the uteroplacental circulation. Phenylephrine and ephedrine are the most commonly used drugs and possibly the safest in the treatment of hypotension associated with regional anesthesia. Maternal heart rate can be used as a guide to therapy when using phenylephrine or ephedrine. However, in situations such as shock, if one vasopressor is believed to have a clear benefit compared with another, the clinician should not hesitate to use the most beneficial drug while monitoring fetal well-being. Many patients with septic shock have relative adrenal insufficiency. Some investigators recommend intravenous hydrocortisone (200–300 mg/d in 3–4 doses) only if the basal serum cortisol level is less than 150 μg/L or if the cortisol level fails to increase by 90 μg/L after adrenocorticotropic hormone (ACTH) stimulation, whereas others treat all patients with corticosteroids.[18] In a multicenter randomized controlled trial, hydrocortisone did not improve survival, although hydrocortisone hastened reversal of shock in patients in whom shock was reversed.[24]

The cause of shock should also be aggressively managed. Septic shock is treated with antibiotics and control of the source of sepsis. Blunt curettage of the infected uterus or aspiration or surgical drainage of pelvic abscesses may be required.

Postpartum hemorrhage remains one of the leading causes of preventable maternal mortality both in the developed and the developing world. Initial assessment of a bleeding patient requires monitoring blood pressure, pulse, capillary refill, mental status, and urinary output.[19] Severe hemorrhage is associated with peripheral vascular constriction, depression of mental status, and severe hypotension leading to multiorgan failure.[25] In postpartum hemorrhage, correction of coagulopathy and thrombocytopenia is vital. When medical therapy is unsuccessful, surgical approaches to postpartum hemorrhage are often considered. These may include uterine curettage aceration repair, balloon tamponade, emboliza-tion, compressive suture techniques, uterine or hypogastric artery ligation, and ultimately hyster-ectomy as a last resort. Blood and blood products should be transfused based on coagulation profile and massive transfusion protocol (MTP) activated. Most trauma centers have an MTP in place. Burte-ow and colleagues[26] have successfully used 6:4:1 (red blood cells/fresh-frozen plasma/platelets) for immediate resuscitation in massive obstetric hemorrhage in their obstetric unit. Recombinant activated Factor VII has recently become avail-able. Initial reports of its use in women with exsan-guinating obstetric hemorrhage are encouraging. It is extremely expensive and should only be considered when conventional therapy fails.[19]

Hypertensive Crisis

Arterial pressure greater than 160/110 mm Hg in preeclampsia can result in pulmonary edema, seizures, intracerebral hemorrhage, and requires rapid blood pressure control. Intravenous labetalol 20 mg can be given initially followed by a 40-mg dose and 2 80-mg doses at 10-minute intervals until blood pressure is controlled or a cumulative dose of 300 mg is reached. Once initial blood pressure is controlled, a continuous infusion at a rate of 0.5 to 2 mg/min of labetalol can be used instead of inter-mittent dosing. As delivery is the ultimate treatment of resistant gestational hypertension, it may obviate the need to use continuous infusions in many cases. Another effective intravenous agent, hydral-azine, is administered at a dose of 5 to 10 mg every 20 minutes (maximum of 40 mg) until blood pres-sure is controlled. Reduction of pressure to normal levels (<140/90 mm Hg) should be avoided as it may compromise placental perfusion. Hyperten-sion refractory to these drugs is an indication for intravenous nitroglycerin (10–100 µg/min) or sodium nitroprusside (2–8 µg/min). Prolonged use of nitroglycerin may lead to methemoglobi-nemia. Cyanide toxicity in the mother and fetus may occur with sodium nitroprusside, limiting its use to less than 4 hours and only as a last resort.

Peripartum Cardiomyopathy

Even in the absence of preexisting heart disease, cardiac failure may occur as a result of peripartum cardiomyopathy (PCCM). PCCM is defined as cardiomyopathy that develops in the last month of gestation or in the first 5 months in the post-partum period without any identifiable cause.[27,28] The incidence is 1:3000 to 1:15,000 live births in the United States. Pathogenesis is poorly under-stood. However, infections and immunologic and nutritional causes have been implicated. Clinical

presentation includes the usual signs and symp-toms of heart failure. Diagnosis is based on clinical presentation of congestive heart failure and objec-tive evidence of left ventricular systolic dysfunc-tion. Early diagnosis and initiation of treatment are essential to optimize the outcome of the partu-rient. Medical management comprises sodium restriction, loop diuretics, afterload reducing agents (hydralazine, nitrates), and digoxin. Angiotensin-converting enzyme (ACE) inhibitors and angiotensin receptor blockers should be avoided during pregnancy because of severe adverse neonatal effects and can be substituted for by hydralazine and nitrates during pregnancy. Some ACE inhibitors can be used in the post-partum period even in women who are breast feeding. Patients with persistent left ventricular abnormalities have a poor prognosis.[29]

If medical therapy fails, patients may then be treated with mechanical circulatory support devices and (or) cardiac transplantation. Mechan-ical assist devices can be used as a bridge to recovery or a bridge to transplantation.[29–31]

Cardiopulmonary Resuscitation in Pregnancy

During cardiopulmonary resuscitation in preg-nancy, the team needs to follow the revised 2005 American Heart Association guidelines with modi-fications to compensate for the altered anatomy and physiology of pregnancy as outlined later. The major modifications include (1) prompt airway management, (2) special attention to lateral displacement of uterus and avoidance of aorto-caval compression, (3) optimal performance of chest compressions in the lateral decubitus posi-tion, (4) caution in the use of sodium bicarbonate as it may not cross the placenta quickly enough to reverse fetal acidosis, and (5) early consider-ation of perimortem cesarean delivery to optimize CPR and survival of mother and baby.[32,33]

Amiodarone has a large iodine load and may have an adverse effect on fetal thyroid function; however, advantages should be weighed against this risk of fetal thyroid dysfunction and the drug used if it is considered to be the best option. Vaso-pressin can be cleared more quickly starting mid pregnancy and may need to be substituted with epinephrine.

Perimortem Cesarean Delivery

Perimortem cesarean deliveries were recommen-ded in 1986.[34] Katz and colleagues[34] recommen-ded a 4-minute rule from the maternal arrest to the initiation of the cesarean delivery, with the fetus being delivered within 5 minutes. This approach was promoted principally on fetal grounds to allow the potential salvage of a viable fetus. The timing of delivery was based on theoretic considerations such as oxygen consumption, and prevention of neurologic injury. Since the initial description by Katz and colleagues,[35] numerous case reports have described often dramatic reversal of the maternal hemodynamic collapse, even in refractory situations. If initial resuscitation is not effective during cardiac arrest in pregnancy, delivering the fetus within 5 minutes may facilitate maternal and fetal survival. The 5-minute rule from arrest to delivery is now recommended by the American Heart Association when the intrauterine gestation is greater than 24 weeks (the cut-off for fetal viability).

RESPIRATORY FAILURE

Numerous insults can lead to acute lung injury and ARDS. ARDS is a form of respiratory failure characterized by acute hypoxemia and increased alveolar-capillary permeability resulting from diffuse pulmonary inflammation. Risk factors for ARDS can be classified into 4 main categories: (1) sepsis from pulmonary or nonpulmonary sources, (2) major trauma, (3) transfusion with multiple-unit blood products, and (4) aspiration of gastric contents. Eighty-five percent of ARDS cases result from 1 of these risk factors and sepsis accounts for up to 50% of all cases.[36] Risk factors for ARDS in pregnant patients can be divided into causes that are unique to pregnancy and those that are not unique to pregnancy as outlined in **Box 2**.

In cases of ARDS and obstructive lung disease, achieving normocapnea leads to more volutrauma, biotrauma, and atelectrauma. The current goals of ventilation are permissive hypercapnea, and maintaining the pH between 7.25 and 7.35. This is accomplished predominantly by the use of small tidal volumes. It is not unusual to allow a Pa_{CO_2} of 60 mm Hg or higher. In pregnancy there are no clear-cut data on the role of permissive hypercapnea. There are a few short-term animal experiments evaluating the effects of hypercapnia on uteroplacental blood flow but no long-term studies. The hypercapnia was induced rapidly without providing time for changes in the compensatory mechanisms to bring the pH to more normal levels. On the contrary, in an anaesthetized sheep model, Walker and colleagues[37] found no significant changes in uterine blood flow even when the maternal Pa_{CO_2} reached 60 mm Hg. At greater than 60 mm Hg Pa_{CO_2} they noted increased uterine vascular resistance, resulting in decreased uterine blood flow. There are no human data regarding the effect of permissive hypoventilation on uteroplacental and umbilical blood flow. Human

---

Box 2
Causes of ARDS

Unique to pregnancy

　Preeclampsia/eclampsia

　Tocolytic-induced pulmonary edema

　Aspiration of gastric contents

　Chorioamnionitis

　Amniotic fluid embolism

　Placental abruption

　Obstetric hemorrhage-related cause

　Endometritis

　Retained placental products

　Septic abortion

Not unique to pregnancy

　Sepsis

　Pneumonia

　Severe trauma

　Multiple transfusions

　Aspiration of gastric contents

　Acute pancreatitis

　Fat emboli

　Near drowning

Data from Katz VL, Dotters DJ, Droegemueller W. Perimortem cesarean delivery. Obstet Gynecol 1986;68:571–76.

---

extrapolation of animal data may not be valid for multiple reasons. The permissive hypoventilation as applied to patients with ARDS is not a sudden change in minute ventilation, but a gradual change while monitoring the patient. The ARDS net protocol provides guidance with regard to the rapidity of CO_2 accumulation and the pH change.[38] Sodium bicarbonate infusions can be given to compensate for severe acidosis without causing maternal alkalosis. There are no published studies investigating the use of low tidal volumes in the treatment of pregnant patients with acute lung injury and ARDS. However, a fetal maternal gradient of Pa_{CO_2} is around 10 to 13 mm Hg, resulting in a higher Pa_{CO_2} in the fetus and a potential for fetal acidosis, an increase in intracranial pressure, and a right shift in the hemoglobin dissociation curve. In addition, hypercapnia in the first 72 hours of life may lead to retinopathy of prematurity. Although bicarbonate infusion can reverse maternal acidosis, the rate of transfer of these ions across the placenta is not well studied and varies between species. It is possible that the rate of transfer of bicarbonate to the human fetus may not occur fast enough to correct fetal acidosis. The proven efficacy of a low tidal volume strategy in nonpregnant patients with ARDS provides strong support for its universal use.[39] In managing the ARDS patients, the authors routinely use small tidal volumes, permissive hypoventilation (up to $Paco_2$ of 60 mm Hg) while closely monitoring the fetal status with the biophysical profile.

Data on fetal oxygenation are derived from sheep models and are discussed by Tomimatsu and colleagues.[40] Oxygen levels should be closely monitored in pregnancy and kept higher than in nonpregnant women, especially in patients with acute changes in oxygenation who may not have a normal placental oxygen transport. Oxygen tension levels should be monitored rather than oxygen saturations because it is the difference in Pao_2 at the placental level that determines oxygen transfer.

Another caveat to keep in mind is that positive pressure ventilation and the application of positive end expiratory pressure increase intrathoracic pressure and decrease venous return. In a pregnant patient, these effects remain true and may be worsened by compression of the inferior vena cava by the gravid uterus, which may reduce venous return further and lead to a decreased urine output.

Management of respiratory failure in pregnancy is similar to management in nonpregnant women, although being mindful of the normal physiologic changes that occur in the parturient. Protective mechanical ventilation using smaller tidal volumes, elevation of the head of the bed to prevent ventilator-associated pneumonia, and routine use of spontaneous awakening trials and spontaneous breathing trials minimize complications caused by mechanical ventilation.

ACUTE RENAL FAILURE

Creatinine clearance is increased in pregnancy to 120 to 160 mL/min and serum creatinine level decreases to 0.4−0.7 mg/dL. Acute renal failure comprises oliguria, azotemia, and metabolic acidosis. It has become rare in the developed world with an incidence of approximately 1:15,000, but continues to be associated with significant mortality and long-term morbidity. The most common cause of renal failure in pregnancy is preeclampsia. Other pregnancy-specific causes include acute fatty liver of pregnancy, thrombotic thrombocytopenic purpura, amniotic fluid embolism, infection, sepsis, intravascular volume depletion, obstruction, or idiopathic causes.[6]

The initial management of renal failure is similar to nonpregnant patients. Nephrotoxins (aminoglycosides, radiocontrast dye) should be avoided if possible. Drugs should be dosed based on renal function with particular attention to magnesium. Dopamine has been administered for both prevention and treatment of acute renal failure in critically ill patients. However, clinical studies have not demonstrated the efficacy of this approach and it is not recommended for routine use for either prophylaxis or treatment of acute renal failure.[41] Initiation of dialysis seems to be safe when indicated. Indications for dialysis include intravascular volume overload, hyperkalemia refractory to medical management, metabolic acidosis, or symptomatic uremia.

SUMMARY

Critical illness may complicate any pregnancy. Obstetricians must be familiar with the issues pertaining to care of pregnant women with multiple organ failure. Many obstetric disorders may mimic medical disorders. Once the correct diagnosis is made, the obstetrician and the intensivists must decide whether delivery will alter the natural history of the disease process and improve maternal survival. If the maternal condition is expected to improve after delivery, then the decision to deliver vaginally or by cesarean section must be made. Fetal viability should obviously be taken into consideration. Hypovolemia, hypotension, and respiratory failure are treated while preparations are made to deliver the fetus. Timely delivery improves not only maternal outcome but also fetal outcome. No efforts should be spared in the management of critically ill obstetric patients because their outcomes are often dramatically better than expected from the initial severity of illness.

REFERENCES

1. Naylor DF Jr, Olson MM. Critical care obstetrics and gynecology. Crit Care Clin 2003;19:127−49.
2. Price LC, Slack A, Nelson-Piercy C. Aims of obstetric critical care management. Best Pract Res Clin Obstet Gynaecol 2008;22:775−99.
3. Soubra SH, Guntupalli KK. Critical illness in pregnancy: an overview. Crit Care Med 2005;33:S248−55.
4. Cartin-Ceba R, Gajic O, Iyer VN, et al. Fetal outcomes of critically ill pregnant women admitted to the intensive care unit for nonobstetric causes. Crit Care Med 2008;36:2746−51.
5. Lewis G, editor. Saving mother's lives: reviewing maternal death to make motherhood safer (2003−2005). London: Confidential Enquiry into Maternal and Child Health; 2007.
6. Galvagno SM Jr, Camann W. Sepsis and acute renal failure in pregnancy. Anesth Analg 2009;108:572−5.

7. Karnad DR, Guntupalli KK. Critical illness and pregnancy: review of a global problem. Crit Care Clin 2004;20:555–76, vii.

8. Afessa B, Green B, Delke I, et al. Systemic inflammatory response syndrome, organ failure, and outcome in critically ill obstetric patients treated in an ICU. Chest 2001;120:1271–7.

9. Zeeman GG, Wendel GD Jr, Cunningham FG. A blueprint for obstetric critical care. Am J Obstet Gynecol 2003;188:532–6.

10. McKay DB, Josephson MA. Pregnancy in recipients of solid organs—effects on mother and child. N Engl J Med 2006;354:1281–93.

11. Walters WA, Ford JB, Sullivan EA, et al. Maternal deaths in Australia. Med J Aust 2002; 176:413–4.

12. Johnson MD. Cardiopulmonary resuscitation. In: Gambling DR, Douglas MJ, editors. Obstetric anesthesia and uncommon disorders. Philadelphia: WB Saunders; 1998. p. 51–74.

13. Rees GA, Willis BA. Resuscitation in late pregnancy. Anaesthesia 1988;43:347–9.

14. Gilbert ES, Harmon JS. Manual of high risk pregnancy & delivery. 3rd edition. St Louis (MO): Mosby; 2003.

15. Di Gregoria R. Vasopressin use in the NYC REMAC protocols: a teaching reference. New York: Regional Emergency Medical Services Council of New York City; 2001.

16. Cummins RO. Cardiac arrest associated with pregnancy. In: Cummins R, Hazinski M, Field J, editors. The reference textbook. Dallas (TX): American Heart Association; 2003. p. 143–58.

17. Abbrescia K, Sheridan B. Complications of second and third trimester pregnancies. Emerg Med Clin North Am 2003;21:695–710, vii.

18. Annane D, Bellissant E, Cavaillon JM. Septic shock. Lancet 2005;365:63–78.

19. Cohen WR. Hemorrhagic shock in obstetrics. J Perinat Med 2006;34:263–71.

20. Fujitani S, Baldisseri MR. Hemodynamic assessment in a pregnant and peripartum patient. Crit Care Med 2005;33:S354–61.

21. Otero RM, Nguyen HB, Huang DT, et al. Early goal-directed therapy in severe sepsis and septic shock revisited: concepts, controversies, and contemporary findings. Chest 2006;130:1579–95.

22. Harvey S, Harrison DA, Singer M, et al. Assessment of the clinical effectiveness of pulmonary artery catheters in management of patients in intensive care (PAC-Man): a randomised controlled trial. Lancet 2005;366:472–7.

23. Finfer S, Bellomo R, Boyce N, et al. A comparison of albumin and saline for fluid resuscitation in the intensive care unit. N Engl J Med 2004;350: 2247–56.

24. Sprung CL, Annane D, Keh D, et al. Hydrocortisone therapy for patients with septic shock. N Engl J Med 2008;358:111–24.

25. Porreco RP, Stettler RW. Surgical remedies for postpartum hemorrhage. Clin Obstet Gynecol 2010;53 182–95.

26. Burtelow M, Riley E, Druzin M, et al. How we treat management of life-threatening primary postpartum hemorrhage with a standardized massive transfusion protocol. Transfusion 2007;47:1564–72.

27. Lapinsky SE, Kruczynski K, Seaward GR, et al. Critical care management of the obstetric patient. Can J Anaesth 1997;44:325–9.

28. Murali S, Baldisseri MR. Peripartum cardiomyopathy. Crit Care Med 2005;33:S340–6.

29. Moioli M, Valenzano MM, Bentivoglio G, et al. Peripartum cardiomyopathy. Arch Gynecol Obstet 2010;281:183–8.

30. Goland S, Modi K, Bitar F, et al. Clinical profile and predictors of complications in peripartum cardiomyopathy. J Card Fail 2009;15:645–50.

31. Zimmerman H, Bose R, Smith R, et al. Treatment of peripartum cardiomyopathy with mechanical assist devices and cardiac transplantation. Ann Thorac Surg 2010;89:1211–7.

32. American Heart Association. Part 10-8: Cardiac arrest associated with pregnancy. Cir J Am Heart Assoc 2005;112:150–3.

33. Suresh MS, LaToya MC, Munnur U. Cardiopulmonary resuscitation and the parturient. Best Pract Res Clin Obstet Gynaecol 2010;24:383–400.

34. Katz VL, Dotters DJ, Droegemueller W. Perimortem cesarean delivery. Obstet Gynecol 1986;68:571–6.

35. Katz V, Balderston K, DeFreest M. Perimortem cesarean delivery: were our assumptions correct? Am J Obstet Gynecol 2005;192:1916–20.

36. Bandi VD, Munnur U, Matthay MA. Acute lung injury and acute respiratory distress syndrome in pregnancy. Crit Care Clin 2004;20:577–607.

37. Walker AM, Oakes GK, Ehrenkranz R, et al. Effects of hypercapnia on uterine and umbilical circulations in conscious pregnant sheep. J Appl Physiol 1976 41:727–33.

38. Ventilation with lower tidal volumes as compared with traditional tidal volumes for acute lung injury and the acute respiratory distress syndrome. The Acute Respiratory Distress Syndrome Network. N Engl J Med 2000;342:1301–8.

39. Campbell LA, Klocke RA. Implications for the pregnant patient. Am J Respir Crit Care Med 2001;163:1051–4.

40. Tomimatsu T, Pena JP, Longo LD. Fetal cerebral oxygenation: the role of maternal hyperoxia with supplemental CO_2 in sheep. Am J Obstet Gynecol 2007;196(4):359, e1–5.

41. Thadhani R, Pascual M, Bonventre JV. Acute renal failure. N Engl J Med 1996;334:1448–60.

Interventional Chest Procedures in Pregnancy

Ross K. Morgan, MD, FRCPI[a],*, Armin Ernst, MD[b]

KEYWORDS

- Interventional pulmonology • Pregnancy • Bronchoscopy
- Pleural intervention

Interventional pulmonology is a growing field that encompasses diagnostic and therapeutic bronchoscopic procedures as well as pleural interventions. Although many of these interventions have been performed by pulmonary physicians and others for a long time, the discipline of interventional pulmonology has only really been defined in the past decade.[1] Since then, older techniques have been refined and exciting new technologies have emerged that have extended the reach and application of the instruments used.[1,2] With this has come an increasing awareness of the need for training and competency assessment within the subspecialty as well as quality control and comparative effectiveness research.[3]

The main areas within pulmonary medicine for which these interventions have a role are in malignant and nonmalignant airway disease, pleural effusion, pneumothorax, and artificial airways. As a result of social, educational, and medical progress, many women are choosing to have children later in life and so it is likely that lung disease for which bronchoscopy and pleural procedures are indicated will become increasingly represented in women of child-bearing years. The techniques used in interventional pulmonology are presented in **Table 1** but the available skills are dependent on local competencies and practice environment. In general, when therapeutic intervention is necessary in pregnancy, bronchoscopy and pleural intubation offer a relatively safe alternative to radiologic or surgical options.

There are no data from well-designed prospective trials to guide recommendations for interventional pulmonary procedures in pregnancy.[4] However, there are several published series for related procedures in gastroenterology and practice guidelines for endoscopy in the pregnant patient have been published.[5–8] The recommendations provided in this article are based on critical review of reported case series and opinion from recognized experts, as well as personal observations.

THE LUNGS IN PREGNANCY

Clinicians who perform pulmonary interventions during pregnancy should have good knowledge of the mechanical and physiologic changes that occur and be aware of the particular risks associated with medications and other tools used during the procedure (eg, ionizing radiation exposure to the mother and fetus).

CHANGES TO THE AIRWAY

The Mallampati classification is a simple grading system that uses a visual scale of mouth opening and has been found to predict the degree of difficulty for oral intubation.[9] Mallampati class 1 is present when the soft palate, uvula, and pillars are visible, class 2 when the soft palate and base of the uvula are visible, class 3 when only the soft palate is visible, and class 4 when only the hard palate is visible (**Fig. 1**). The incidence of failed intubation has been reported in obstetric patients to be up to 8 times higher than in general surgery.[10,11] One potential mechanism for this is a hormone-mediated increase in pharyngeal

a Department of Respiratory Medicine, Beaumont Hospital, Dublin 9, Ireland
b Interventional Pulmonology, Beth Israel Deaconess Medical Center, Harvard Medical School, One Deaconess Road, Deaconess Building- 201, Boston, MA 02215, USA
* Corresponding author.
E-mail address: rossmorgan@beaumont.ie

Clin Chest Med 32 (2011) 61–74
doi:10.1016/j.ccm.2010.10.007
0272-5231/11/$ — see front matter © 2011 Elsevier Inc. All rights reserved.

Table 1
Interventional pulmonary procedures: indications, contraindications and risks

Pleural	Indications for Pleural Space Drainage in Pregnant Patients	General Contraindications to All Procedures
Transthoracic pleural ultrasound	Fluid: diagnosis and symptom relief in large effusion, hemothorax, empyema, complicated parapneumonic effusions, chylothorax	Lack of patient cooperation
Thoracentesis		Lack of appropriate facilities
Pleural manometry		Lack of appropriate consent from patient or representative
Chest tube placement		Inexperienced operator working without direct supervision
Pleurodesis	Air: large or symptomatic spontaneous pneumothorax, chest trauma, patient on mechanical ventilation, unstable patient	
Pleuroscopy		
Indwelling pleural catheter placement		
Airway	**Indications for Bronchoscopy in Pregnancy**	**Increased Risk of Complications**
Diagnostic	To assess airway patency	Recent myocardial infarction or unstable angina
Endobronchial biopsy, bronchoalveolar lavage, cytology brush, protected specimen brush, transbronchial biopsy, transbronchial needle aspiration	To investigate hemoptysis, unexplained cough, localized wheeze, stridor, or suspected airway trauma	Uncontrolled arrhythmia
		Refractory hypoxia
	To investigate suspected lung cancer	Hemodynamic instability
Endobronchial ultrasound (EBUS) linear probe	To sample mediastinal lymphadenopathy	Partial tracheal obstruction
Radial probe EBUS	To obtain microbiologic samples in suspected pulmonary infections	Unstable bronchial asthma
Autofluorescence bronchoscopy		Increased bleeding risk: severe coagulopathy; uremia; pulmonary hypertension; superior vena cava obstruction
Electromagnetic navigational bronchoscopy	To obtain samples from the lungs of patients with diffuse or focal infiltrates on chest radiographs	Respiratory failure requiring mechanical ventilation
Image-guided (fluoroscopic) transbronchial lung biopsy	To evaluate problems associated with endotracheal tubes	High positive end-expiratory pressure
Airway	**Indications in Pregnancy**	**Specific Contraindications for Rigid Bronchoscopy**
Therapeutic	Management of massive hemoptysis	Cervical spine instability
Rigid bronchoscopy with dilatation or tumor debridement	Removal of retained secretions or mucous plugs	Maxillofacial trauma
Airway ablative techniques: cryotherapy, cryorecanalization, argon plasma photocoagulation, electrocautery, laser, microdebrider	Foreign body extraction	Obstructing oral or laryngeal disease
	Resection of airway tumor	Severe head and neck deformity
Photodynamic therapy	Relief of tracheobronchial obstruction	
Balloon bronchoplasty	Management of airway fistula	
Foreign body extraction	To assist with difficult intubations	
Airway stenting		
Endobronchial brachytherapy		
Bronchial thermoplasty		
Bronchoscopic lung volume reduction		
Percutaneous dilatational tracheostomy		

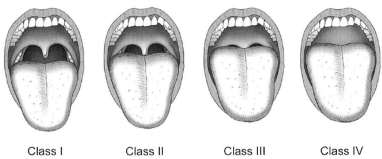

| Class I | Class II | Class III | Class IV |

Fig. 1. The Mallampati classification for difficult laryngoscopy and intubation. (*From* Nuckton TJ, Glidden DV, Browner WS, et al. Physical examination: Mallampati score as an independent predictor of obstructive sleep apnea. Sleep 2006;29(7):903–8; with permission.)

edema. This is reflected by an increase in Mallampati score as pregnancy progresses as detected in a study of 242 women assessed at 12 weeks and again at term.[12] In this study the number of grade 4 cases by 38 weeks' gestation had increased by 34%.[12] In addition nasal symptoms and congestion are more common during pregnancy with several ultrastructural changes including mucus gland hypertrophy evident.[13,14] This may influence ability to perform bronchoscopy safely through the nasal route; the nasal route is not used during pregnancy in our institutions.

PULMONARY RESPONSE TO PREGNANCY

Normal pregnancy is associated with adaptations to maternal pulmonary physiology in response to both hormonal and mechanical factors.[15] Early pregnancy is associated with dyspnea secondary to hyperventilation and this effect seems to be mediated by progesterone, which increases minute ventilation primarily because of an increased sensitivity of the respiratory center to P_{CO_2}.[16] Later in pregnancy, the anatomic effects of the pregnancy come to the fore as the gravid uterus enlarges out of the pelvis, elevating the diaphragms and resulting in a decrease in functional residual capacity and residual volume. The reduction in lung volumes is off set to some degree by an increase in the anterior-posterior diameter of the chest.[17]

The caliber of the large airway also changes as lung volumes decrease in later pregnancy, which may affect airway resistance. Although these changes to pulmonary physiology are well described, overall there is a balance between the factors that affect airway resistance and lung volumes, and so in practice these changes are not usually of great clinical significance. There are certain lung diseases that seem to present

more frequently, such as complications and presentations of lymphangioleiomyomatosis.[18,19]

HEMODYNAMIC EFFECTS OF PREGNANCY

Adaptive circulatory responses also occur in pregnancy and result in an increase in cardiac output and circulating blood volume by approximately 2 L.[11] Compression of the inferior vena cava (IVC) by gravid uterus in the recumbent position leads to a reduction in cardiac preload and consequent reduction in cardiac output leading to hypotension.[20] This can be exacerbated by procedural-related sedation and vasodilatation, which may combine to cause a reduction in blood flow to the placenta and fetal distress. After 28 weeks the left lateral position should be used from the outset of the procedure; alternatively the semi-seating position should be used.

SYMPTOMS OF LUNG DISEASE IN PREGNANCY

During a normal pregnancy and without any lung disease, a significant number of pregnant women complain of breathlessness, and this number increases as the pregnancy progresses. In a study of 62 normal pregnancies, Milne and colleagues[21] plotted the incidence, severity, and time course of dyspnea. This study revealed that 50% of patients complained of this symptom before 20 weeks and almost 80% by term. Dyspnea in this setting probably relates to individual adaptation and perception of the hyperventilation that accompanies pregnancy. This needs to be considered when evaluating and treating patients who present with lung disease during pregnancy (eg, small pleural effusion), and should be distinguished from pathologic causes of breathlessness.

INDICATIONS FOR BRONCHOSCOPIC PROCEDURES IN PREGNANCY

The indications for diagnostic bronchoscopy in pregnancy are the same as those in nonpregnant patients and include the assessment of endobronchial symptoms such as hemoptysis and localized wheeze or abnormalities on chest imaging. Chest radiograph findings that warrant a bronchoscopic examination include pulmonary mass, recurring pulmonary infiltrates, persistent atelectasis, mediastinal adenopathy, and diffuse parenchymal lung disease.[4,22] To minimize inappropriate procedures, particularly in pregnant women, it is important to have knowledge of the limitations of the bronchoscope. Examples of situations where flexible bronchoscopy may not be helpful include evaluation of a solitary pulmonary nodule, isolated pleural effusion, uncomplicated pneumonia, and chronic cough. Respiratory toilette is occasionally indicated when there are difficult secretion retention problems and lobar atelectasis, particularly of the left lower lobe. However, as a general rule, postural drainage, cough, and suction of secretions are often sufficient and should be considered first-line treatment. Indications for therapeutic bronchoscopy in pregnancy include foreign body removal, massive hemoptysis, and central airway stenosis.[2] Other situations where bronchoscopy is helpful are in the performance of difficult intubation and to assess and treat complications of the endotracheal tube in mechanically ventilated patients. The range of interventional pulmonary procedures, indications, contraindications, and risks are outlined in **Table 1**.

PULMONARY PROCEDURES IN PREGNANCY
General Considerations

The first consideration should always be whether the procedure can be safely delayed until late in the pregnancy, or even deferred until after delivery. This requires determination of the risk-benefit of the intervention, including the risk of a delayed diagnosis or intervention on maternal and fetal well-being. When a procedure is to be performed, it should always be in collaboration with a multidisciplinary team that includes the bronchoscopist, obstetrician, neonatologist, thoracic surgeon, and anesthesiologist as appropriate.[23] The diagnostic approach with the highest diagnostic yield and the lowest maternal and fetal risk should be chosen.

Informed Consent

Before performing the procedure, the rationale, risks, benefits, and alternatives to the procedure as well as the planned sedation should be discussed with the patient with particular emphasis on balancing the risks of lack or delay in diagnosis or treatment with fetal safety and all questions should be answered. In nonurgent cases, involvement of the patient's obstetrician in this process may place the mother at ease and allay her anxieties. In the rare emergency situations, implied consent may be acceptable when the patient is unable to provide explicit consent because of altered mental status.

Preparation

As with routine bronchoscopy, a medical history should document known allergies and problems with procedural sedation in the past. A physical examination with special attention to the upper airway should be performed. The upper airway including the nose undergoes several changes that can result in more difficult intubation.[10,12] If signs suggesting a difficult airway are identified alternatives to procedural sedation should be considered in consultation with the anesthesiologist.[24] Intravenous access should be established in all cases. Because of the susceptibility of the pregnant patient to hypotension, particularly as pregnancy progresses, preprocedural hydration may be considered in patients who are kept fasting for more than 4 hours.

Aspiration of gastric contents during procedural anesthesia is a rare although well-described and much-feared complication. Because of increased aspiration risk in pregnancy, some investigators have recommended administration of medications that improve gastroesophageal sphincter tone and reduce gastric volume such as metoclopramide before gastrointestinal endoscopy.[8,25,26] There is no evidence to support the use of such agents before bronchoscopy.

Supplemental oxygen should be provided to maintain oxygen reserves and prevent hypoxemia caused by hypoventilation. Without supplemental oxygen a significant decrease in arterial oxygen pressure has been shown to occur during flexible bronchoscopy, with decreases in arterial oxygen tension (Pao_2) of around 15 mm Hg during the procedure common.[25,26] This can be even more pronounced if bronchoalveolar lavage is performed.[27] Although it may be assumed (because of the affinity of fetal hemoglobin for oxygen) that fetal desaturation is not likely in the absence of maternal respiratory depression, it is reasonable to maintain higher maternal oxygen saturations (eg, >96%) than would normally be tolerated routinely in nonpregnant patients (>90%).[22]

The equipment necessary to perform the procedure and to deal with possible complications should be available. This includes suction to manage vomiting or oral secretions, oropharyngeal airways, and equipment for endotracheal intubation. Reversal agents, fluids, and advanced cardiac life-support medications and a defibrillator should also be available.

Positioning

In the late second and third trimester, the gravid uterus can compress the IVC when the mother is in the supine position and the resultant reduction in preload can cause hypotension.[20] This may be exacerbated by vasodilating medications used during the procedure. Left lateral displacement of the uterus relieves this compression of the IVC and thereby reduces the risk of maternal hypotension and consequent risks of placental hypoperfusion and fetal hypoxemia. Displacement is achieved by placing a wedge or pillow under the right hip, creating a pelvic tilt to the left. When this is not possible, a sitting position is an alternative as it also helps avoid caval compression.

Monitoring

Mother

Proper monitoring of the mother's response to medications and to the procedure is crucial. This requires knowledge of the risks of procedural sedation and the intervention (see **Table 1**; **Table 2**). The principal concerns are hypoventilation and resulting hypoxemia, cardiac arrhythmias, loss of airway protection, and possible gastric aspiration. The mother's blood pressure should be measured at frequent regular intervals and respiratory rate, oxygen saturation, and heart rate/cardiac rhythm should be monitored continuously.[8,28,29] Several studies have determined that supplemental oxygen does not reliably prevent hypoxemia and delays the detection of respiratory depression, as the oxygen saturation levels may not actually decrease until a prolonged period of hypoventilation has occurred.[30,31] Capnography, which measures changes in the end-tidal carbon dioxide levels and which is more sensitive than pulse oximetry for detecting respiratory depression, has been suggested as a useful adjunct in procedural sedation but does not have a routine role to date.[32]

Fetus

In general, it is reasonable to assume that if the mother is tolerating the procedure well, the fetus should not be in any distress. Before 28 weeks, expert opinion suggests that efforts at intraprocedural monitoring of fetal heart rate can be unreliable, difficult to interpret because of fetal heart rate variability, and largely uninformative.[33] This may lead to further anxiety and prolongation of the procedure. Some institutions have anesthesia protocols in pregnancy that require fetal monitoring during the procedure but overall it is usually unnecessary for routine bronchoscopy, in particular before fetal viability, around 24 weeks' gestation.

Procedural Sedation

Procedural sedation involves the use of short-acting analgesic and sedative medications that enable clinicians to perform procedures effectively. Relative contraindications to sedation may include older age, significant medical comorbidities that increase patient susceptibility to the cardiorespiratory depressant effects of sedatives, and signs of a difficult airway. Before proceeding with procedural sedation in pregnancy, the clinician and patient must agree that the potential benefits of the sedation and analgesia outweigh the risks. Outside of the pregnancy, comorbidities that increase the risk of sedation include heart failure, chronic obstructive pulmonary disease, neuromuscular disease, dehydration, and anemia.

As the ventilatory response to sedatives may be exaggerated in pregnancy and the consequences of hypoxemia greater, common sense dictates that a conservative approach to sedation should be adopted to reduce these. This should include giving a lower starting dose, redosing medications at less frequent intervals and avoiding optional medications as well as maintaining sedation for the shortest period necessary to perform the procedure.

MEDICATIONS USED IN PULMONARY PROCEDURES DURING PREGNANCY

Recommendations for drugs used during procedures in pregnancy are based mainly on observational studies and expert opinion. There are no published guidelines for bronchoscopy but the American Society for Gastrointestinal Endoscopy have published recommendations for the choice of medications during pregnancy and lactation that serve as a useful guide,[8] and there are several case series in the endoscopy literature that have shown that procedural sedation is not associated with adverse fetal outcomes.[5,6] The US Food and Drug Administration (FDA) lists 5 categories of drugs with regard to safety during pregnancy from A (safest) to X (to be avoided). Category A classification requires that controlled studies have been performed that demonstrate there is

Table 2
Safety and recommendations for commonly used medication in procedural sedation and anesthesia

Drug	FDA Category	Properties/Risks	Recommendations
Lidocaine	B	Crosses placental and blood-brain barrier Nonteratogenic in first trimester Risks: seizures; arrhythmias; methemoglobinemia	Use lowest dose necessary to provide effective topical anesthesia Total dose should not exceed 300 mg or 4.5 mg/kg As absorption may be increased in pregnancy consider having patient gargle and spit out rather than swallow
Meperidine	B	Nonteratogenic opiate Metabolized to long half-life opiate so can accumulate with repetitive doses	It is preferred over morphine and fentanyl, which cross the fetal blood-brain barrier more rapidly Use lowest dose that achieves analgesia
Naloxone	B	Rapidly acting opiate antagonist crosses the placenta within 2 min of intravenous administration Not teratogenic May precipitate acute withdrawal in mothers dependent on opiates	Not for routine use Use if needed for hypotension, unresponsiveness or respiratory depression Potential for resedation as it is rapidly metabolized
Propofol	B	Short-acting anesthetic that causes deep sedation Risk of maternal respiratory depression Crosses placental barrier and associated with neonatal neurologic depression	Anesthesiologist should be in attendance because of the narrow therapeutic index and the importance of close monitoring
Fentanyl	C	Synthetic narcotic agonist Fentanyl is not teratogenic Risks of hypoxia and placental hypoperfusion from hypotension	Seems safe in low doses
Flumazenil	C	Safety profile in humans not studied Not teratogenic in mice May precipitate seizures in patients using benzodiazepines chronically	Reserve for maternal benzodiazepine overdose only
Midazolam	D	Category D as related to diazepam, which may cause cleft palate and neurobehavioral problems in neonate Midazolam has not been reported to be associated with congenital abnormalities	Midazolam is the preferred benzodiazepine when sedation with meperidine is inadequate Should be avoided in the first trimester if possible

Category B: there are no adequate and well-controlled studies in pregnant women and animal studies have revealed no evidence of harm to the fetus or adequate and well-controlled studies in pregnant women have failed to demonstrate a risk to the fetus but animal studies have shown an adverse effect. Category C: there are no adequate and well-controlled studies in pregnant women but animal studies have either not been performed or have revealed an adverse effect. Category D: studies in pregnant women have demonstrated a risk to the fetus; however, the benefits of therapy may be acceptable despite the risk.

no risk to humans, obviously a difficult standard for most medications to reach.

For the drugs used in procedural sedation and anesthesia, the data are limited, confined to case reports in humans, consensus opinion, pharmacologic observations or (frequently weak) animal data, and none of the agents are in the class A category. The FDA classification may be of limited value when determining the safety of a once-off administration and the risk of these medications must be weighed on a case-by-case basis, taking account of the need for patient comfort and safety, as well as the need to complete the procedure with desirable outcome.

The risks of maternal distress during procedures and the consequences of having to abandon the intervention because of maternal intolerance as a result of inadequate sedation need to be considered. In general, if the procedure is clinically necessary, then so is the procedural sedation. The target level for most procedures is anxiolysis or mild sedation, and this can be achieved by using the lowest possible dose, avoiding use of optional medication, and having the procedure performed by the most experienced operator to ensure timely completion.[32] An overview of the medications used in procedural sedation in the pulmonary procedures unit is provided in **Box 1**. These medications should be used with caution close to labor and delivery as they may result in neonatal withdrawal.

For procedural sedation in lactating women, fentanyl is preferred to meperidine as opiate anesthetic because it does not reach pharmacologically significant concentrations in breast milk and therefore breastfeeding may be continued without interruption after administration. By contrast, midazolam accumulates in breast milk and can lead to respiratory depression in the infant.[29] Infants should therefore not be breastfed for at least 4 hours after maternal midazolam administration and at the end of this time the breast milk should be pumped and discarded before breastfeeding recommences.[29]

The indications for prophylactic antibiotic use have been rationalized recently and are now limited to situations where the mucosa will be breached in patients with prosthetic heart valves, previous infective endocarditis, some types of congenital heart disease, and patients who develop valvopathy after cardiac transplant.[34] The recommended agents are amoxicillin, ampicillin, or clindamycin, all of which are considered safe throughout pregnancy.

RISKS OF BRONCHOSCOPY IN PREGNANCY

The risks of bronchoscopy in pregnancy are from the procedure and the procedural sedation. Most adverse effects of diagnostic bronchoscopy are caused by the medication used, the threshold for which is lowered in pregnancy; medication may cause depressed mental status, hypoxemia, hypoventilation, bronchospasm, loss of airway protection, gastric aspiration, cardiac arrhythmias, and seizures. In particular dosing of lidocaine should be minimized (see **Table 2**). Although these risks are in common with standard procedure, they are aggravated because of the mechanical and physiologic adaptations in pregnancy as previously outlined. Sedation-related risks to the fetus include teratogenesis when given during the first trimester as well as hypoxia, hypoperfusion, and induction of premature labor.[29,35] Procedure-related complications depend on how invasive the procedure is and the modalities used but include hypoxemia, hypertension, bronchospasm, respiratory distress, vagally mediated hypotension, pulmonary hemorrhage, and pneumothorax.

SPECIAL ISSUES
Diagnostic Tools

The emergence of bedside ultrasound to guide pleural procedures is a welcome development as it is safe, quickly learnt, and is associated with a reduction in the complications of thoracentesis.[36,37] In pregnancy in particular, where the gravid uterus displaces the abdominal contents and diaphragm, transthoracic ultrasound is even more useful in the evaluation of the pleural fluid and in enhancing safety in pleural effusion

---

Box 1
Causes of pleural effusion in pregnancy

Transudative

Physiologic

Pulmonary embolism

Peripartum cardiomyopathy

Preeclampsia/HELLP (HELLP is an abbreviation of the main findings: hemolytic anemia, elevated liver enzymes, and low platelet count)

Ovarian hyperstimulation syndrome

Meigs syndrome

Pseudo-Meigs syndrome

Urinothorax

Pulmonary edema

Exudative

Parapneumonic

Tuberculosis

Chylothorax; lymphangioleiomyomatosis

Ectopic pregnancy

Malignancy

Trophoblastic disease

Drug-related (eg, nitrofurantoin)

Connective tissue disease (eg, lupus pleuritis)

Sarcoidosis

Pancreatitis/pancreatic pseudocyst

drainage. In the airway, endobronchial ultrasound (EBUS), has emerged as one of the most useful adjuncts to the flexible bronchoscope.[2] The linear probe EBUS scope, by providing the ability to see outside the airway and perform transbronchial needle aspiration of adjacent tissue, has revolutionized the assessment of mediastinal adenopathy and staging of lung cancer (**Fig. 2**). The radial EBUS probe, which is inserted through the working channel of the bronchoscope has been shown to be useful in inspection of the airway wall and for guiding sampling of peripheral lung nodules. The use of EBUS has not been formally evaluated but ultrasound is considered safe for use in pregnancy.

When hemostasis is required after bronchoscopic biopsy, this can normally be controlled by staying in wedge position, suctioning to produce tamponade, and instillation of cold saline. Epinephrine is a category C drug in pregnancy as it causes a decrease in uterine blood flow. It is usually not necessary for hemostasis and its safety, when used in the airway at low volumes of 1:20,000 solution, has not been studied. However, when epinephrine is considered the best option to control significant bleeding, the benefit of its use outweighs the small risk of decreased uterine blood flow.

Fluoroscopy

Ionizing radiation exposure is associated with growth retardation and fetal anomalies as well as pregnancy loss, and thus the safety of radiological investigations is a common concern of clinicians and patients. However, the perception of that risk is often higher than the actual risk posed by radiation exposure in pregnancy,[38] and the effect of a missed or delayed diagnosis on the mother and her pregnancy needs to be considered.[39] There is no evidence of an increased risk to the fetus at doses less than 50 mGy (5 rad)[40] and a chest radiograph results in exposure to 20 mrad for posterior-anterior film.

Situations for which fluoroscopy is considered during bronchoscopy may arise in the performance of transbronchial biopsies and in airway stent placement. We do not use fluoroscopy routinely in these circumstances and would not consider using it in pregnancy in particular because no evidence base exists.[41] However, the safety of using fluoroscopy in 65 pregnant women undergoing endoscopic retrograde cholangiopancreatography (ERCP), where the radiation source is closer to the fetus, has been reported.[42]

If fluoroscopy is to be used, consultation with a radiologist or radiation safety officer should be considered to minimize exposure. The fetus should be shielded from the ionizing radiation by placement of lead shields under the pelvis and lower abdomen, and measurement of radiation exposure to the uterus should be considered. Radiation exposure is reduced during fluoroscopy by modifying the exposure time, beam size, and imaging area. Brief snapshots of fluoroscopy should be used to confirm forceps or wire position, and taking of fluoroscopy images that use additional radiation should be avoided if possible.

A   **B**

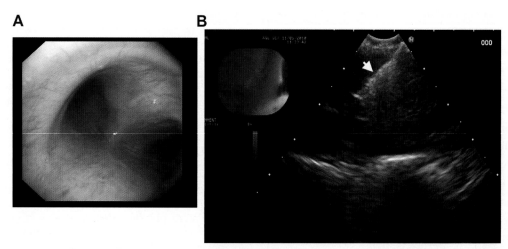

Fig. 2. Airway endoscopic (*A*) and endobronchial ultrasound view (*B*) displaying needle aspiration of enlarged station 7 lymph node (arrow shows needle within the lymph node) in a 36-year-old pregnant woman presenting at 29 weeks with cough. The lymph node aspirate found adenocarcinoma. The patient was delivered at 35 weeks of a healthy infant and commenced combined chemoradiation for locally advanced (stage IIIa) non–small cell lung cancer.

Therapeutic Tools

Central airway obstruction caused by benign or malignant masses can present in the pregnant patient and may require emergency management (**Fig. 3**).[43,44] The interventional bronchoscopist has an array of tools to assist in relieving the obstruction, and the tool chosen depends on the location (trachea vs main bronchi) and type (intraluminal, extraluminal, or mixed) of obstruction.[43] Modalities used in therapeutic bronchoscopy are listed in **Fig. 1** and, in practice, a combined approach is often used (eg, tumor debridement followed by airway stenting). Although some of these tools can be used safely with the flexible bronchoscope, the rigid bronchoscope and accompanying airway stabilization is often preferable and may be mandated by the clinical scenario (eg, respiratory failure, stridor).

Electrocautery and argon plasma photocoagulation (APC) are widely used in airway interventions with rare reported complications of hemorrhage, airway perforation, or airway fires (for APC). There is no published experience or evidence base for use of these therapeutic bronchoscopic interventions in pregnancy where amniotic fluid can conduct electrical current to the fetus. Data for use of electrocautery when used for sphincterotomy and hemostasis in ERCP during pregnancy would suggest that it is relatively safe.[42] Care should be taken to place the grounding pad in such a position that the uterus is not between it and the electrical catheter and bipolar electrocautery should be used to minimize this risk of stray currents going through the fetus. Laser bronchoscopy may be associated with systemic gas embolization,[45,46] and more recently life-threatening gas embolism occurring as a complication of bronchoscopic application of APC has been described.[47]

Although there are no published data on the use of these modalities, it may be appropriate to reserve their use for the pregnant patient in whom airway ablation of central stenosis is required in favor of mechanical debridement with rigid bronchoscope, forceps, and microdebrider as the preferable option initially. There is no particular contraindication to cryotherapy, which is a safe method without risk of airway perforation and minimal risk of systemic effects although its effects in the airway are delayed and the patient is subjected to the risk of repeat clear-out procedures. Other airway tumor ablative techniques with delayed effect such as photodynamic therapy and endobronchial brachytherapy are contraindicated because of unacceptable or unknown fetal risk and the presence of reasonable alternatives. Whole-lung lavage performed therapeutically for pulmonary alveolar proteinosis has been reported and seems to be safe when performed in an expert center.[48] Overall, therapeutic airway interventions are infrequently required in pregnant women and referral to expert centers is recommended.

PLEURAL DISEASE IN PREGNANCY

Pleural effusion and pneumothorax may present in pregnancy and the causes and management of the mother are generally no different from other patients with these conditions. Many pregnancy-related conditions associated with pleural effusions are particular to women of child-bearing age including gestational trophoblastic disease, ovarian hyperstimulation syndrome, and peripartum cardiomyopathy (see **Box 1**).

Small pleural effusions are commonly detected by ultrasound during pregnancy and in the immediate postpartum period and likely reflect an increase in blood volume and reduced colloid osmotic pressure during pregnancy.[49,50] In 47

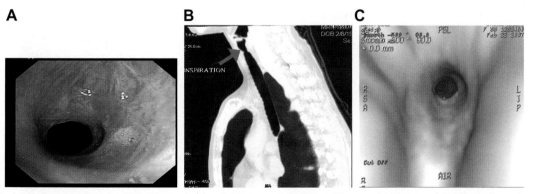

Fig. 3. Relux-associated subglottic tracheal stricture presenting in a 30-year-old woman. (*A*) Airway bronchoscopic view. (*B*) Sagittal computed tomography view with subglottic short-segment stenosis demonstrated (*arrow*). (*C*) Appearance on virtual bronchoscopy with three-dimensional computed tomography reconstruction.

healthy pregnant women, Kocijancic and colleagues[50] reported that a small layer of effusion in the costodiaphragmatic recess was visible in almost 2 out of 3 women and was bilateral in 40%. Such small effusions do not require further evaluation but in the presence of symptoms and larger effusion, further evaluation is required.

Pleural interventions offered by pulmonary procedures and indications for drainage of the pleural space are included in **Table 1**. Sampling of pleural fluid by thoracentesis is indicated in the presence of unexplained effusion (diagnostic) or in the presence of symptoms and a large effusion (therapeutic). The procedure is generally safe when performed by a competent operator and the major complication is inadvertent puncture of the abdominal viscera or the lung, resulting in pneumothorax, which occurs in up to 12% of blind thoracentesis procedures.[37]

In recent years the use of bedside ultrasound performed by the pulmonologist to evaluate suspected pleural effusion and guide thoracentesis and other pleural interventions has become standard in many institutions.[36,51] Advantages of this approach include that it is readily learnt, easy to use, portable, and allows real-time imaging (**Fig. 4**). In addition, pleural ultrasound can provide an alternate diagnosis (eg, elevated hemidiaphragm mimicking pleural effusion on chest radiograph) and does not expose the operator or patient to radiation.[52] The use of pleural ultrasound is associated with a higher sensitivity for identifying pleural fluid and reduces the dry-tap or inadequate specimen collection rate. Near misses are also avoided (eg, splenic puncture) as the rate of pneumothorax after thoracentesis is lower.[51] Ultrasound can be very informative in the

management of parapneumonic effusion; it distinguishes between simple free-flowing effusion and a complex effusion with loculations, fibrinous debris, strands, and pleural thickening, and predicts the need for surgical intervention.[53] Although the usefulness of pleural ultrasound has not been formally studied in pregnancy, these features are clearly desirable in the pregnant patient and it makes intuitive sense that ultrasound be used particularly in the last trimester when the gravid uterus enlarges and distorts normal chest anatomic landmarks.

Measurement of pleural pressure during thoracentesis by pleural manometry is easily performed and may be useful in distinguishing patients with lung entrapment from trapped lung and in minimizing the risk of reexpansion pulmonary edema when large volumes of pleural fluid are removed.[36]

Whenchest tube drainage is required for complicated pleural space infection, evidence supports the use of small drains placed over wires using the Seldinger technique as being significantly less painful to endure than larger (>24F) tubes and providing similar clinical outcomes when proper tube maintenance including regular flushing is performed.[36,54,55] The use of intrapleural fibrinolytics is of questionable benefit in assisting pleural fluid drainage but should be avoided during pregnancy; pregnancy has been considered a contraindication to enrolment in trials.[36,56] Video-assisted thoracoscopic surgery (VATS) decortication should be considered early in the course of complicated pleural empyema. It is associated with faster clinical resolution and reduced length of stay.[57]

Thoracoscopy performed under local anesthesia and procedural sedation by the

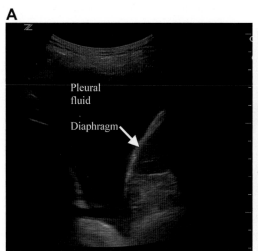
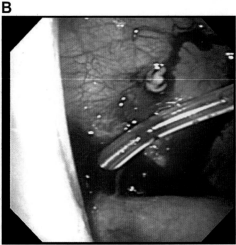

Fig. 4. Pleural effusion on transthoracic ultrasound and pleuroscopic view with chest tube in situ (*A, B*).

pulmonologist has not been reported in pregnancy.[58] This technique is used in the investigation of exudative pleural effusion and growth in medical thoracoscopy has been partially fuelled recently with the development of the semi-rigid pleuroscope. Pleuroscopy is particularly useful for guiding pleural biopsy when pleural malignancy is suspected, as the yield of cytology from the pleural fluid is low.[59] Tuberculous pleuritis, another major differential for an unexplained exudative effusion, can be most accurately assessed by this method. However, where pleuroscopy is unavailable and in countries with high prevalence of this disease, a combination of pleural fluid microbiology and biochemistry (adenosine deaminase and lymphocyte/neutrophil ratio) in addition to closed pleural biopsy has a diagnostic accuracy reaching 93%.[60] The role of the closed pleural biopsy outside this setting is declining.

PNEUMOTHORAX

Spontaneous pneumothorax may occur as a primary event in pregnant women with normal underlying lungs (primary) or in women with chronic underlying lung disease (eg, cystic fibrosis, emphysema, lymphangioleiomyomatosis). Management should follow standard protocols for drainage, which is indicated in larger symptomatic primary pneumothorax, at first by aspiration at the second intercostal space in the midclavicular line or with chest tube placement in the event of large symptomatic or secondary pneumothorax. Ultrasound is not generally useful in directing chest tube drainage in pneumothorax, however drains are usually placed high in the axilla and therefore the opportunities for tube misplacement here are limited when performed by experienced operators. Small-bore tubes are again favored over large-bore tubes as they are as effective and more tolerable for the patient.[61,62] In the presence of persistent air leak or recurrent pneumothorax in pregnancy, VATS with mechanical pleurodesis is a valid alternative to thoracotomy with pleurectomy and should not be delayed.[63,64] It can be safely performed in pregnancy as confirmed by several published series.[65,66]

Chemical pleurodesis has not been formally studied in pregnancy. Although talc may be safe, it should probably be avoided because of concerns of acute lung injury and possible systemic absorption of material, at least with the graded talc used in the United States. Other agents that are commonly used for pleurodesis in the management of malignant pleural effusion, such as bleomycin and tetracycline, should be avoided during pregnancy whenever possible because of a high likelihood of fetal risk.

Box 2
General principles of bronchoscopy in pregnancy

Flexible diagnostic bronchoscopy can be safely performed during pregnancy.

Always have a strong indication and defer bronchoscopy to the second trimester if possible.

A multidisciplinary team approach involving the obstetrician, pharmacologist, and anesthesiologist is recommended. If these are not available consider referral to a specialized center.

After midpregnancy, position pregnant patients in left pelvic tilt or left lateral position to avoid vena caval or aortic compression.

Use lowest effective dose of sedative medications, and where possible use medications with the best safety profile.

Supplemental oxygen to maintain saturations greater than 95% is suggested.

Continuous pulse oximetry and cardiac monitoring is recommended with intermittent blood pressure monitoring during the procedure. Capnography is not required routinely.

The presence of fetal heart sounds should be confirmed before sedation is begun and after the procedure but continuous fetal monitoring is not necessary in most cases in particular before the third trimester.

Minimize procedure time and abandon procedure if poorly tolerated or goals cannot be achieved.

Fluoroscopy is not recommended for transbronchial biopsy but when used, care should be taken to minimize radiation exposure to the fetus and risks to the mother.

When required, bipolar electrocautery is preferred over monopolar cautery. The grounding pad should be placed to minimize the flow of electrical current through the amniotic fluid.

Obstetric support should be available in the event of a pregnancy-related complication.

SUMMARY

Interventional pulmonary procedures encompassing bronchoscopy and pleural procedures are often indicated and have been safely performed during pregnancy. Important goals of these interventions are effective performance; maximizing maternal comfort and acceptance, and minimizing fetal risk. There have been no studies of pulmonary interventions performed in pregnancy and safety and usefulness is not known. As a consequence, when delaying the diagnostic or therapeutic intervention does not affect disease course or pregnancy outcome and does not complicate labor and delivery, procedures can be deferred until the postpartum period. Any physician who performs procedures in pregnancy should be aware of the physiologic changes that occur, the risks of the medications used for mother and fetus, and have the expertise to provide airway stabilization and manage other complications. The principles of pulmonary interventions are outlined in **Box 2**. Alternatives to bronchoscopy such as enhanced three-dimensional computed tomography reconstruction and virtual bronchoscopy should be considered but they have attendant risks of radiation exposure that need to be balanced. With the increasing number of diagnostic and therapeutic modalities on offer to the procedural pulmonologist and in the absence of studies of efficacy and safety, it is particularly important that decisions on interventions in pregnancy are taken as part of a multidisciplinary process with engagement of the radiologist, obstetrician, anesthesiologist, pharmacist, and thoracic surgeon where appropriate.

REFERENCES

1. Bolliger CT, Mathur PN, Beamis JF, et al. ERS/ATS statement on interventional pulmonology. European Respiratory Society/American Thoracic Society. Eur Respir J 2002;19(2):356–73.
2. Wahidi MM, Herth FJ, Ernst A. State of the art: interventional pulmonology. Chest 2007;131(1):261–74.
3. Ernst A, Simoff M, Ost D, et al. A multi-center, prospective, advanced diagnostic bronchoscopy outcomes registry. Chest 2010;138(1):165–70.
4. Bahhady IJ, Ernst A. Risks of and recommendations for flexible bronchoscopy in pregnancy: a review. Chest 2004;126(6):1974–81.
5. Cappell MS, Colon VJ, Sidhom OA. A study at 10 medical centers of the safety and efficacy of 48 flexible sigmoidoscopies and 8 colonoscopies during pregnancy with follow-up of fetal outcome and with comparison to control groups. Dig Dis Sci 1996; 41(12):2353–61.
6. Cappell MS, Colon VJ, Sidhom OA. A study of eight medical centers of the safety and clinical efficacy of esophagogastroduodenoscopy in 83 pregnant females with follow-up of fetal outcome with comparison control groups. Am J Gastroenterol 1996;91(2) 348–54.
7. Cappell MS. Sedation and analgesia for gastrointestinal endoscopy during pregnancy. Gastrointest Endosc Clin N Am 2006;16(1):1–31.
8. Qureshi WA, Rajan E, Adler DG, et al. ASGE guideline: guidelines for endoscopy in pregnant and lactating women. Gastrointest Endosc 2005;61(3): 357–62.
9. Mallampati SR, Gatt SP, Gugino LD, et al. A clinical sign to predict difficult tracheal intubation: a prospective study. Can Anaesth Soc J 1985; 32(4):429–34.
10. Kuczkowski KM, Reisner LS, Benumof JL. Airway problems and new solutions for the obstetric patient. J Clin Anesth 2003;15(7):552–63.
11. Rizk NW, Kalassian KG, Gilligan T, et al. Obstetric complications in pulmonary and critical care medicine. Chest 1996;110(3):791–809.
12. Pilkington S, Carli F, Dakin MJ, et al. Increase in Mallampati score during pregnancy. Br J Anaesth 1995; 74(6):638–42.
13. Bende M, Hallgarde M, Sjogren U, et al. Nasal congestion during pregnancy. Clin Otolaryngol Allied Sci 1989;14(5):385–7.
14. Toppozada H, Michaels L, Toppozada M, et al. The human respiratory nasal mucosa in pregnancy. An electron microscopic and histochemical study. J Laryngol Otol 1982;96(7):613–26.
15. Milne JA. The respiratory response to pregnancy. Postgrad Med J 1979;55(643):318–24.
16. Skatrud JB, Dempsey JA, Kaiser DG. Ventilatory response to medroxyprogesterone acetate in normal subjects: time course and mechanism. J Appl Physiol 1978;44(6):393–44.
17. Bonica JJ. Maternal respiratory changes during pregnancy and parturition. Clin Anesth 1974;10(2): 1–19.
18. Johnson SR, Tattersfield AE. Clinical experience of lymphangioleiomyomatosis in the UK. Thorax 2000; 55(12):1052–7.
19. Warren SE, Lee D, Martin V, et al. Pulmonary lymphangiomyomatosis causing bilateral pneumothorax during pregnancy. Ann Thorac Surg 1993; 55(4):998–1000.
20. Kinsella SM, Lohmann G. Supine hypotensive syndrome. Obstet Gynecol 1994;83(5 Pt 1):774–88.
21. Milne JA, Howie AD, Pack AI. Dyspnoea during normal pregnancy. Br J Obstet Gynaecol 1978; 85(4):260–3.
22. British Thoracic Society Bronchoscopy Guidelines Committee, a Subcommittee of Standards of Care Committee of British Thoracic Society. British

Thoracic Society guidelines on diagnostic flexible bronchoscopy. Thorax 2001;56(Suppl 1):i1−21.

23. Abu-Hiljeh M. Pulmonary procedures during pregnancy. In: Bourjeily G, Rosene-Montella K, editors. Respiratory medicine. New York (NY): Humana Press; 2009. p. 313.

24. Pare PD, Donevan RE, Nelems JM. Clues to unrecognized upper airway obstruction. Can Med Assoc J 1982;127(1):39−41.

25. Albertini R, Harrel JH, Moser KM. Letter: hypoxemia during fiberoptic bronchoscopy. Chest 1974;65(1): 117−8.

26. Matsushima Y, Jones RL, King EG, et al. Alterations in pulmonary mechanics and gas exchange during routine fiberoptic bronchoscopy. Chest 1984;86(2):184−8.

27. Pirozynski M, Sliwinski P, Radwan L, et al. Bronchoalveolar lavage: comparison of three commonly used procedures. Respiration 1991;58(2):72−6.

28. Gilinsky NH, Muthunayagam N. Gastrointestinal endoscopy in pregnant and lactating women: emerging standard of care to guide decision-making. Obstet Gynecol Surv 2006;61(12):791−9.

29. Iqbal MM, Sobhan T, Ryals T. Effects of commonly used benzodiazepines on the fetus, the neonate, and the nursing infant. Psychiatr Serv 2002;53(1):39−49.

30. McQuillen KK, Steele DW. Capnography during sedation/analgesia in the pediatric emergency department. Pediatr Emerg Care 2000;16(6):401−4.

31. Miner JR, Heegaard W, Plummer D. End-tidal carbon dioxide monitoring during procedural sedation. Acad Emerg Med 2002;9(4):275−80.

32. Practice guidelines for sedation and analgesia by non-anesthesiologists. A report by the American Society of Anesthesiologists Task Force on Sedation and Analgesia by Non-Anesthesiologists. Anesthesiology 1996;84(2):459−71.

33. Schwartz N, Young BK. Intrapartum fetal monitoring today. J Perinat Med 2006;34(2):99−107.

34. Wilson W, Taubert KA, Gewitz M, et al. Prevention of infective endocarditis: guidelines from the American Heart Association: a guideline from the American Heart Association Rheumatic Fever, Endocarditis, and Kawasaki Disease Committee, Council on Cardiovascular Disease in the Young, and the Council on Clinical Cardiology, Council on Cardiovascular Surgery and Anesthesia, and the Quality of Care and Outcomes Research Interdisciplinary Working Group. Circulation 2007;116(15):1736−54.

35. Gin T. Propofol during pregnancy. Acta Anaesthesiol Sin 1994;32(2):127−32.

36. Feller-Kopman D. Therapeutic thoracentesis: the role of ultrasound and pleural manometry. Curr Opin Pulm Med 2007;13(4):312−8.

37. Grogan DR, Irwin RS, Channick R, et al. Complications associated with thoracentesis. A prospective, randomized study comparing three different methods. Arch Intern Med 1990;150(4):873−7.

38. Ratnapalan S, Bona N, Chandra K, et al. Physicians' perceptions of teratogenic risk associated with radiography and CT during early pregnancy. AJR Am J Roentgenol 2004;182(5):1107−9.

39. McCollough CH, Schueler BA, Atwell TD, et al. Radiation exposure and pregnancy: when should we be concerned? Radiographics 2007;27(4):909−17.

40. Brent RL. The effect of embryonic and fetal exposure to x-ray, microwaves, and ultrasound: counseling the pregnant and nonpregnant patient about these risks. Semin Oncol 1989;16(5):347−68.

41. Anders GT, Johnson JE, Bush BA, et al. Transbronchial biopsy without fluoroscopy. A seven-year perspective. Chest 1988;94(3):557−60.

42. Tang SJ, Mayo MJ, Rodriguez-Frias E, et al. Safety and utility of ERCP during pregnancy. Gastrointest Endosc 2009;69(3 Pt 1):453−61.

43. Ernst A, Feller-Kopman D, Becker HD, et al. Central airway obstruction. Am J Respir Crit Care Med 2004; 169(12):1278−97.

44. Kuczkowski KM, Benumof JL. Subglottic tracheal stenosis in pregnancy: anaesthetic implications. Anaesth Intensive Care 2003;31(5):576−7.

45. Peachey T, Eason J, Moxham J, et al. Systemic air embolism during laser bronchoscopy. Anaesthesia 1988;43(10):872−5.

46. Tellides G, Ugurlu BS, Kim RW, et al. Pathogenesis of systemic air embolism during bronchoscopic Nd:YAG laser operations. Ann Thorac Surg 1998; 65(4):930−4.

47. Reddy C, Majid A, Michaud G, et al. Gas embolism following bronchoscopic argon plasma coagulation: a case series. Chest 2008;134(5):1066−9.

48. Jankowich MD, Wahidi MM, Feller-Kopman D. Pulmonary alveolar proteinosis diagnosed in pregnancy and managed with whole lung lavage. J Bronchol 2006;13:204−6.

49. Gourgoulianis KI, Karantanas AH, Molyvdas PA. Peripartum pleural effusion. Chest 1997;111(5): 1467−8.

50. Kocijancic I, Pusenjak S, Kocijancic K, et al. Sonographic detection of physiologic pleural fluid in normal pregnant women. J Clin Ultrasound 2005; 33(2):63−6.

51. Feller-Kopman D. Ultrasound-guided thoracentesis. Chest 2006;129(6):1709−14.

52. Diacon AH, Brutsche MH, Soler M. Accuracy of pleural puncture sites: a prospective comparison of clinical examination with ultrasound. Chest 2003; 123(2):436−41.

53. Chen KY, Liaw YS, Wang HC, et al. Sonographic septation: a useful prognostic indicator of acute thoracic empyema. J Ultrasound Med 2000;19(12):837−43.

54. Colice GL, Curtis A, Deslauriers J, et al. Medical and surgical treatment of parapneumonic effusions: an evidence-based guideline. Chest 2000;118(4): 1158−71.

55. Rahman NM, Maskell NA, Davies CW, et al. The relationship between chest tube size and clinical outcome in pleural infection. Chest 2010;137(3):536–43.

56. Maskell NA, Davies CW, Nunn AJ, et al. UK controlled trial of intrapleural streptokinase for pleural infection. N Engl J Med 2005;352(9):865–74.

57. Wait MA, Sharma S, Hohn J, et al. A randomized trial of empyema therapy. Chest 1997;111(6):1548–51.

58. Loddenkemper R. Thoracoscopy—state of the art. Eur Respir J 1998;11(1):213–21.

59. Rodriguez-Panadero F, Janssen JP, Astoul P. Thoracoscopy: general overview and place in the diagnosis and management of pleural effusion. Eur Respir J 2006;28(2):409–22.

60. Diacon AH, Van de Wal BW, Wyser C, et al. Diagnostic tools in tuberculous pleurisy: a direct comparative study. Eur Respir J 2003;22(4):589–91.

61. Baumann MH, Strange C, Heffner JE, et al. Management of spontaneous pneumothorax: an American College of Chest Physicians Delphi consensus statement. Chest 2001;119(2):590–602.

62. Horsley A, Jones L, White J, et al. Efficacy and complications of small-bore, wire-guided chest drains. Chest 2006;130(6):1857–63.

63. Chan P, Clarke P, Daniel FJ, et al. Efficacy study of video-assisted thoracoscopic surgery pleurodesis for spontaneous pneumothorax. Ann Thorac Surg 2001;71(2):452–4.

64. Mouroux J, Elkaim D, Padovani B, et al. Video-assisted thoracoscopic treatment of spontaneous pneumothorax: technique and results of one hundred cases. J Thorac Cardiovasc Surg 1996;112(2). 385–91.

65. Reid CJ, Burgin GA. Video-assisted thoracoscopic surgical pleurodesis for persistent spontaneous pneumothorax in late pregnancy. Anaesth Intensive Care 2000;28(2):208–10.

66. Sills ES, Meinecke HM, Dixson GR, et al. Management approach for recurrent spontaneous pneumothorax in consecutive pregnancies based on clinical and radiographic findings. J Cardiothorac Surg 2006;1:35.

Smoking and Smoking Cessation in Pregnancy

Susan Murin, MD, MSc[a,b],*, Rokhsara Rafii, MD, MPH[a,b], Kathryn Bilello, MD[c]

KEYWORDS

• Tobacco • Smoking • Pregnancy • Women

Smoking during pregnancy is among the leading preventable causes of adverse maternal and fetal outcomes. Because only a minority of smoking women of childbearing age manage to quit smoking when they become pregnant, smoking among young women is the primary determinant of the prevalence of smoking during pregnancy. Smoking among women of childbearing age is associated with reduced fertility, increased complications of pregnancy such as placenta previa and placental abruption, and a variety of adverse fetal outcomes such as stillbirth, low birth weight (LBW), and small for gestational age (SGA). In addition, there is increasing evidence of adverse effects on offspring including increased risk of sudden infant death syndrome (SIDS), reduced lung function, increased incidence of neurocognitive disorders, and increased risk of tobacco addiction and obesity. Pregnancy represents a unique motivation for smoking cessation, and more women quit smoking during pregnancy than at any other time in their lives. However, most women smoking at conception continue to smoke, and relapse rates after parturition are high. Guidelines for smoking cessation during pregnancy have been developed to guide health care professionals in their efforts to help women who are pregnant to cease smoking. This article reviews the epidemiology of smoking during pregnancy; the adverse effects of smoking on the mother, fetus, and offspring; and recommended approaches to smoking cessation for pregnant women.

EPIDEMIOLOGY OF SMOKING AND SMOKING CESSATION IN PREGNANCY

Smoking Among Women of Reproductive Age

Smoking among women of reproductive age has decreased in the United States. In 1965, 38% of women aged 18 to 24 years smoked, as did 44% of women aged 25 to 44 years.[1] In 2000, these percentages decreased to 25% and 23%, respectively.[1] In the past decade, smoking rates among women of reproductive age have reached a plateau. According to the 2006 Behavioral Risk Factor Surveillance System (BRFSS), 22.4% of women of reproductive age (18–44 years) were current smokers.[2] Findings from the Global Youth Tobacco Survey show an increase in smoking among young girls compared with adult women, raising the possibility that, worldwide, smoking among women of childbearing age may increase in the future.[3]

Smoking During Pregnancy: US Trends

Smoking prevalence during pregnancy is usually based on self-reported information (taken from birth certificates and questionnaires) and probably underestimates the true prevalence of smoking. Studies validating smoking status during pregnancy using cotinine measurements have shown underestimation of smoking by as much as 25%.[4] Smoking prevalence during pregnancy in the United States has fallen, and this decrease is attributable more to the overall decline in smoking

The authors have nothing to disclose.

a Division of Pulmonary, Critical Care and Sleep Medicine, UC Davis School of Medicine, 4150 V Street, Suite 3400, Sacramento, CA 95817, USA

b VA Northern California Healthcare System, CA, USA

c Department of Medicine, University of California, San Francisco-Fresno Program, 2823 Fresno Street, Fresno, CA 93721, USA

* Corresponding author. Division of Pulmonary, Critical Care and Sleep Medicine, UC Davis School of Medicine, 4150 V Street, Suite 3400, Sacramento, CA 95817.

E-mail address: susan.murin@ucdmc.ucdavis.edu

Clin Chest Med 32 (2011) 75–91
doi:10.1016/j.ccm.2010.11.004
0272-5231/11/$ — see front matter © Published by Elsevier Inc.

initiation rates among women of childbearing age than to an increased rate of smoking cessation during pregnancy. According to BRFSS data collected yearly from 1987 to 1996, the smoking initiation rate among women aged 18 to 44 years decreased significantly from 44.1% in 1987 to 38.2% in 1996.[5] In the same 10-year interval, the prevalence of current smoking also decreased significantly among both pregnant women (from 16.3% to 11.8%) and nonpregnant women (from 26.7% to 23.6%). In contrast, the percentage of women who had quit smoking changed minimally between 1987 and 1996 among both pregnant women (from 26.3% to 25.2%) and nonpregnant women (from 16.3% to 14.4%). Using data collected on birth certificates reported by 49 states and the District of Columbia, smoking during pregnancy decreased from 18.4% in 1990 to 11.4% in 2002.[6] The highest percentage of women who smoked during pregnancy was seen in Kentucky (24.4%) and the lowest in Utah (7.0%).

The most recent trends examining smoking during pregnancy used data from the Pregnancy Risk Assessment Monitoring System (PRAMS) from 31 sites covering the years 2000 to 2005.[7] These 31 sites represented approximately 54% of the live births in 2005. Based on aggregated data from 16 sites for which data were available for all 6 years, the prevalence of smoking during the 3 months before pregnancy did not change significantly (22.3% in 2000 to 21.5% in 2005). However, the prevalence of smoking during pregnancy did decrease significantly (from 15.2% in 2000 to 13.8% in 2005). There was marked spread among the sites, with prevalence of smoking during pregnancy in 2005 ranging from 35.7% in West Virginia to 5.2% in New York City.

Smoking During Pregnancy: International Trends

Most of the international information on smoking during pregnancy comes from developed countries where smoking trends parallel those seen in the United States. In Canada, cigarette smoking during pregnancy decreased from 31% in 1992[8] to 12% in 2002.[9] The prevalence of smoking during pregnancy among Danish women decreased from 22% in 1997 to 16% in 2005.[10] In Australia, the percentage of women reporting smoking during pregnancy decreased from 23% in 2001 to 20% in 2004.[11] In contrast, in Japan, where male smokers historically have outnumbered female smokers, the prevalence of smoking among women of childbearing age and among pregnant women has increased significantly. The prevalence of smoking among women in their

20s increased from 10.7% in 1994 to 19.2% in 2004[12]; the prevalence of smoking during pregnancy nearly doubled as well, going from 5.6% in 1991 to 10.0% in 2001.[13] The targeting of new markets by the tobacco industry in eastern European and Asian countries raises concern that the prevalence of smoking among young women and pregnant women in these regions will increase in the future.[14–16]

Factors Associated with Smoking During Pregnancy

Maternal smoking prevalence differs according to age, race, education, and socioeconomic status (SES). Higher smoking rates are consistently reported among younger pregnant women (adolescents and 18–24 years old). Review of yearly birth certificates from 1990 to 2002 showed that for every year from 1996 to 2001, girls and women aged 15 to 19 years had the highest percentage of smoking during pregnancy. In 2002, the percentage of maternal smokers aged 15 to 19 years (16.7%) was the same for women aged 20 to 24 years, with the highest percentage reported among women aged 18 to 19 years (18.2%). United States birth statistics from 2005 showed that 16.6% of mothers aged 15 to 19 years smoked and 18.6% of mothers aged 20 to 24 years smoked, whereas only 11.5% of mothers aged 25 to 29 years and 7.1% of mothers aged 30 to 39 years smoked during pregnancy.[17]

Although overall pregnancy-related smoking rates have decreased over time, rates among young women have increased. From 1987 to 1996, the smoking prevalence rate among pregnant 18 to 20 year olds increased from 13.4% to 15.3%.[5] The prevalence of smoking among white non-Hispanic women aged 20 to 24 years increased significantly, from 30.0% in 2000 to 32.8% in 2005.[7] In Denmark, although the overall prevalence of women who smoked during pregnancy decreased, among women younger than 20 years, the prevalence of pregnancy-related smoking increased from 37% in 1997 to 43% in 2005.[10] In Japan, the prevalence of smoking among young women in their 20s increased from 10.7% in 1994 to 19.2% in 2004, with a doubling of smoking prevalence among pregnant women seen in the same time interval.[12,13]

Race and ethnicity influence smoking rates during pregnancy. A study of trends in pregnancy-related smoking rates in the United States from 1987 to 1996 showed that white mothers smoke more than nonwhite mothers (11.9% vs 8.5% in 1996).[5] In 2005, prevalence of smoking during pregnancy was highest among Alaska Natives (36.3%) and

American Indians (20.6%) and lowest among Hispanic women (4.0%) and Asian/Pacific Islanders (5.4%).[7] Prevalence among white non-Hispanic women was 18.5% and 10.1% among black non-Hispanic women.[7]

Lower SES and lack of education have been associated with higher pregnancy-related smoking rates. In the United States, only 1.8% of mothers who completed college reported smoking during 2005 in contrast to 20.2% of mothers with less than a high school education.[17] A systematic review of 9 cohort studies of the determinants of smoking during pregnancy consistently identified lower SES and less education as risk factors for smoking during pregnancy.[18] PRAMS data from 2005 showed that, compared with nonsmokers, women who smoked during pregnancy were more likely to have 12 years of education or less, have an annual income of less than $15,000, and be enrolled in Medicaid.[7] Other factors associated with a higher likelihood of smoking during pregnancy include being unmarried, having an unplanned pregnancy, having a partner who smokes, higher nicotine addiction, early age at smoking initiation, and increased parity.[7,18–20]

Smoking Cessation During Pregnancy

In spite of the known adverse effects of smoking on fetal health, most smokers who become pregnant continue smoking, and most of those who do quit resume smoking after delivery. Cessation rates by cigarette smokers after becoming aware of their pregnancy vary according to time period and geographic region. A systematic review of 9 cohort studies from 8 European countries and Australia reported quit rates ranging from 11.5% to 48%.[18] A cross-sectional survey from Japan reported that 66.5% of women who had smoked before pregnancy quit.[21] Data reported by the BRFSS between 1987 and 1996 showed that the percentage of women who quit smoking during pregnancy remained stable at around 25% (26.3% in 1987 vs 25.2% in 1996).[5] The most recent trends in the United States do show improvement in smoking cessation rates during pregnancy, with the percentage of smokers who quit during pregnancy climbing to 45% (43.9% in 2000 vs 45.7% in 2005).[7] However, relapse rates among women who abstain from smoking during pregnancy are high, with most women resuming smoking by 6 months after parturition.[7,20–22] According to PRAMS data from 2000 to 2005, the percentage of quitters who relapsed after delivery remained in excess of 50% (50.3% in 2000 vs 51.4% in 2005).[7]

Most women smokers who successfully abstain from smoking throughout pregnancy have quit on their own shortly after discovering their pregnancy and before their first prenatal visit.[22] Factors associated with continued smoking during pregnancy versus quitting have been examined. Women who quit smoking during pregnancy are more likely to have more years of education, less poverty, be married, have a planned pregnancy, and be a first-time mother.[7,20,22,23] In the United States, Hispanic women are more likely to quit smoking during pregnancy compared with other ethnic groups.[7,23] Intensity of nicotine addiction and cohabitation with a smoker are strong determinants of continued smoking during pregnancy as well as relapse after delivery. Women who were lighter smokers, started smoking at an older age, and had smoked for fewer years at the time of conception were more likely to quit.[7,18,22,23] Partner's smoking habits play a significant role in the ability to refrain from smoking during and after pregnancy.[18–22] In a multivariate analysis of factors associated with continued smoking during pregnancy, living with a partner who smokes was associated with double the risk of smoking during pregnancy (odds ratio [OR] 2.3) compared with living with a nonsmoker.[19] In a large longitudinal cohort study of maternal smoking in the United States, women who lived with another smoker were 4 times as likely to relapse after delivery as women who did not live with another smoker.[20]

ADVERSE EFFECTS OF SMOKING ON MOTHER, FETUS, AND OFFSPRING

Since the middle of the twentieth century, researchers have been studying the adverse effects of smoking tobacco during pregnancy.[24] Smoking exerts indirect adverse effects on the fetus by altering umbilical blood flow and direct effects through placental transfer of toxins to the fetus.[25,26] Cigarette smoke is made up of more than 4000 compounds, which include a variety of harmful chemicals such as nicotine, carbon monoxide, tar, benzene, and heavy metals.[27,28] Of these chemicals, an ever-increasing body of evidence implicates nicotine as causing the most harm to the fetus.[28]

Because of its high lipid solubility, nicotine (and its main metabolite, cotinine) readily crosses the placental tissue into the fetal bloodstream.[25] When nicotine is measured in the amniotic fluid and fetal plasma, the fetus is found to have greater exposure to nicotine than the smoking mother.[25] Animal models have indicated that nicotine has neuroteratogenic effects during development, including induction of mitotic arrest, cell death, and decreased central nervous system cell number.[25] Evidence from human studies has linked fetal exposure to tobacco smoke to complications during pregnancy, adverse effects on growth, abnormal neurodevelopment (manifesting later as conduct disorders, propensity to addiction, and decreased cognitive and learning skills), as well as lasting adverse effects on the respiratory system.[25] This article highlights the adverse effects tobacco smoke has on the mother, her fetus, and residual effects in her offspring.

Delayed Conception and Infertility

Epidemiologic studies have provided evidence of a dose-related effect of smoking on conception, with a delay in conception of about 2 months.[29] Tobacco can cause DNA and chromosomal damage to human germinal cells, oocytes, and spermatozoa.[29] Chemicals in cigarette smoke also accelerate follicular depletion and reduce the number of oocytes in a dose-related fashion, which is clinically manifested by a reduction in the age of menopause by about 2 years among smokers, thus shortening the span of the woman's fertile years.[29]

A growing number of studies support the association between smoking and a delay in conception and infertility. A meta-analysis performed by Augood and colleagues[30] found a 60% increased risk of infertility among smoking women (OR 1.60, 95% confidence interval [CI] 1.34–1.91). A reduced OR of becoming pregnant was also noted for smokers in a meta-analysis of women undergoing in vitro fertilization treatment (OR 0.66, 95% CI 0.49–0.88).[30] The adverse effects of smoking on fertility seem to be reversible. Former smokers seem to have comparable rates of infertility with those who never smoked.[30]

Complications During Pregnancy

The effects of tobacco smoke become tangible and clinically apparent before the birth of the fetus. Tobacco can adversely affect the woman's ability to carry a pregnancy to term without complications.[31] In a meta-analysis performed by Castles and colleagues,[31] smoking during pregnancy was strongly associated with an increased risk for abruption of placenta, ectopic pregnancy, and preterm premature rupture of the membrane. After reviewing the data reported in 34 studies, the authors conclude that the OR among smokers for the outcomes mentioned earlier ranged from 1.6 to 1.91. The OR for preeclampsia was 0.51. The explanation for this seemingly protective finding remains unclear. Theories proposed include that the plasma volume expands less in pregnant smokers than in pregnant nonsmokers, that the thiocyanate found in tobacco smoke has a hypotensive effect, and that nicotine has an inhibitory effect on the production of fetal thromboxane A2, a potent vasoconstrictor. Nevertheless, this likely benefit is outnumbered by the risk of pregnancy-related complications that tobacco smoke presents.

The risk of stillbirths among pregnant smokers has also been investigated in the last several years. In a review of the Missouri maternally linked cohort data files spanning from 1978 to 1997, the rate of stillbirths (defined by in utero fetal death at ≥ 20 weeks) climbed with increasing tobacco use.[32] Furthermore, smoking mothers were about 50% more likely to experience intrapartum (occurrence during labor) fetal death than their nonsmoking counterparts.[32]

The same investigators also assessed the effect of prenatal smoking among women of advanced maternal age. Women were divided into 2 age groups (<35 years of age, or ≥ 35 years of age). Compared with nonsmoking younger gravidas, younger (group aged <35 years) smoking mothers had a 30% greater likelihood of stillbirth (both antepartum and intrapartum). The adjusted hazard ratios (AHR) for the smokers greater than age 35 years were 2.6 (antepartum) and 3.2 (intrapartum) compared with the younger nonsmoker referent group.[33] Thus, when adjusted for confounders, increasing age appeared to be an important modifier in the relationship between in utero fetal exposure to tobacco smoke and stillbirths, particularly intrapartum stillbirths.

An increased risk was noted in the other end of the age spectrum: adolescence. Pregnant adolescents already have an increased risk for adverse birth outcomes, including preterm birth, LBW, fetal growth restriction, late fetal death, and infant mortality.[34] After adjusting for maternal race, body mass index (BMI), prenatal care received, fetal sex, and year of birth, the investigators found the risk for intrapartum stillbirth among smoking adolescents less than 15 years of age to be twice the risk for older adolescent and mature mothers. Based on the AHR, the risk of intrapartum stillbirth among smokers decreased as maternal age increased (AHR of 4.0 for mothers <15 years of age, AHR of 1.5 for mothers aged 15–19 years, and AHR of 1.8 for mothers aged 20–24 years). These studies are in concordance with others that report an increased risk of stillbirths among smoking mothers, and point to a particular need for smoking cessation interventions at both ends of the maternal age spectrum.

LBW and SGA

In 1957, Simpson[24] reported an adverse relationship between maternal smoking and birth weight. The association between tobacco smoke exposure and infant LBW and SGA has since been confirmed in numerous studies, and has been attributed to intrauterine growth retardation rather than preterm delivery.[35–37] LBW, less than 2500 g, is one of the most reported complications of tobacco smoke in the literature. Cigarette smoking is the single most important factor affecting birth weight in developed countries.[27,36]

Women who smoke are 2 to 3 times more likely to deliver an LBW infant than their nonsmoking counterparts, with an average decrease in their baby's weight of 150 to 300 g at birth.[35,38] Smokers also have an increased risk for an SGA infant, with a relative risk ranging from 1.3 to 10.0.[1] In a recent population-based analysis among smoking and nonsmoking mothers, maternal tobacco use was an independent predictor of SGA (<10th percentile for gestational age).[39] A disproportionate increase in SGA remained when compounded with additional maternal nutritional and uteroplacental constraints such as maternal underweight and essential hypertension.[39] Studies have shown a statistically significant dose-response relationship between the number of cigarettes smoked by the mother and the risk of LBW and SGA.[1,35,40] This dose-response relationship seems to be more pronounced among older (≥30 years) mothers.[35] Both maternal and paternal smoking is associated with LBW, with maternal smoking having a greater effect.[27]

In a prospective study of the offspring of 1518 women, anthropometric measurements (including birth weight, crown-heel length, ponderal index) were less affected when women stopped smoking during their pregnancy compared with those who continued to smoke throughout pregnancy.[1,41] It is not yet fully understood at what point during pregnancy a mother can quit smoking and avoid the increased risks of LBW and SGA. Most studies have shown that those who quit in the first trimester can achieve the same lower relative risk of LBW and SGA than those who never smoked during pregnancy, whereas others show the greatest effect occurring during the third trimester.[1,38,40,42] These findings highlight the importance of continued smoking cessation interventions throughout pregnancy.

SIDS

SIDS has been linked repeatedly with maternal smoking. SIDS is one of the leading causes of death among infants 1 month to 1 year of age in the United States.[27,43] Multiple risk factors have been identified, and the incidence of SIDS declined in developed nations in the 1990s thanks to an aggressive Back to Sleep public health campaign advising parents to lay sleeping infants on their back.[27] Given the success of this intervention, maternal smoking has now become a major risk factor for SIDS.

There are many hypotheses as to the cause of SIDS and the role tobacco plays. It is believed that the immediate cause of death in SIDS is functional and affects the cardiorespiratory system.[44] One theory is that these infants have an abnormal arousal or respiratory control mechanism.[44] Additional reports reveal evidence that nicotine may affect the ventilatory response to hypoxia, that there is impairment of the peripheral autonomic nervous system, and that there is an absent adrenomedullary response to hypoxia after nicotine exposure.[44,45]

The relationship between tobacco smoke and SIDS has been reviewed extensively in the literature as well as by federal agencies and the World Health Organization.[27] In a large systematic review conducted by Anderson and Cook,[44] it was determined that maternal smoking doubles the risk of SIDS, and that the data point to a causal relationship between SIDS and postnatal exposure to tobacco smoke. A report by the National Cancer Institute/California Environmental Protection Agency concludes that, after a review of the literature, a causal relationship between maternal smoking and SIDS is implied.[46] Additional investigations have quantified smoking and found a significant dose-response relationship between smoking and SIDS, and one study found that the risk of SIDS was reduced with smoking cessation during pregnancy.[27]

Behavior and Cognitive Function

The effect of nicotine on neurotransmitters

Smoking-induced changes in utero to the fetal central nervous system may lead to the long-term development of learning, memory, and attention deficits.[25] Once nicotine has entered the fetal bloodstream, it binds to nicotinic acetylcholine receptors (nAChRs), which are present in the fetal brain as early as 4 to 5 weeks of gestation.[25] Following binding and activation by nicotine, the nAChR can influence the expression of several neurotransmitters in the peripheral and central nervous system, including acetylcholine, dopamine, norepinephrine, epinephrine, serotonin, glutamate, and γ-aminobutyric acid.[25]

Catecholamines have been implicated in drug addiction and affective disorders, behavioral and cognitive functions regulated in the prefrontal cortex, and response to stress.[25] Both increases and decreases in catecholamines have been noted in the animal offspring following nicotine exposure during gestation.[25] In humans, the effects of smoking on catecholamines during pregnancy are still being scrutinized. Amniotic fluid of smokers has been shown to contain higher levels of norepinephrine and epinephrine during the third trimester compared with nonsmokers, suggesting fetal adrenergic activation.[25] Furthermore, levels of epinephrine in the umbilical artery cord blood were found to be decreased among smokers compared with nonsmokers following birth.[47] Such alterations point to a likely sympathetic nervous system dysfunction. Further studies are needed to better understand this imbalance of neurotransmitters and their clinical relevance.

Maternal smoking during pregnancy has also been associated with an increased rate of mood and conduct disorders in the offspring.[25,48] This link has spurred an increasing interest in the effect of nicotine on the serotonin system. After being exposed prenatally to nicotine, neonatal and juvenile rats were found to have decreased serotonin turnover in certain regions of the brain.[25] At birth and in adolescence, both an increased density of serotonin transporter (SERT) and decreased density of SERT binding sites in the cortex have been reported in animals exposed to prenatal nicotine.[25] These studies propose that nicotine has long-lasting effects on the fetal neurotransmitter system, lasting even into adulthood. The myriad interactions of nicotine on the neurotransmitter systems contribute to understanding of the gross implications on fetal development that seem to extend into adulthood.

Attention-deficit disorder/hyperactivity

The effect of prenatal and postnatal tobacco smoke on behavioral and cognitive functions has been reported increasingly in the past 2 decades. Studies of children whose mothers smoked during pregnancy have repeatedly shown an increased rate of behavior problems compared with children of nonsmoking mothers.[27,28] Weitzman and colleagues[49] investigated the possible association between maternal smoking and behavioral problems among 2256 children aged 4 to 11 years. They found that maternal smoking (prenatal, postnatal, and combined) had an independent association with an increase in behavioral problems (eg, anxiety, depression, antisocial behavior, and hyperactivity). In addition, smoking a pack or more per day was independently associated with a twofold increase in extreme behavior problem scores compared with children of mothers who did not smoke.[49]

Fergusson and colleagues[50] set out to replicate these findings while controlling for confounders believed to be limitations in the study by Weitzman and colleagues.[49] Using longitudinal data, they assessed the relationship between maternal smoking and conduct and attention-deficit disorders on a cohort of 1265 children in New Zealand. Overall, they concluded that smoking during pregnancy increases the risk of conduct and attention-deficit disorders among the offspring with a greater significant association for smoking during, rather than after, pregnancy. Reports have continued to be published, including a systematic analysis of 24 studies of children born to mothers who smoked prenatally, with findings consistent with an increased risk of attention-deficit hyperactivity disorder–related disorders.[51] Because of methodological limitations and variations among the literature, further studies are needed to fully understand the relationship between perinatal tobacco exposure and behavioral disorders among offspring.

Cognitive impairments

Studies on cognitive development among children exposed to tobacco smoke perinatally are conflicting because confounders in this area of research are particularly difficult to control for. Women who smoke during pregnancy tend be of lower SES, and differ in other health-related behaviors, personality, and childrearing approaches.[52]

Among studies that attempted to control for potential confounders, several have found a dose-dependent relationship.[53–55] In a prospective follow-up study of 400 families in upstate New York, Olds and colleagues[56] found a decline in Stanford-Binet scores of 4.35 points among 3- and 4-year-old children of smokers compared with those of nonsmokers. This finding was assessed after controlling for confounders such as social class, maternal education and intelligence quotient (IQ), and qualities of caregiving.[56] Conversely, Fergusson and Lloyd[57] found that, after controlling for SES and features of home environment, intellectual differences among 8 and 10 year olds were lost when comparing those exposed to prenatal tobacco with those who were not.[57] Differences in study methodology as well as in age of the children studied may account for the different findings. In a recent cohort analysis performed by Lundberg and colleagues,[58] sons of smoking mothers had an increased risk of poor intellectual performance compared with sons of nonsmoking mothers. However, this finding was lost once familial factors such as birth order and maternal age were controlled for. Thus, further research is needed in this field to better understand the role pre- and postnatal tobacco smoke plays in the cognitive and intellectual performance among offspring.

Addiction: use of tobacco among offspring

When adolescent rats are given the opportunity, those exposed prenatally to nicotine will self-administer larger amounts than rats that were not exposed to nicotine.[28] Results from human analyses indicate that prenatal tobacco smoke is associated with a higher likelihood of offspring smoking later in life.

In a retrospective study of 2 cohorts conducted by Kandel and colleagues,[59] prenatal smoking increased the odds of smoking among daughters fourfold. Cornelius and colleagues[60] studied a cohort of 589 10 year olds who were followed since their gestation. Offspring who were exposed to greater than half a pack per day were 5.5 times more likely to have experimented with smoking tobacco. In a 30-year prospective study (sample size 1248), Buka and colleagues[61] evaluated the link between prenatal tobacco smoke and smoking among the offspring. When adjusted for SES, maternal age at pregnancy, offspring gender, and age at time of interview, the investigators report a twofold statistically significant increase between mothers who smoked 1 pack or more per day during pregnancy and offspring nicotine dependence.

There are several proposed mechanisms to support the association between prenatal tobacco use and the predilection for tobacco use among the offspring. One such hypothesis is that in utero nicotine exposure causes embryologic changes that lead to an increase in the number of nicotine receptors, which may increase susceptibility for tobacco use later in life.[60] Another mechanism is that the association can be the result of the disruption that nicotine exposure causes on fetal brain development. Nicotine receptors (which are present early in fetal development), are stimulated and thus upregulated by nicotine.[45] This upregulation causes a premature switch from cell replication to differentiation, and the changes this leads to in fetal brain development can have lasting behavioral effects that become evident later in life. There is also the possibility that mothers who smoke may pass on a genetic predisposition to their offspring.[61]

Prenatal Smoking and Child Overweight

Recent research indicates that prenatal smoking is associated with overweight and obesity among offspring later in life. The strength of this relationship, as well as the effect of confounders such as maternal weight and social differences, still need to be better understood.

Oken and colleagues[62] studied the association of perinatal tobacco smoke and child overweight in a prospective cohort study. Women of singleton birth in Massachusetts were enrolled at gestational age less than 22 weeks, and were interviewed during prenatal care visits, at delivery, and at 6 months and 3 years after parturition. Both BMI and various skinfold measurements were obtained, and potential confounders such as maternal education, race/ethnicity, income, and child diet were adjusted for. Maternal early pregnancy smoking (smoking during the 3 months before learning of pregnancy) was strongly associated with offspring being overweight by age 3 years, with an adjusted OR for overweight of 2.2 compared with those of mothers who never smoked. In addition, children of mothers who had quit smoking before pregnancy were not more overweight compared with children of never smokers (OR of 1.0). The small sample size of women who smoked past their first trimester did not allow for multivariable analysis of exposure.[62]

Some of the same investigators conducted a meta-analysis of the existing literature to better understand the link between prenatal tobacco exposure and childhood adiposity.[63] Fourteen studies were ultimately eligible, included 84,563 children, and represented pregnancies from 1958 to 2002 among low- and non–low-income populations residing in North America, Europe, and Australia. Children of mothers who smoked during pregnancy were at increased risk for being overweight (adjusted OR 1.5) compared with children of those who did not smoke during pregnancy. Most studies adjusted for maternal weight, fetal growth, and SES. Among studies that included quantitative measurements of prenatal tobacco smoke, a dose-response relationship was consistently evident. Furthermore, in several studies, smoking throughout pregnancy was associated with a greater risk for child overweight than smoking only during early pregnancy.[63] Thus, despite a wide range of populations and after adjusting for certain confounders, the literature suggests that exposure to prenatal tobacco smoke increases the risk for childhood overweight.

To date, the association between prenatal tobacco exposure and offspring overweight is not fully understood. A hypothesized mechanism is that fetal exposure to nicotine leads to changes in the catecholaminergic system associated with the brain's reward system, or that nicotine directly affects the hypothalamic centers that direct appetite and eating behavior.[45,62,64] A better understanding of the relationship between prenatal tobacco exposure and overweight in children can offer valuable insight into the fight against the current childhood obesity epidemic.

Respiratory Illness and Lung Function in Offspring

Studies have shown an increase in respiratory illnesses among infants and children of smoking mothers. The effects of prenatal nicotine exposure have been studied in both animal models and humans. In a national British study of 12,743 children, Taylor and Wadsworth[65] found a significant increase in bronchitis and hospital admissions for lower respiratory tract illnesses in the first 5 years of life among those born to mothers who smoked during pregnancy. Smoking after birth did not influence the rate of hospital admissions for respiratory illnesses, thus suggesting a significant prenatal effect on outcome. Other studies have had similar findings, with prenatal (and not postnatal) exposure to nicotine being associated with increased number of respiratory illnesses among the offspring.[66]

There is also some evidence that maternal smoking increases the risk of childhood asthma. In a population-based cohort study, 58,842 singleton births were followed by means of registries from birth until the age of 7 years.[67] The primary outcome was asthma, and adjustments were made for gender, birth order, maternal age, marital status, and maternal occupation (used as an indicator for SES). Maternal smoking increased the risk of asthma, with an adjusted OR of 1.23 for light (<10 cigarettes per day) and 1.35 for heavy (>10 cigarettes per day) smoking.[67]

Evidence also shows a correlation between perinatal tobacco smoke and decreased lung function among infants as well as among school-age children. Hanrahan and colleagues[68] showed that infants whose mothers smoked during pregnancy had decreased functional flow rates at functional residual capacity compared with those whose mothers did not smoke during pregnancy. Cunningham and colleagues[69] furthered this assessment by comparing spirometry results among children age 8 to 12 years whose mothers did not smoke during or after pregnancy, smoked during pregnancy and not after, smoked during and after pregnancy, and did not smoke during pregnancy but did so later. After adjusting for certain confounders, the investigators found that children whose mothers smoked during pregnancy had slight but statistically significant deficits, the largest of which were a 5.2% decrease in forced expiratory flow at 25% to 75% and 6.8% in forced expiratory flow at 65% to 75%. The spirometry values among children whose mothers smoked only after pregnancy were not significantly different from those of nonsmokers. Thus, it seems that there is not only an association

with prenatal smoking and decreased lung function among offspring, but that this may have a lasting effect, at least until early adolescence.

In animal models, the neonatal lung manifests maternal nicotine exposure by hypoplasia, decreased elastin in the parenchyma, and increased alveolar volume, which suggests emphysemalike changes.[70] Nicotine receptors are present in bronchial smooth muscle, submucosal glands, bronchial epithelial cells, and vascular endothelial cells. Work by Sekhon and colleagues[66] showed that maternal nicotine exposure greatly increases α-7 nACHR subunit expression in airway epithelial cells, increases collagen gene expression and collagen staining in airway and alveolar walls, and increases type II cells in newborn rhesus monkeys. Nicotine may therefore directly stimulate α-7 nACHR–bearing fibroblasts to lay down an increased amount of connective tissue, leading to increased airway wall thickness.

Sekhon and colleagues[71] were able to identify an increase in collagen mRNA and protein expression following nicotine exposure throughout the lung. The investigators propose that this accumulation of excess collagen may play an important role in the decrease in fixed lung volume found in the nicotine-exposed neonatal lung. Furthermore, increased collagen content may also explain the decrease in functional residual capacity and decrease in lung compliance found in infants subjected to prenatal tobacco exposure.[71] The collagen accumulation and airway wall dimensions discovered by the investigators were more prominent in the peripheral rather than central airways. Because changes in peripheral airways produce greater alterations in airway resistance and maximum expiratory flow rates than those in central airways, this provides insight into why the spirometry measurements discussed earlier among children exposed to tobacco prenatally were decreased compared with their non–nicotine-exposed cohorts.[71]

SMOKING CESSATION AND PREGNANCY

Given the well-documented adverse effects of smoking during pregnancy, efforts to reduce the prevalence of smoking among pregnant women are critically important. Women are uniquely motivated to quit during pregnancy; they are more likely to quit during pregnancy than at any other point in their lives.[1] However, tobacco addiction is a chronic disorder, and most women smoking when they become pregnant continue to smoke. The United States Public Health Service has estimated that if all women ceased smoking during pregnancy, the cumulative benefits would be

Box 1
Components of the 5 A's approach

1. Ask. All pregnant women should be questioned about smoking status at each visit. Because of the stigma against smoking in pregnancy, there is greater risk of deception about smoking behavior in this population.[78,79] A more nuanced approach, using multiple-choice questions about smoking rather than Yes/No questions, has been shown to increase disclosure, and is recommended.[74] An example of appropriate multiple-choice questions is provided in **Box 2**.
2. Advise. Women who smoke should be given clear, strong, direct, and personalized advice to cease smoking, emphasizing the potential benefits to mother and fetus. Self-help materials (discussed later) should be offered. The combination of brief counseling and simple self-help materials increase quit rates by 30% to 70% compared with simple advice to quit.[77]
3. Assess. Smokers' readiness to quit smoking should be assessed at each prenatal visit. It is suggested that this be framed as readiness to quit within the next 30 days. If yes, assistance with cessation should be provided (see #4). For those patients who are not yet ready to quit, nonjudgmental encouragement should be provided, and obstacles to cessation identified and, if possible, addressed. Motivational interviewing may be helpful in moving patients toward cessation readiness.
4. Assist. Patients who express a willingness to quit should be encouraged to set a quit date and counseled about strategies for a successful quit attempt. Although even minimal counseling has been shown to improve quit rates, more extensive counseling is superior and the USDHHS PHS guidelines recommend that more than minimal counseling be provided to pregnant women. As part of the counseling intervention, women should be encouraged to review past quit attempts to identify and remedy reasons why they may not have been successful, and to anticipate challenges and identify strategies for coping with them. Specific concerns raised by patients about the quitting process should be addressed, and patients should be encouraged to seek social support for their quit attempt from family, friends, and others. Self-help materials should be provided, and the patient directed to other available resources that might help in the quit attempt (additional individual or group counseling, cognitive behavioral therapy, quit helplines).
5. Arrange. Follow-up visits to assess and support the cessation effort should be arranged.

Box 2
An example of appropriate multiple-choice questions about smoking status

Which of the following best describes your cigarette smoking?

- I smoke regularly now, about the same as before finding out I was pregnant
- I smoke regularly now, but have cut down since I found out I was pregnant
- I smoke every once in a while
- I have quit smoking since finding out I was pregnant
- I was not smoking around the time I found out I was pregnant, and I do not currently smoke cigarettes[74]

substantial, with an 11% reduction in stillbirths and a 5% reduction in newborn deaths.[72] Although most women who quit during pregnancy resume smoking after delivery, some do remain abstinent. Pregnancy thus provides a window of opportunity for smoking cessation that should be maximally exploited by health care workers.

Tobacco dependence is considered a chronic but treatable condition. Cessation is difficult but achievable, and smoking cessation interventions in pregnancy have been shown to reduce the proportion of women who continue to smoke and to reduce the complications associated with smoking.[73] Extensive, evidence-based, well-referenced guidelines for smoking cessation have been published and are readily available.[74,75] Although most recommendations are applicable to all smoking patients, pregnant women are considered a special population for which there is some variation from standard recommendations, chiefly concerning the role of pharmacotherapy in cessation efforts. Recommendations specifically tailored to the pregnant smoker are included in the United States Department of Health and Human Services (USDHHS) Public Health Service (PHS) Clinical Practice Guideline *Treating Tobacco Use and Dependence: 2008 Update*,[74] as well as in a Committee Opinion of the American College of Obstetricians and Gynecologists.[75] A brief overview of smoking cessation during pregnancy, largely drawn from these sources, is provided later.

Timing of Cessation

Smoking cessation before conception is ideal. Quitting before pregnancy offers the greatest potential benefits to mother and fetus, and also presents the broadest range of cessation options because there are no concerns about the potential adverse effects to the fetus of including medications in the cessation

Table 1
Key features of the published randomized clinical trials of efficacy and safety of NRT use during pregnancy

Study	Year Published	Design	Subjects	Intervention	Outcomes	Chemical Confirmation?	Results	Comments
Wisborg et al[89]	2000	RCT, single blind, placebo controlled	Pregnant, smoking ≥10 cigarettes/d after first trimester	Patch (N = 124) vs placebo patch (N = 126). All subjects received counseling	Continuous abstinence, abstinence at various visits, birth weight, gestational age	Salivary cotinine	Continuous abstinence 21% in NRT vs 19% in placebo group. No significant differences in other endpoints	Compliance very low in both groups. Abstinence lower in both groups than in patients not enrolled in trial
Kapur et al[84]	2001	RCT, double-blind, placebo controlled	Pregnant, smoking ≥15 cigarettes/d	Patch (N = 17) vs placebo patch (N = 13)	Cessation rate, time point unclear	Serum and salivary cotinine	23.5% cessation vs 0% but P = .11	Study underpowered
Hegaard et al[86]	2003	Prospective, randomized by birth dates	Pregnant, daily smokers	Intervention with multimodal program (individual counseling and invitation to cessation group with option of nicotine patch and/or gum) (N = 327) vs usual care (N = 320)	Self-reported cessation rate and combined self-reported cessation plus low salivary cotinine	Salivary cotinine	Cessation with low cotinine 7% in intervention vs 2.2% in control group (P = .004). No significant differences in birth weight	Only 75 of 327 women in intervention arm elected to receive NRT

Hotham et al[90]	2006	Prospective, randomized pilot study	Pregnant, smoking ≥15 cigarettes/d	Counseling plus nicotine free patch (N = 20) vs counseling only (N = 20)	Abstinence at delivery	Exhaled carbon monoxide and salivary cotinine	15% vs 0% cessation; 35% vs 25% had a reduction in cotinine level from baseline	Low compliance with treatment. No patients had cotinine levels on patch that were higher than baseline
Pollak et al[87]	2007	Prospective, randomized, open label	Pregnant, smoking >5 cigarettes/d	CBT plus NRT (patch, gum, or lozenge) N = 122 vs CBT alone (N = 59)	7-day point prevalence self-reported, chemically confirmed abstinence at various time points	Exhaled carbon monoxide and salivary cotinine	18% vs 7% abstinent at 38 wk gestation (P = .04) but no difference 3 mo after parturition	Study terminated prematurely caused by/because of higher rate of adverse birth outcomes in treatment arm
Oncken et al[88]	2008	Prospective, randomized, placebo controlled, single blind	Pregnant, smoking ≥1 cigarettes/d	Nicotine gum (N = 100) vs placebo (N = 94). All subjects received brief counseling	7-day point prevalence self-reported, chemically confirmed abstinence; birth weight, others	Exhaled carbon monoxide and urinary cotinine; other tobacco alkaloids	Study terminated early because of lack of efficacy. 18% vs 14.9% abstinent at 34 wk gestation (P = .56)	Statistically significant increases in birth weight and gestational age in NRT group

Abbreviations: CBT, cognitive behavioral therapy; RCT, randomized controlled trial.

effort. Women of childbearing age, particularly those who are contemplating pregnancy, should be encouraged to quit, and offered assistance with doing so. Although for smoking cessation during pregnancy the adage "the sooner the better" applies, quitting at any time during pregnancy is better than not quitting at all. Even quitting later in pregnancy is associated with a reduction in complications, especially LBW.[76]

Approach to Smoking Cessation

The 5 A's approach to smoking cessation is broadly endorsed. The 5 A's approach has been adapted for pregnant women.[75,77] The components of this approach are detailed in **Box 1**; **Box 2**.

Self-help Materials

Self-help materials are materials that can be used alone. The most common self-help materials are written materials such as booklets, but videos, computer-based interventions, audiocassettes, and recorded telephone messages are also in this category. Although self-help materials are generally considered only marginally effective in aiding smoking cessation, a 2008 systematic review and meta-analysis of self-help materials for smoking cessation in pregnancy found that they were associated with a pooled ratio of 1.834 for cessation in this population.[80] Self-help materials that are tailored to pregnancy have been shown to be associated with a significantly higher quit rate than general materials.[81] Materials may also be tailored to the patient's age group, educational level, or cultural group. There is no evidence that self-help materials of greater intensity are associated with higher quit rates than lower intensity interventions.[80]

Counseling

A variety of psychosocial interventions to support smoking cessation have been studied, including informational counseling, cognitive behavior therapy (intended to identify and modify faulty or distorted negative thinking styles and the maladaptive behaviors associated with those thinking styles), and motivational interviewing (a question-and-answer method of interviewing intended to increase the patient's motivation to change). The themes that emerge from this literature are that trained counselors are more effective than untrained counselors, heavier smokers seem to be more resistant to the effects of counseling and other interventions than are lighter smokers, and that counseling of any extent is more effective than usual care, usually defined as simple advice to quit and brief (<3 minutes) counseling.

The USDHHS guidelines recommend that "…because of the serious risks of smoking to the pregnant smoker and the fetus, whenever possible pregnant smokers should be offered person-to-person psychosocial interventions that exceed minimal advice to quit."[74] No specific counseling approach is recommended, and it is not clear that, once counseling is more than minimal, additional benefit is derived from more intensive interventions.

Pharmacologic Therapies

Among nonpregnant smokers, the efficacy of nicotine replacement therapy (NRT) and other pharmacotherapies is well established and pharmacotherapy is recommended as part of usual care. However, pharmacotherapy as an aid for smoking cessation during pregnancy remains controversial; the evidence base to guide decision making in this area is minimal, and neither safety nor efficacy has been proved. There are numerous concerns about NRT during pregnancy. Because nicotine is considered to be the primary agent of the injurious effects of smoking on the fetus, prescribing nicotine carries risk of the same adverse outcomes as smoking, including congenital malformations, LBW, and preterm delivery. It is unknown whether the different pharmacokinetics of constant-rate nicotine delivery, such as from the nicotine patch, carry different risks of harm than the intermittent dosing that results from smoking and intermittent forms of NRT (gum, lozenge, inhaler, nasal spray). Theoretically, during a period of NRT, the fetus could be exposed to higher levels of nicotine than from smoking if the dose used for replacement therapy exceeded that obtained from smoking, or if active smoking continued during NRT. However, in those trials that have monitored baseline cotinine levels and cotinine levels on NRT, this has not been the case. Although guidelines have suggested that practitioners consider monitoring blood nicotine levels in pregnant women prescribed NRT,[82] this is not common practice.

One potential benefit to NRT is allowing the fetus a more gradual withdrawal from nicotine than might occur with abrupt smoking cessation, which may cause physiologic stress to the fetus.[83,84] This topic of NRT during pregnancy was recently and comprehensively reviewed.[85] To date, there have been only 6 published randomized clinical trials of efficacy and safety of NRT use during pregnancy. Key features of these trials are summarized in **Table 1** and several are discussed here in greater detail.

The largest study to date was that of Hegaard and colleagues.[86] This prospective quasi-randomized, unblinded study compared intervention (individual counseling plus invitation to join a cessation program with optional NRT) versus usual care (standard counseling). The study showed a substantial benefit to intervention compared with usual care, with an OR for cessation of 4.2 in the intervention group. Cotinine validated cessation rates were 7% in the intervention group and 2% in the control group. Low caffeine consumption, years of education, lack of exposure to passive smoking outside the home, and previous quit attempts were positively associated with cessation. However, only a minority of women in the intervention arm (87 of 327) elected to participate in the intensive smoking cessation program. Of those who did, 75 (86%) used NRT as either patch, gum, or patch plus gum. Their self-reported cessation rate was 14.4% versus 5% in the control group, and the outcome of self-reported cessation plus cotinine less than 30 ng/ml was also significantly better for intervention versus control patients (7% vs 2.2%). There was no difference in birth outcomes. Although this study supports the efficacy of a multimodal intervention including NRT to promote cessation among pregnant smokers, it also indicates a lack of enthusiasm for such therapy among pregnant smokers.

A large, open-label randomized trial comparing cognitive behavioral therapy plus NRT (patch, gum, or lozenge) with cognitive behavioral therapy alone found a nearly threefold increase in biochemically validated smoking cessation at multiple time points.[87] However, study recruitment was suspended because interim analysis found a higher rate of negative birth outcomes (prematurity, neonatal intensive care unit admission, SGA, abruption, fetal demise) in the NRT arm. However, randomization in the groups resulted in a much higher proportion of women with a history of previous preterm birth in the NRT arm (32% vs 12%), which may have contributed to this difference in outcome. The benefit of the pharmacologic intervention in this study did not persist after parturition. Cotinine levels were measured and were higher in women with adverse fetal outcomes than in those without, and lower in those on NRT than in continued smokers.

Most recently, a randomized, double blind, placebo-controlled study of NRT (nicotine gum) versus placebo was performed. Subjects had to be smoking only 1 cigarette per day at enrollment, although the average was 18/d. All subjects received individualized counseling. Compliance was low in both groups, with an average of only ~3 pieces of gum used per day per subject. The study terminated early because of lack of efficacy

at interim analysis; biochemically confirmed abstinence rates were not significantly different for NRT versus usual care groups, 18% versus 14.9% abstinent at 34 weeks' gestation (*P* = .56). However, birth weights and gestational age were both greater with NRT than placebo.[88]

Cumulatively, the trials of NRT in pregnancy show that quit rates are low among women still smoking at the end of the first trimester whether or not intervention is offered, that pregnant women are not eager to use NRT during pregnancy, and that there are substantial difficulties inherent in intervention studies in pregnant women.

Without definitive evidence on which to base recommendations, current guidelines are based on expert opinion and call for judgment on the part of the treating clinician. The USDHHS guidelines state: "Although the use of NRT exposes pregnant women to nicotine, smoking exposes them to nicotine plus numerous other chemicals that are injurious to the woman and fetus. These concerns must be considered in the context of inconclusive evidence that cessation medications boost abstinence rates in pregnant smokers." The American College of Obstetricians and Gynecologists (ACOG) recommends that NRT should be used only when the potential benefits outweigh the unknown risks.[75]

The safety and efficacy of other pharmacotherapies for smoking cessation are unknown. ACOG suggests that bupropion may be considered during pregnancy and lactation when nonpharmacologic therapies fail,[75] and the USDHHS guidelines state that "Bupropion SR should be used during pregnancy only if the increased likelihood of smoking abstinence, with its potential benefits, outweighs the risk of bupropion SR treatment and potential concomitant smoking."[74]

SUMMARY

Smoking during pregnancy is a leading cause of adverse maternal and fetal outcomes and causes a variety of lasting ill effects in offspring. Most women who are smoking at conception continue to smoke during pregnancy. Although fewer women now smoke during pregnancy than during past decades, most of this gain has been caused by reduced smoking prevalence among young women rather than improved rates of cessation among pregnant women, and troubling trends in smoking among youth suggest that smoking during pregnancy will continue to be a major public health issue. Smoking during pregnancy is most prevalent among young, uneducated women, and partner smoking is a major risk factor for both smoking during pregnancy and resuming smoking afterward among those who have quit. All pregnant women should be assessed for smoking status, advised to quit, and offered assistance in doing so at all prenatal visits. Counseling and self-help materials are the cornerstones of cessation, and the role of NRT and other pharmacologic approaches in cessation remains unclear. Further research is needed into optimal approaches to smoking cessation for pregnant women to reduce the myriad adverse effects of smoking during pregnancy on mother, fetus, and offspring, and for relapse prevention for those women who do manage to quit smoking during pregnancy.

REFERENCES

1. Women and smoking: a report of the surgeon general. Washington, DC: US Department of Health and Human Services, Public Health Service; 2001.
2. Centers for Disease Control and Prevention (CDC). Smoking prevalence among women of reproductive age—United States, 2006. MMWR Morb Mortal Wkly Rep 2008;57(31):849—52.
3. Warren CW, Jones NR, Peruga A, et al. Global youth tobacco surveillance, 2000—2007. MMWR Surveill Summ 2008;57(1):1—28.
4. Shipton D, Tappin DM, Vadiveloo T, et al. Reliability of self reported smoking status by pregnant women for estimating smoking prevalence: a retrospective, cross sectional study. BMJ 2009;339:b4347.
5. Ebrahim SH, Floyd RL, Merritt RK 2nd, et al. Trends in pregnancy-related smoking rates in the United States, 1987—1996. JAMA 2000;283(3):361—6.
6. Centers for Disease Control and Prevention (CDC). Smoking during pregnancy—United States, 1990—2002. MMWR Morb Mortal Wkly Rep 2004; 53(39):911—5.
7. Tong VT, Jones JR, Dietz PM, et al. Trends in smoking before, during, and after pregnancy - Pregnancy Risk Assessment Monitoring System (PRAMS), United States, 31 sites, 2000—2005. MMWR Surveill Summ 2009;58(4):1—29.
8. Dodds L. Prevalence of smoking among pregnant women in Nova Scotia from 1988 to 1992. CMAJ 1995;152(2):185—90.
9. Chan B, Einarson A, Koren G. Effectiveness of bupropion for smoking cessation during pregnancy. J Addict Dis 2005;24(2):19—23.
10. Jensen DM, Korsholm L, Ovesen P, et al. Adverse pregnancy outcome in women with mild glucose intolerance: is there a clinically meaningful threshold value for glucose? Acta Obstet Gynecol Scand 2008;87(1):59—62.
11. Laws P, Hilder L. Australia's mothers and babies 2006. Perinatal statistics series no. 22. Sydney (Australia): AIHW National Perinatal Statistics Unit: 2006; 2008. PER 46.
12. Annual Report of the National Nutrition Survey Japan. Tokyo: Ministry of Health, Labour and Welfare; 2003.
13. Surveys on the growth of infants and preschool children Japan. Tokyo: Ministry of Health, Labour and Welfare; 2000.
14. Some like it "light." Women and smoking in the European Union. Brussels (Belgium): European Network for Smoking Prevention; 1999.
15. WHO framework convention on tobacco control. 205. Geneva (Switzerland): WHO; 2003.
16. Warren CW, Jones NR, Eriksen MP, et al. Patterns of global tobacco use in young people and implications for future chronic disease burden in adults. Lancet 2006;367(9512):749—53.
17. Martin JA, Hamilton BE, Sutton PD, et al. Births: final data for 2005. Natl Vital Stat Rep 2007;56(6):1—103.
18. Lu Y, Tong S, Oldenburg B. Determinants of smoking and cessation during and after pregnancy. Health Promot Int 2001;16(4):355—65.
19. Penn G, Owen L. Factors associated with continued smoking during pregnancy: analysis of sociodemographic, pregnancy and smoking-related factors. Drug Alcohol Rev 2002;21(1):17—25.
20. Kahn RS, Certain L, Whitaker RC. A reexamination of smoking before, during, and after pregnancy. Am J Public Health 2002;92(11):1801—8.
21. Kaneko A, Kaneita Y, Yokoyama E, et al. Smoking trends before, during, and after pregnancy among women and their spouses. Pediatr Int 2008;50(3): 367—75.
22. Solomon L, Quinn V. Spontaneous quitting: self-initiated smoking cessation in early pregnancy. Nicotine Tob Res 2004;6(Suppl 2):S203—16.
23. Yu SM, Park CH, Schwalberg RH. Factors associated with smoking cessation among U.S. pregnant women. Matern Child Health J 2002;6(2):89—97.
24. Simpson WJ. A preliminary report on cigarette smoking and the incidence of prematurity. Am J Obstet Gynecol 1957;73(4):807—15.
25. Shea AK, Steiner M. Cigarette smoking during pregnancy. Nicotine Tob Res 2008;10(2):267—78.
26. Albuquerque CA, Smith KR, Johnson C, et al. Influence of maternal tobacco smoking during pregnancy on uterine, umbilical and fetal cerebral artery blood flows. Early Hum Dev 2004;80(1):31—42.
27. DiFranza JR, Aligne CA, Weitzman M. Prenatal and postnatal environmental tobacco smoke exposure and children's health. Pediatrics 2004;113(Suppl 4): 1007—15.
28. Blood-Siegfried J, Rende EK. The long-term effects of prenatal nicotine exposure on neurologic development. J Midwifery Womens Health 2010;55(2): 143—52.
29. Zenzes MT. Smoking and reproduction: gene damage to human gametes and embryos. Hum Reprod Update 2000;6(2):122—31.

30. Augood C, Duckitt K, Templeton AA. Smoking and female infertility: a systematic review and meta-analysis. Hum Reprod 1998;13(6):1532–9.

31. Castles A, Adams EK, Melvin CL, et al. Effects of smoking during pregnancy. Five meta-analyses. Am J Prev Med 1999;16(3):208–15.

32. Aliyu MH, Salihu HM, Wilson RE, et al. Prenatal smoking and risk of intrapartum stillbirth. Arch Environ Occup Health 2007;62(2):87–92.

33. Aliyu MH, Salihu HM, Wilson RE, et al. The risk of intrapartum stillbirth among smokers of advanced maternal age. Arch Gynecol Obstet 2008;278(1): 39–45.

34. Aliyu MH, Salihu HM, Alio AP, et al. Prenatal smoking among adolescents and risk of fetal demise before and during labor. J Pediatr Adolesc Gynecol 2010; 23:129–35.

35. Windham GC, Hopkins B, Fenster L, et al. Prenatal active or passive tobacco smoke exposure and the risk of preterm delivery or low birth weight. Epidemiology 2000;11(4):427–33.

36. Kramer MS. Determinants of low birth weight: methodological assessment and meta-analysis. Bull World Health Organ 1987;65(5):663.

37. Kramer MS. Socioeconomic determinants of intrauterine growth retardation. Eur J Clin Nutr 1998;52-(Suppl 1):S29–32 [discussion: S32–3].

38. Vardavas CI, Chatzi L, Patelarou E, et al. Smoking and smoking cessation during early pregnancy and its effect on adverse pregnancy outcomes and fetal growth. Eur J Pediatr 2010;169(6):741–8.

39. Aagaard-Tillery KM, Porter TF, Lane RH, et al. In utero tobacco exposure is associated with modified effects of maternal factors on fetal growth. Am J Obstet Gynecol 2008;198(1):66, e61–6.

40. Lieberman E, Gremy I, Lang JM, et al. Low birthweight at term and the timing of fetal exposure to maternal smoking. Am J Public Health 1994;84(7): 1127–31.

41. Cliver SP, Goldenberg RL, Cutter GR, et al. The effect of cigarette smoking on neonatal anthropometric measurements. Obstet Gynecol 1995;85(4): 625–30.

42. Polakowski LL, Akinbami LJ, Mendola P. Prenratal smoking cessation and the risk of delivering preterm and small-for-gestational-age newborns. Obstet Gynecol 2009;114(2 Pt 1):318–25.

43. Martin JA, Kung HC, Mathews TJ, et al. Annual summary of vital statistics: 2006. Pediatrics 2008; 121(4):788–801.

44. Anderson HR, Cook DG. Passive smoking and sudden infant death syndrome: review of the epidemiological evidence. Thorax 1997;52(11): 1003–9.

45. Slotkin TA. Fetal nicotine or cocaine exposure: which one is worse? J Pharmacol Exp Ther 1998;285(3): 931–45.

46. California Environmental Protection Agency, National Cancer Institute (US). Health effects of exposure to environmental tobacco smoke: the report of the California Environmental Protection Agency. Oakland (CA). Bethesda (MD): US Department of Health and Human Services, Public Health Service, National Institutes of Health. California Environmental Protection Agency, Office of Environmental Health Hazard Assessment, Reproductive and Cancer Hazard Assessment Section, Air Toxicology and Epidemiology Section; 1999.

47. Oncken CA, Henry KM, Campbell WA, et al. Effect of maternal smoking on fetal catecholamine concentrations at birth. Pediatr Res 2003;53(1):119–24.

48. Fergusson DM, Woodward LJ, Horwood LJ. Maternal smoking during pregnancy and psychiatric adjustment in late adolescence. Arch Gen Psychiatry 1998;55(8):721–7.

49. Weitzman M, Gortmaker S, Sobol A. Maternal smoking and behavior problems of children. Pediatrics 1992;90(3):342–9.

50. Fergusson DM, Horwood LJ, Lynskey MT. Maternal smoking before and after pregnancy: effects on behavioral outcomes in middle childhood. Pediatrics 1993;92(6):815–22.

51. Linnet KM, Dalsgaard S, Obel C, et al. Maternal lifestyle factors in pregnancy risk of attention deficit hyperactivity disorder and associated behaviors: review of the current evidence. Am J Psychiatry 2003;160(6):1028–40.

52. Olds DL, Henderson CR Jr, Tatelbaum R. Prevention of intellectual impairment in children of women who smoke cigarettes during pregnancy. Pediatrics 1994;93(2):228–33.

53. McCartney JS, Fried PA, Watkinson B. Central auditory processing in school-age children prenatally exposed to cigarette smoke. Neurotoxicol Teratol 1994;16(3):269–76.

54. Fried PA, Watkinson B, Gray R. Differential effects on cognitive functioning in 9- to 12-year olds prenatally exposed to cigarettes and marihuana. Neurotoxicol Teratol 1998;20(3):293–306.

55. Obel C, Henriksen TB, Hedegaard M, et al. Smoking during pregnancy and babbling abilities of the 8-month-old infant. Paediatr Perinat Epidemiol 1998; 12(1):37–48.

56. Olds DL, Henderson CR Jr, Tatelbaum R. Intellectual impairment in children of women who smoke cigarettes during pregnancy. Pediatrics 1994;93(2):221–7.

57. Fergusson DM, Lloyd M. Smoking during pregnancy and its effects on child cognitive ability from the ages of 8 to 12 years. Paediatr Perinat Epidemiol 1991;5(2):189–200.

58. Lundgren F, Chattingius S, D'Onofrio B, et al. Maternal smoking during pregnancy and intellectual performance in young adult Swedish male offspring. Paediatr Perinat Epidemiol 2010;24(1):79–87.

59. Kandel DB, Wu P, Davies M. Maternal smoking during pregnancy and smoking by adolescent daughters. Am J Public Health 1994;84(9): 1407–13.

60. Cornelius MD, Leech SL, Goldschmidt L, et al. Prenatal tobacco exposure: is it a risk factor for early tobacco experimentation? Nicotine Tob Res 2000; 2(1):45–52.

61. Buka SL, Shenassa ED, Niaura R. Elevated risk of tobacco dependence among offspring of mothers who smoked during pregnancy: a 30-year prospective study. Am J Psychiatry 2003;160(11): 1978–84.

62. Oken E, Huh SY, Taveras EM, et al. Associations of maternal prenatal smoking with child adiposity and blood pressure. Obes Res 2005;13(11):2021–8.

63. Oken E, Levitan EB, Gillman MW. Maternal smoking during pregnancy and child overweight: systematic review and meta-analysis. Int J Obes (Lond) 2008; 32(2):201–10.

64. von Kries R, Toschke AM, Koletzko B, et al. Maternal smoking during pregnancy and childhood obesity. Am J Epidemiol 2002;156(10):954.

65. Taylor B, Wadsworth J. Maternal smoking during pregnancy and lower respiratory tract illness in early life. Arch Dis Child 1987;62(8):786–91.

66. Sekhon HS, Jia Y, Raab R, et al. Prenatal nicotine increases pulmonary alpha7 nicotinic receptor expression and alters fetal lung development in monkeys. J Clin Invest 1999;103(5):637–47.

67. Jaakkola JJ, Gissler M. Maternal smoking in pregnancy, fetal development, and childhood asthma. Am J Public Health 2004;94(1):136–40.

68. Hanrahan JP, Tager IB, Segal MR, et al. The effect of maternal smoking during pregnancy on early infant lung function. Am Rev Respir Dis 1992;145(5): 1129–35.

69. Cunningham J, Dockery DW, Speizer FE. Maternal smoking during pregnancy as a predictor of lung function in children. Am J Epidemiol 1994;139(12): 1139–52.

70. Hafstrom O, Milerad J, Sandberg KL, et al. Cardiorespiratory effects of nicotine exposure during development. Respir Physiol Neurobiol 2005;149(1–3): 325–41.

71. Sekhon HS, Keller JA, Proskocil BJ, et al. Maternal nicotine exposure upregulates collagen gene expression in fetal monkey lung. Association with alpha7 nicotinic acetylcholine receptors. Am J Respir Cell Mol Biol 2002;26(1):31–41.

72. The health consequences of smoking: a report of the surgeon general. Atlanta (GA): US Department of Health and Human Services, Center for Disease Control and Prevention; 2004.

73. Lumley J, Oliver SS, Chamberlain C, et al. Interventions for promoting smoking cessation during pregnancy. Cochrane Database Syst Rev 2004;4: CD001055.

74. Fiore M. United States. Tobacco use and dependence guideline panel. Treating tobacco use and dependence: 2008 update. 2008 update. Rockville (MD): US Department of Health and Human Services, Public Health Service; 2008.

75. ACOG Committee on Health Care for Underserved Women, ACOG Committee on Obstetric Practice. ACOG committee opinion. Number 316, October 2005. Smoking cessation during pregnancy. Obstet Gynecol 2005;106(4):883–8.

76. Bernstein IM, Mongeon JA, Badger GJ, et al. Maternal smoking and its association with birth weight. Obstet Gynecol 2005;106(5 Pt 1):986–91.

77. Melvin CL, Dolan-Mullen P, Windsor RA, et al. Recommended cessation counselling for pregnant women who smoke: a review of the evidence. Tob Control 2000;9(Suppl 3):III80–4.

78. Kendrick JS, Zahniser SC, Miller N, et al. Integrating smoking cessation into routine public prenatal care: the Smoking Cessation in Pregnancy project. Am J Public Health 1995;85(2):217–22.

79. Moore L, Campbell R, Whelan A, et al. Self help smoking cessation in pregnancy: cluster randomised controlled trial. BMJ 2002;325(7377):1383.

80. Naughton F, Prevost AT, Sutton S. Self-help smoking cessation interventions in pregnancy: a systematic review and meta-analysis. Addiction 2008;103(4): 566–79.

81. Windsor RA, Cutter G, Morris J, et al. The effectiveness of smoking cessation methods for smokers in public health maternity clinics: a randomized trial. Am J Public Health 1985;75(12):1389–92.

82. Fiore M. United States. Tobacco use and dependence guideline panel. Treating tobacco use and dependence. Rockville (MD): US Department of Health and Human Services, Public Health Service; 2000.

83. Selby P, Kapur B, Hackman R, et al. No one asked the baby – an ethical issue in placebo-controlled trials in pregnant smokers. Can J Clin Pharmacol 2005;12(2):e180–1.

84. Kapur B, Hackman R, Selby P, et al. Randomized, double-blind, placebo-controlled trial of nicotine replacement therapy in pregnancy. Curr Ther Res 2001;62(4):274–8.

85. Forest S. Controversy and evidence about nicotine replacement therapy in pregnancy. MCN Am J Matern Child Nurs 2010;35(2):89–95.

86. Hegaard HK, Kjaergaard H, Moller LF, et al. Multimodal intervention raises smoking cessation rate during pregnancy. Acta Obstet Gynecol Scand 2003;82(9):813–9.

87. Pollak KI, Oncken CA, Lipkus IM, et al. Nicotine replacement and behavioral therapy for smoking cessation in pregnancy. Am J Prev Med 2007;33(4):297–305.

88. Oncken C, Dornelas E, Greene J, et al. Nicotine gum for pregnant smokers: a randomized controlled trial. Obstet Gynecol 2008;112(4): 859–67.

89. Wisborg K, Henriksen TB, Jespersen LB, et al. Nicotine patches for pregnant smokers: a randomized controlled study. Obstet Gynecol 2000;96(6): 967–71.

90. Hotham ED, Gilbert AL, Atkinson ER. A randomised-controlled pilot study using nicotine patches with pregnant women. Addict Behav 2006;31(4): 641–8.

Asthma in Pregnancy

Vanessa E. Murphy, BMedChem (Hons), PhD[a,b,*],
Peter G. Gibson, MBBS (Hons), FRACP[a,b,c]

KEYWORDS

- Asthma • Pregnancy • Exacerbation
- Inhaled corticosteroid

ASTHMA DURING PREGNANCY

What is the Prevalence of Asthma During Pregnancy?

The burden of asthma in pregnancy is increasing worldwide,[1,2] with European estimates of at least 4% of women having asthma,[3] and at least 8% of women in antenatal clinics in the United Kingdom having asthma.[4] Increases in asthma prevalence have also been reported in the United States[1] from around 3% to more than 8% since 1994.[2] In Australia the prevalence of asthma in pregnancy is 12%.[5] As the most common respiratory disorder to complicate pregnancy, asthma represents a significant public health issue. Adequate asthma treatment and careful management is the key to a successful pregnancy outcome for these mothers and babies.

Can Changes in Asthma Be Expected in Pregnancy?

Most women with asthma experience a change in their disease control while pregnant. While for one-third this is an improvement, for at least one-third of women it is a worsening.[6,7] These changes are unpredictable from woman to woman and from pregnancy to pregnancy,[8] necessitating careful regular review of asthma during pregnancy. In the 1980s, subjective questionnaires completed by a large prospective cohort of 330 pregnant women in the United States provided evidence of the "one-third hypothesis," indicating that among women who rated their asthma as having worsened, symptoms of wheeze and sleep and activity limitation due to asthma were significantly increased between 25 and 32 weeks' gestation.[7] Among women reporting an improvement, however, there was a decrease in wheeze and little change in sleep/activity interference. These observations suggested that asthma control (wheezing, nocturnal asthma, activity limitation) is altered in the latter stages of pregnancy.

Until recently, few studies had assessed asthma changes during pregnancy using objective measures.[9–11] Studies in the 1970s and 1980s among small cohorts of women found no pregnancy-related changes in lung function measured by spirometry in either asthmatic or non-asthmatic women.[9,11] Juniper and colleagues[9,12] described an overall improvement in methacholine airway responsiveness in the second trimester compared with preconception; however, no relationship with serum progesterone or estriol concentrations was found. Peak expiratory flow values have recently been analyzed throughout pregnancy and have been found to increase with each trimester in a cohort of 43 women with asthma.[13] It is possible that the increase in progesterone with advancing gestation contributes to cyclic adenosine monophosphate (cAMP)-induced

Funding support: V.E.M. is funded by an Australian Research Training Fellowship (Part-Time) from the National Health and Medical Research Council.
The authors have nothing to disclose.
[a] Centre for Asthma and Respiratory Diseases, University of Newcastle and Hunter Medical Research Institute, Locked Bag 1, HRMC, Newcastle, New South Wales 2310, Australia
[b] Department of Respiratory and Sleep Medicine, John Hunter Hospital, Locked Bag 1, HRMC, Newcastle, New South Wales 2310, Australia
[c] Woolcock Institute of Medical Research, 431 Glebe Point Road, Glebe (Sydney), New South Wales 2037, Australia
* Corresponding author. Department of Respiratory and Sleep Medicine, John Hunter Hospital, Locked Bag 1, HRMC, Newcastle, New South Wales 2310, Australia.
E-mail address: vanessa.murphy@newcastle.edu.au

Clin Chest Med 32 (2011) 93–110
doi:10.1016/j.ccm.2010.10.001
0272-5231/11/$ — see front matter © 2011 Elsevier Inc. All rights reserved.

bronchodilation, thereby improving asthma and peak flow.[13] Also recently analyzed were changes in asthma severity from a cohort of 641 pregnant women with asthma, for whom medication use and asthma symptoms had been recorded several times through the second half of pregnancy.[14] Severity before pregnancy and in each month of pregnancy was described as intermittent, mild persistent, or moderate/severe, according to the Global Initiative for Asthma (GINA) guidelines. There was little evidence of any pregnancy-specific changes in asthma severity when data were stratified by prepregnancy severity rating; however, the measure of severity as a GINA category lacks sensitivity. The only group that had a significant change was the mild persistent group, where severity was reduced in months 6 and 9 compared with the second month. Among the factors analyzed (race, age, atopic status, prepregnancy asthma severity, body mass index [BMI], parity, fetal sex, smoking, and use of medication according to guidelines), only the prepregnancy severity and medication use was related to changes in asthma severity during pregnancy, with prepregnancy status predicting worse asthma in pregnancy, and lack of appropriate medication use being related to more severe asthma in pregnancy.[14]

A potentially useful objective marker of airway inflammation in asthma is fractional exhaled nitric oxide (FENO). In a small cross-sectional study, Tamasi and colleagues[15] found that FENO was not altered by pregnancy itself, but among pregnant women with asthma FENO was correlated with the level of asthma control. Unfortunately measures of FENO were not taken prospectively through pregnancy, so any effect of the stage of pregnancy on this inflammatory marker is unknown. Further studies are required to elucidate the predictors for clinically relevant changes in asthma control during pregnancy.

What are the Risk Factors for Asthma Exacerbations During Pregnancy?

Exacerbations are an important clinical feature of asthma and when severe, may require hospitalization. During pregnancy, around 5.8% of women are hospitalized with an exacerbation of asthma,[16] with some studies reporting more than 20% of women having exacerbations requiring medical intervention, including hospitalization, unscheduled doctor visits, and use of emergency therapy.[17,18] Even among well-managed cohorts, the exacerbation rate is high.[18,19] In Australia, 36% of women had a severe exacerbation requiring medical intervention for asthma during

pregnancy and a further 19% had a mild exacerbation during pregnancy.[19]

While exacerbations may occur at any time during gestation, they appear to be more common in the late second trimester.[6,19–21] A Canadian study found that visits to the emergency department for asthma exacerbations was clearly distinct from visits for other reasons, peaking in the second trimester and falling as gestation advanced.[22] Asthma exacerbations are unlikely to occur during labor and delivery[7,23–25]; however, one study described 46% of women with severe asthma having symptoms during labor.[18]

Women with severe asthma are most likely to experience exacerbations in pregnancy.[6,18,19,26] In one study, severe exacerbations requiring medical intervention occurred among 8% of women with mild asthma, 47% of women with moderate asthma, and 65% of women with severe asthma.[19] Women with severe exacerbations in pregnancy have significantly lower asthma-specific quality of life, which may be a more sensitive measure of limitations due to asthma than symptoms alone.[27] The effects of atopy, sinusitis, and gastroesophageal reflux on exacerbations require further investigation, as these conditions may worsen in pregnancy leading to an exacerbation of asthma.[28] Other risk factors for exacerbation during pregnancy include inadequate prenatal care,[29,30] obesity,[14,31] and lack of appropriate treatment with inhaled corticosteroids.[19–21,32] Almost one-third of women self-reported nonadherence to prescribed inhaled corticosteroid (ICS) medication before a severe exacerbation.[19] In Finland, the risk of having an exacerbation was reduced by more than 75% among women who were regular users of ICS.[21] More recent data demonstrated a higher rate of emergency department and physician visits during pregnancy among women who did not use ICS before pregnancy.[32] Improvements in asthma management that address the issue of ICS nonadherence may reduce the exacerbation rate among pregnant women.

There are limited data addressing the causal factors of severe asthma exacerbations during pregnancy; however, several studies have suggested that respiratory tract viral infections may be common contributors,[19,20,33,34] as they are in children and nonpregnant adults.[35] Viral infection was the most common self-reported cause of severe asthma exacerbations, reported by 34% of women.[19] Pregnant women may be more susceptible to viral infection, due to changes in cell-mediated immunity during pregnancy.[6] Pregnant women and those with asthma are certainly 2 groups with significantly increased susceptibility to infection with influenza strains, including seasonal and H1N1 influenza.[36,37] In the early stages of the H1N1 pandemic in the United States, 7% of hospitalized patients were pregnant, with 22% of these women also having asthma.[36] In total 9% of all admissions to intensive care units and 16% of all deaths were among pregnant women, indicating that both the prevalence of illness and its severity is increased with pregnancy.[36] Specific studies of cohorts of pregnant women have shown that those with asthma were more likely to have an upper respiratory tract or urinary tract infection during pregnancy than those without asthma, with severe asthma being associated with significantly more infections than mild asthma.[38] However, this evidence comes from a retrospective study relying on self-report of infection, and further evaluation using a prospective study design with objective confirmation of viral infection and specific identification of the viruses responsible may provide useful data. A study from New York suggested that prevention of infection may improve asthma symptoms among pregnant women, demonstrating an improvement in asthma symptoms during pregnancy among 50% of women who received an influenza vaccine, compared with improvement among only 15% of women not receiving the vaccine.[39]

What are the Mechanisms for Changes in Asthma During Pregnancy?

Over the years the involvement of hormones, altered immune function, and fetal sex in pregnancy-related changes in asthma have been proposed as mechanisms. Increases in maternal hormones during pregnancy may contribute to physiologic changes that result in improved asthma, for example, the promotion of anti-inflammatory effects by the increase in serum free cortisol.[34,40] Progesterone may contribute to improved asthma via increased minute ventilation,[41] smooth muscle relaxation,[42] or cAMP-induced bronchodilation.[13] On the other hand, progesterone may contribute to worsening asthma via changes in β_2-adrenoreceptor responsiveness and airway inflammation.[43] Among nonpregnant women, a high proportion of asthmatics have an abnormal concentration of either progesterone or estradiol compared with nonasthmatics,[44] which may explain why the progression of asthma during pregnancy differs between women.

A novel marker of the immunotolerance of pregnancy is heat shock protein (Hsp) 70, which is decreased in the circulation of healthy pregnant women as compared with nonpregnant adults.[45,46] Women with asthma have higher levels of Hsp70 than their nonasthmatic counterparts;

however, the role of this marker in chronic inflammation of asthma and its potential relationship with perinatal outcomes of these pregnancies requires further investigation.[46] Other alterations in the maternal immune system during pregnancy such as a suppression of cell-mediated immunity, and the development of a predominantly Th2 cytokine environment, which is essential for fetal survival,[47] may contribute to changes in asthma. Th2 cytokine polarization typical of allergic asthma may be heightened by the Th2 polarization of pregnancy. The placenta has a very high Th2:Th1 cytokine ratio, which was further elevated in samples collected from women with asthma who did not use ICS treatment during pregnancy.[48] In a cross-sectional analysis, interleukin (IL)-4 and interferon-γ—producing T-lymphocyte subsets were found to be significantly increased in pregnant women with asthma, compared with healthy pregnant women and nonpregnant asthmatic women.[49] However, this was not related to whether women perceived their asthma to have improved or worsened during pregnancy.[49] In a recent study, there was no evidence of enhanced lymphocyte activation among pregnant women with asthma as compared with healthy pregnant women.[50] In addition, no differences in maternal IL-6, IL-8, eotaxin, and RANTES concentrations were found in the peripheral blood of pregnant women with asthma in the third trimester, compared with pregnant controls.[51] However, bronchial epithelial cells demonstrated increased production of IL-8 and sICAM-1 in the presence of plasma from pregnant women with asthma, and results were suggestive of an increased chemotactic capacity,[52] which may be a mechanism contributing to worsening asthma in some pregnant women.

It has been hypothesized that the progression of maternal asthma symptoms in pregnancy may be influenced by the sex of the fetus.[53–56] Recently, Bakhireva and colleagues[57] demonstrated that women pregnant with a female fetus had a higher incidence of hospitalization for asthma during pregnancy. However, other reports do not support this association.[8,22,58] The largest study in this area of more than 10,000 asthmatic pregnancies in Quebec found no differences between women pregnant with male and female fetuses with regard to the occurrence of severe exacerbations, or the use of ICS or short-acting β_2-agonist (SABA) treatment.[58]

CHANGES IN ASTHMA AFFECT BOTH MOTHER AND BABY

In addition to the effect of pregnancy on asthma, it has been well described that asthma affects a wide range of pregnancy outcomes, related to both the mother (**Table 1**) and the neonate (**Table 2**). However, there is conflicting evidence in the literature regarding these effects, possibly due to sizeable variation in study design, sample size, and confounding factors in each published report. Many of the studies reporting increased risk of perinatal complications with asthma have been large database studies, whereas many of the studies not finding increased risks have been among smaller, yet better managed cohorts of pregnant women. It is possible and likely that better management of asthma improves outcomes among pregnant women; however, smaller clinical studies may also lack the power to detect increased risks in this population.

Is Asthma Associated with Poor Maternal Outcomes in Pregnancy?

In several prospective and retrospective cohort studies, pregnant women with asthma have been identified as being at increased risk of pregnancy-induced hypertension (PIH) or pree-clampsia.[21,25,59−69] For example, in Finland, 15% of women with asthma developed preeclampsia compared with 5% of women without asthma, with the rate even higher at 25% among women using oral steroids.[25] A relationship between oral steroid use, but not ICS use, and the development of PIH was also described by a case-control study.[70] Another study found that women with moderate to severe symptoms during pregnancy were at increased risk of preeclampsia, suggestive of a role of active maternal inflammation,[68] while others have described an association with reduced lung function.[71]

However, there are also numerous reports from prospective[23,38,72−74] and retrospective cohort studies[75,76] that do not find an increased risk of preeclampsia or PIH among pregnant women with asthma. In particular, a study of 486 pregnant women with actively managed asthma and 486 matched controls demonstrated no increased risk on this and other perinatal complications,[73] suggesting that asthma that is well controlled does not have significant adverse effects on either the mother or baby.

There is no evidence that asthma exacerbations in pregnancy are associated with an increased risk of preeclampsia.[16,21,70,73,74] In other studies, exacerbations prior to pregnancy increased the risk of PIH and pre-eclampsia,[70,77] suggesting that the underlying severity of asthma is an important factor.

Together, these studies suggest that severity, rather than control or exacerbations, may be related to the increased risk of preeclampsia in asthmatic women, possibly due to a common pathogenesis of the 2 diseases, such as mast cell infiltration into the smooth muscle of both the lungs and myometrium.[78] Preeclampsia has been associated with airway hyperresponsiveness.[78] Measurements in postpartum women with and without asthma indicated that those with a history of preeclampsia required significantly less methacholine to produce a 20% decrease in lung function, compared with women with previously normotensive pregnancies. Vascular hyperreactivity is another potential mechanism leading to changes in uteroplacental blood flow observed in vitro in placentas from women with moderate and severe asthma[79] and women with preeclampsia.[80]

Few studies have been specifically designed to test an association between maternal asthma and gestational diabetes. However, many large studies have examined this outcome, along with others, and have concluded that there is no increased risk in women with asthma.[21,23,25,38,59,66,72−74] Some studies[62,65,69,76] did find an increased risk

---

Table 1
Cohort studies examining the risk of maternal complications of pregnancy with asthma

| Maternal Outcome | Number of Studies | | Association of Outcome with Asthma Exacerbations in Pregnancy |
	Increased Risk with Maternal Asthma[a]	No Effect of Maternal Asthma[a]	
Preeclampsia or pregnancy-induced hypertension	13[21,25,59−69]	7[23,38,72−76]	No
C section	13[4,25,61,62,64,65,69,72,74,76,81−83]	3[23,66,75]	No
Gestational diabetes	4[62,65,69,76]	9[21,23,25,38,59,66,72−74]	No

[a] Compared with women without asthma.

Table 2
Cohort studies examining the risk of fetal and neonatal complications with maternal asthma

Fetal/Neonatal Outcome	Number of Cohort Studies		Association of Outcome with Asthma Exacerbations in Pregnancy
	Increased Risk with Maternal Asthma[a]	No Effect of Maternal Asthma[a]	
Congenital malformations	3[61,109,110]	8[4,17,21,23,64,72,73,76]	Yes
Perinatal mortality	3[60,88,108]	9[5,21,23,25,69,72–74,82]	No
Preterm labor or delivery	11[59,60,61,64,65,69,72,76,86,87,98]	7[5,17,21,23,38,73,75]	Yes
Low birth weight or intrauterine growth restriction	13[4,5,23,56,59,60,61,64,76,81,83,85,86]	8[26,38,66,72,73,82,87,88]	Yes
Neonatal sepsis	1[72]	1[4]	No
Transient tachypnea of the newborn	3[4,61,121]	1[72]	No

[a] Compared with women without asthma.

of gestational diabetes, and in one of these the increased risk occurred in oral steroid–dependent asthmatics only.[76]

Is Asthma Associated with Increased Medical Intervention During Labor and Delivery?

Many studies of both prospective and retrospective design have concluded that maternal asthma is a risk factor for delivery by cesarean (C) section.[4,25,61,62,64,65,69,72,74,76,81–83] However, the majority of these studies have described either total C sections or elective C sections only, with one study specifically showing an increase in C sections for fetal distress.[76] Although there was an increase in total C sections among mothers with asthma, Dombrowski and colleagues[72] found no increase in C sections for fetal distress compared with mothers without asthma. Similarly, Clark and colleagues[4] showed an increase in elective C sections among women with asthma, but no increase in emergency C sections. In the large Swedish Medical Birth Registry study, the increased risk remained after excluding women with medical conditions associated with C delivery, such as preeclampsia, premature rupture of membranes, and gestational diabetes.[62] Some studies have found an increase in complications such as placental abruption[62,84] and premature rupture of membranes,[69,76] which may contribute to the higher rate of C sections among women with asthma.

Is Asthma Associated with Poor Neonatal Outcomes?

The literature has been somewhat divided on the effect of maternal asthma on fetal growth. The majority of cohort studies that report an increased risk of intrauterine growth restriction or low birth weight (<2500 g) among women with asthma have been retrospective in design,[4,5,59,60,61,64,76,81,83,85] with fewer prospective cohorts demonstrating this risk.[23,56,86] However, the majority of studies reporting no increased risk are prospective in design,[26,38,66,72,73,87] with fewer retrospective cohorts finding no risk.[82,88] These findings may indicate a lack of power to detect a risk of fetal growth restriction among smaller prospective studies, or may be related to the level of asthma control among the subjects in these studies, which may be improved by participation in a prospective study.

Two explanations for an increased risk of low birth weight are supported by the current literature. The first is that ICS use protects against this perinatal outcome, and the second is that maternal exacerbations are a risk factor for low birth weight. Data from 4 studies in which women did not use ICS treatment for asthma during pregnancy[60,75,81,88] was combined in a meta-analysis.[89] There was a significantly increased risk of low birth weight in these asthmatic pregnancies compared with pregnancies without asthma (relative risk [RR] 1.55, 95% confidence interval [CI] 1.28, 1.87). Conversely, the meta-analysis of data from 5 studies in which some or all women had used ICS during pregnancy[23,66,73,81,86] demonstrated no significantly increased risk of low birth weight in women with asthma compared with those without asthma (RR 1.19, 95% CI 0.97, 1.45). Olesen and colleagues[85] assessed ICS use using a prescriptions database, and found that birth weights were lower among women who reduced their ICS use during pregnancy as compared with women who increased ICS use during pregnancy.

Data from 3 studies that described exacerbations during pregnancy as recurrent attacks of severe asthma or status asthmaticus,[88] hospitalization for asthma,[23] or acute asthma managed in the emergency department or clinic with nebulized bronchodilators[73] were combined in a meta-analysis.[16] Women who had an asthma exacerbation during pregnancy were at significantly increased risk of having a low birth weight neonate compared with women without asthma (RR 2.54, 95% CI 1.52, 4.25), whereas women without exacerbations were not at increased risk of low birth weight when compared with women without asthma (RR 1.12, 95% CI 0.8, 1.40). This analysis indicates that severe exacerbations increase the risk of low birth weight by more than 2.5-fold in women with asthma during pregnancy. This result is supported by studies that have described the reduction in mean birth weight among these women, finding that compared with women without exacerbations or a nonasthmatic group, severe exacerbations are associated with significant reductions in birth weight of between 56 and 434 g.[17,23,67,90] Recent work has also demonstrated an increased risk of small for gestational age babies among women with moderate or severe asthma, compared with women with mild asthma.[91]

Exacerbations of asthma during pregnancy are associated with an increased risk for low birth weight,[16] with a similar effect size to that of maternal smoking during pregnancy, which doubles the risk of low birth weight.[92] A direct effect of chronic maternal hypoxia on fetal growth via reduced fetal oxygenation, or indirect effects of alterations in placental vascular composition, blood flow, or function are possible mechanisms.[48,56,79,93–97]

Many cohort studies suggest an increased risk of preterm labor or delivery in pregnant women with asthma.[59,60,61,64,65,69,72,76,86,87,98] However, there are also several cohort studies showing no increased risk of preterm labor or delivery with maternal asthma.[5,17,21,23,38,73,75] Some of the larger prospective cohort studies have suggested that the effect of asthma on preterm birth may be related to the use of oral steroids during pregnancy.[72,86,99] The increased odds of preterm delivery was 2.2[72] in one study and 1.1 in another.[86] The effects of severe asthma and/or severe asthma exacerbations are difficult to separate from the effects of the oral steroids themselves. A meta-analysis[16] of 4 studies[21,23,73,88] found that severe exacerbations were not a significant risk factor for preterm delivery. Despite this, a North American study that evaluated asthma control by interview prospectively during pregnancy and postpartum found a higher rate of preterm delivery among women with inadequate asthma control in early pregnancy compared with those with adequate control, and among women who were hospitalized for asthma during pregnancy compared with those not hospitalized.[100] These relationships remained significant after adjustment for confounders such as age, BMI, smoking, and socioeconomic status.[100] A relationship has also been described between lower lung function and premature birth, consistent with the concept that more severe asthma is a risk factor.[71] Reduced lung function may also be a marker of poor control of asthma, which influences preterm delivery via hypoxic mechanisms.[71] The release of inflammatory mediators from the mother as a result of asthma may also be involved,[89] given the association between other active inflammatory diseases such as rheumatoid arthritis and low birth weight or preterm delivery.[101–103]

The risk of preterm labor among women with asthma has been found to be increased among African Americans as compared with white Americans,[104] suggesting that socioeconomic status or ethnicity may be a confounder and risk factor for poor maternal outcomes during asthmatic pregnancies. Similar findings from other studies suggest that poor prenatal care or lack of education about asthma may contribute to adverse perinatal outcomes.[30,69] Another potential mechanism is that a common pathogenic pathway leads to hyperactivity of both the bronchial and myometrial smooth muscle, leading to preterm labor in women with asthma.[87,105,106] One study demonstrated that mothers of premature infants had evidence of airway hyperactivity,[105] but this was not confirmed by another group examining airway responsiveness in mothers of premature or low birth weight children.[107]

Is Asthma Associated with Perinatal Mortality?

Until recently, there were few studies adequately powered to determine the effect of asthma or asthma exacerbations on perinatal mortality.

Before the introduction of ICS treatment for asthma, a study by Gordon and colleagues[88] studied 277 women with actively treated asthma. Sixteen of these women had severe asthma characterized by regular acute attacks or status asthmaticus during pregnancy. Almost 40% of these women had either a spontaneous abortion, fetal death, or neonatal death.[88] Another study in the 1970s that extracted data on 381 women with asthma and more than 112,000 controls from the Norwegian medical birth registry found a significantly higher rate of neonatal mortality with maternal asthma, but no significant increase in still births, perinatal mortality, or infant mortality.[60] In more recent reports, cohort studies examining still birth and perinatal or neonatal mortality in women with asthma have found no increased risk as compared with women without asthma.[5,21,23,25,69,72–74,82] One exception to this was the much larger 2009 study by Canadian investigators Breton and colleagues.[108] Their study showed an increased odds of perinatal mortality (including still birth after 20 weeks' gestation, and neonatal death up to 29 days) among the 13,100 women with asthma compared with the 28,042 women without asthma (odds ratio [OR] 1.35, 95% CI 1.08, 1.67). However, this was no longer significant when adjusted for birth weight and gestational age, suggesting that the higher rates of low birth weight and premature delivery among women with asthma may be contributing to the increased risk of perinatal mortality.[108]

Is Asthma Associated with Congenital Malformations?

The majority of cohort studies on the risk of congenital malformations in women with asthma have shown no increased risk.[4,17,21,23,64,72,73,76] However, it is likely that many were underpowered to detect a difference in rare outcomes such as malformations, and over the last few decades treatments for asthma have changed. Larger and more recent studies suggest that there is an increased risk of congenital anomalies among women with asthma.[61,109,110] Extensive examination of data from administrative databases in Quebec has revealed that pregnant women with asthma have a 30% increased risk of any congenital malformation and a 34% increased risk of a major congenital malformation, compared with women without asthma.[109] The risk for women using antiasthmatic medications in the Swedish Medical Birth Register studies was smaller, at 9%.[110] A case-control study from the United Kingdom has also identified a slight increased risk of any malformations among children of asthmatic mothers (OR 1.10, 95% CI 1.01, 1.20).[111]

It is unclear whether this increased risk is caused by the disease itself or the use of medications, but several clues are emerging. A prescriptions database was used to specifically estimate ICS dose in the first trimester in more than 4500 women with asthma, and a significantly reduced risk of malformations among users of moderate-dose ICS compared with nonusers was described.[112] Further research by this group in a larger cohort of 13,280 asthmatic pregnancies identified a 63% increased risk of malformations among users of high doses of ICS in the first trimester, compared with users of lower doses.[113] This work adds to evidence for the safety of lower doses of ICS, suggesting that doses be minimized to maintain asthma control in order to lessen potential risks of high doses of these medications. Among a cohort of 4344 asthmatic women, severe exacerbations in the first trimester were associated with an increased risk of any malformation as compared with women with no exacerbation of asthma.[114] These data were not supported by the United Kingdom case-control study, which found no relationship between clinically reported exacerbations and congenital malformations.[111]

Specific malformations for which maternal asthma has been found to be a risk factor include malformations of the nervous system (not including spina bifida), respiratory system and digestive system,[109,115] cardiac defects, and orofacial clefts.[110] A case-control study demonstrated that the risk of gastroschisis was increased among women using bronchodilators in the month before conception and during the first trimester, compared with nonusers of medication (adjusted OR 2.06, 95% CI 1.19, 3.59).[115] In a case-control study, pregnant women with asthma who used medication were also at twice the risk of heart defects.[116] Case-control studies have also provided evidence for an increased risk of oral clefts when women used oral steroids during the first trimester of pregnancy.[117,118] However, studies were not specifically conducted in asthmatic women, so the implications for them are unclear.

Studies that have examined the effects of specific asthma treatments on malformations have found no increased risk of malformations among users of budesonide.[119,120] One study described a significant but small increased risk of malformations in women using any drugs for asthma during pregnancy, compared with the rate of malformations in the whole population.[110]

Is Asthma Associated with Neonatal Complications?

There is relatively limited literature examining the relationship between maternal asthma and complications such as neonatal sepsis and transient tachypnea of the newborn. Neonatal sepsis was identified as an adverse outcome in women with mild asthma only[72] while another study did not find an association between asthma and neonatal sepsis, although women were not stratified by asthma severity.[4] In a retrospective cohort study in the United Kingdom, of more than 700 women with asthma and 700 controls without asthma, there was an increased rate of neonatal hospitalizations when mothers had asthma with an increased rate of transient tachypnea of the newborn.[4]

Is Maternal Asthma Associated with Long-Term Changes into Childhood?

Despite the increased risks of perinatal complications in women with asthma, there are few data available on longer-term health outcomes of children with asthmatic mothers. To date, increases in the prevalence of wheeze[121] and respiratory diseases,[122] left-handedness,[123] and mild to moderate intellectual disability[124] have been described. Schatz and colleagues[125] published the only follow-up of infants from a cohort of asthmatic women followed through pregnancy, and found that at 15 months of age, mental and psychomotor developmental outcomes were similar to those in children of nonasthmatic mothers.

Recent analysis has revealed that the children of asthmatic mothers are more at risk of asthma themselves when the mother's asthma is inadequately controlled during pregnancy.[126] In particular, during the first 10 years of life, children were at greater risk of asthma (adjusted OR 1.27, 95% CI 1.06, 1.52) when their mothers had asthma of moderate to severe severity that was also uncontrolled during pregnancy.[126] Asthma was considered uncontrolled when the mothers used high doses of SABA, or had severe exacerbations, including use of oral steroids, emergency department visits, or hospitalizations for asthma in the pregnancy.[127] In addition, children of asthmatic mothers had an 11% increased risk of atopic dermatitis, but this was not associated with maternal asthma severity or control during pregnancy.[127] Infants were more likely to have been prescribed antibiotics in the first 6 months of life when their mothers had asthma.[127] These data indicate that maternal asthma is a risk factor for childhood asthma, and that this risk could be reduced by improvements in asthma control that lead to reduced exacerbations during pregnancy.

BARRIERS TO GOOD ASTHMA MANAGEMENT IN PREGNANCY: DEBUNKING THE MYTHS AND ADDRESSING NEGATIVE HEALTH BEHAVIORS

Do Women Stop Using Asthma Medications While Pregnant?

There is a large body of evidence indicating that pregnant women reduce their use of asthma medications during pregnancy, against the advice of current guidelines or their physician.[28,56,128–130] A 2003 survey of more than 500 women of childbearing age who had asthma indicated that 82% of those who used ICS treatment were concerned about the effects of this medication on the fetus.[131] Despite also having concerns for their own health about the consequences of discontinuing medication, 36% reported that they would discontinue medication use while pregnant, without first seeking advice from their physician.[131]

Recent North American studies using data from prescription databases have confirmed this practice, identifying a significant decrease in prescriptions for asthma medications in early pregnancy as compared with before pregnancy.[32,112,132] When examining the use of asthma medications in the 6 months before and 6 months after the first pregnancy claim in a medical insurance database, Schatz and Leibman[32] demonstrated that of the 16% of women who used ICS before pregnancy, 52% discontinued ICS after pregnancy. The use of SABA was also discontinued in 57% of subjects using them before pregnancy.[32] Another American study found a 13% reduction in prescriptions for SABA, a 23% reduction in ICS, and a 54% reduction in prescriptions for oral steroids compared with the 20 weeks before pregnancy.[132] Blais and colleagues[112] also found that whereas 47.2% of women filled prescriptions for ICS before pregnancy, only 40% did in the first trimester. It is not clear whether these changes reflect changes in the attitudes of pregnant women themselves or to altered prescribing practices of their physicians.

One study did provide evidence of altered treatment of pregnant women with asthma by physicians during emergency department visits. Despite having symptoms and lung function similar to those in a nonpregnant group of women, those who were pregnant were significantly less likely to be treated with oral steroids either in the emergency department or after discharge from hospital.[133] The 2004 clinical guidelines for the treatment of asthma during pregnancy contain lear messages about the safety of medication use (particularly ICS and β_2-agonists) during pregnancy and the importance of vigorous treatment of asthma exacerbations,[28] which may facilitate improvements in the outcome for both mother and baby.

Cessation of medication during pregnancy may have adverse consequences for both mother and baby. The number of emergency department or physician visits for asthma was increased among women who had not taken ICS medication before pregnancy.[32] Conversely, among women who were using ICS before pregnancy, there was a 36% decrease in the number of asthma-related physician visits during pregnancy. It has also been shown that women who did not use ICS during pregnancy are at greater risk of exacerbations.[21] Women who reduced the intensity of their asthma treatment during pregnancy (eg, from ICS use to SABA use) had babies with lower mean birth weight, birth length, and gestational age, compared with women who increased the intensity of asthma treatment during pregnancy.[85] A recent large prospective cohort study found that women who used less medication than was recommended by guidelines for their prepregnancy level of severity had more severe asthma during pregnancy than women who did follow the recommendations of the guidelines.[14] Maintaining good asthma control with appropriate treatments is important for both maternal and fetal health outcomes.

Do Women with Asthma Smoke While Pregnant?

Many cohort studies from around the world have shown that cigarette smoking is more common among pregnant women with asthma than in pregnant women without asthma (**Table 3**).[5,38,61,62,66,74,75,83,134,135] There is even some evidence that smoking rates are higher still among women who do not use medication to treat their asthma.[4,75,112,136] A cohort study of 725 pregnant women identified maternal asthma as a predictor of pregnancy-associated smoking,[137] and another study showed that pregnant smokers were 4 times more likely to have asthma.[138] In a recent Australian study, 34% of pregnant women with asthma were current smokers, and asthmatic women were more likely to be heavier smokers than pregnant women without asthma.[5] Higher rates of passive smoke exposure among pregnant women with asthma (24%) compared with nonasthmatic women (4%) have also been described, but were not significant when considering only the subgroup of nonsmoking women.[66] Recently, a North American analysis of more than 2000 pregnant women with asthma found that 36% of nonsmokers were exposed to passive smoke at home.[139]

Table 3
Cigarette smoking among pregnant women with and without asthma

Study	Country	% Smokers in Asthma Group (%)	% Smokers in No-Asthma Group (%)
Dombrowski et al,[134] 1986	USA	46	28
Stenius-Aarniala et al,[25] 1988	Finland	8.8	16.2
Stenius-Aarniala et al,[21] 1996	Finland	11.5	15.2
Alexander et al,[75] 1998	Canada	34.8	27.3
Minerbi-Codish et al,[38] 1998	Israel	16.8	6.5
Demissie et al,[61] 1998	USA	15.3	12.1
Kurinczuk et al,[135] 1999	Australia	25.3	22.3
Mihrshahi et al,[66] 2003	Australia	30	17
Sheiner et al,[83] 2005	Israel	11.1	4.2
Clark et al,[4] 2007	UK	36.1	36.1
Kallen and Otterblad Olausson,[62] 2007	Sweden	16.3	12.4
Tata et al,[74] 2007	UK	34.3	31.0
Bakhireva et al,[136] 2007	USA and Canada	11.5	8.3
Enriquez et al,[17] 2007	USA	38	27.5
Clifton et al,[5] 2009	Australia	34	28
Murphy et al,[140] 2010	Australia	34	15

In pregnant women with asthma, current and former smokers had higher rates of severe exacerbation than never smokers, and these exacerbations were more severe in current smokers as demonstrated by higher asthma control scores.[140] Another study showed a greater number of symptomatic days and nights of sleep disturbance among active smokers than in nonsmokers with asthma.[139] Smoking is a well-recognized contributor to poor perinatal outcomes. Although the combined effects of maternal smoking and asthma have not been systematically investigated, both smoking and exacerbations are risk factors for low birth weight, so it is possible that smoking further increases the perinatal risks associated with asthma.[139] Smoking cessation programs should be provided to all pregnant women, and particularly those with asthma, and avoidance of triggers, including passive smoke exposure, should be strongly encouraged.[28,141]

Is There Any Relationship Between Asthma in Pregnancy and Anxiety and Depression?

Asthmatic women have a 52% increased risk of suffering depression during pregnancy compared with women without asthma,[74] which is not dependent on medications and was further elevated (twofold increased risk) among women who had exacerbations of asthma during pregnancy.[74] There has also been an increased use of antidepressants reported among women using antiasthmatic drugs during pregnancy.[62]

Psychological stress and anxiety may contribute to worsening of asthma in nonpregnant adults. Among university students, sputum eosinophils following allergen challenge are increased in the final examination week (characterized by significantly higher depression and anxiety scores) compared with mid-semester,[142] demonstrating an interaction between psychological stress and deteriorating airway inflammation in asthma.

Stress, anxiety, and depression may be contributors to worsening asthma during pregnancy. Concerns about the effects of medication use on the baby appear to lead to anxiety and nonadherence among pregnant women with asthma.[128,131] One survey reported that 5% of women with asthma reported feeling sadness, depression, or anxiety, 44% were worried for the baby, 11% were concerned that their stress and worry could lead to asthma attacks, and 7% were fearful of having an asthma attack in public.[128] A randomized controlled trial has demonstrated a potential benefit of relaxation techniques among pregnant women with asthma.[143] Over an 8-week period, there was a significant improvement in FEV_1 (forced expiratory volume in 1 second) among women with asthma who received training in progressive muscle relaxation, compared with women trained in sham exercise. Other benefit of this therapy included an improvement in health-related quality of life and a reduction of anger levels.[143] Improving psychological parameters may have significant effects on lung function during pregnancy.

EFFECTIVE TREATMENT AND MANAGEMENT OF PREGNANT WOMEN WITH ASTHMA

Asthma that is well controlled in pregnancy is less likely to result in adverse outcomes than poorly controlled asthma. Consequently, during pregnancy regular medical review and monitoring of asthma is recommended, and a multidisciplinary approach may be most effective. The goals of management in pregnant women are to minimize asthma symptoms and limitations, prevent exacerbations, and maintain near normal lung function with minimal medication use, thereby ensuring maternal quality of life and normal fetal maturation.[28]

What is the Safety Level of Asthma Treatments in Pregnancy?

In 2004, the National Asthma Education and Prevention Program (NAEPP) released an updated expert panel report on the management of asthma in pregnant women.[28] This report addressed safety concerns of asthma medications in pregnancy, and found that there was a significant amount of reassuring data on the safety of SABA, particularly albuterol.[28] A prospective cohort study found no significant differences in perinatal mortality, congenital malformations, preterm delivery, and low birth weight in asthmatic women who used SABA compared with women who did not use treatment for asthma during pregnancy.[99,144] There are limited data available on the use of long-acting β_2-agonists (LABA) during pregnancy. An epidemiologic study reported no adverse outcomes among 65 women who used salmeterol while pregnant.[145] Current guidelines recommend salmeterol as the preferred LABA used in pregnancy, based on its having been available for a longer period of time in the United States.[28]

The majority of studies addressing the safety of ICS use in pregnancy have examined women using budesonide and consequently, this is the ICS of choice, recommended for use in pregnant women with persistent asthma, following a stepwise approach to achieve asthma control.[2] However, because other ICS drugs have no been shown to be unsafe, women whose asthma was well controlled on other medications could continue to use these during pregnancy.[28,146]

The use of ICS medication for asthma during pregnancy in appropriate doses does not appear to result in any adverse outcomes for the fetus[99]; and although many studies in this area have lacked statistical power,[147] a meta-analysis of recent data (1997–2005) examining the relationship with perinatal outcomes provided further reassurance.[148] By maintaining adequate asthma control, ICS use may actually protect against some adverse outcomes such as low birth weight.[32,89] An adequately powered, large multicenter prospective cohort study found no significant relationships between ICS use during pregnancy and outcomes such as preterm birth at less than 32 weeks' gestation, major malformations, low birth weight, and small for gestational age infants.[99]

Most data on asthma treatment during pregnancy are derived from cohort studies. However, one randomized controlled trial of low-dose budesonide (400 μg/d) versus placebo among patients with recent-onset mild to moderate asthma included a subgroup of 313 pregnant women.[120] The rate of adverse pregnancy outcomes (including spontaneous abortion, neonatal death, and congenital abnormalities) was similar among women using low-dose budesonide or placebo throughout pregnancy. Unfortunately, other important perinatal outcomes such as birth weight were not reported in this study.[120]

Estimates suggest that approximately 2.4% of pregnant women with asthma use oral corticosteroids at some time during pregnancy.[62] The effects of oral steroid use on pregnancy are not well described, due to a lack of information about doses, timing, and length of use. Associations between oral steroid use and preeclampsia,[76,149] preterm delivery,[72,86,99] and reduced birth weight[26,99] have been described. However, it is difficult to separate the effects of the drug from the effects of the exacerbations that necessitated its use. A recent study of more than 113 pregnant women with asthma who used systemic steroids during pregnancy has addressed this question with linear regression analysis, finding that oral steroid use was significantly associated with birth weight, whereas all measures of asthma control (including hospitalizations) were not significantly associated with birth weight.[26]

Asthma should be well managed to avoid the need for rescue oral steroid medication.[146] However, when required for the treatment of a severe exacerbation during pregnancy, the possible risks described are still less than the risks of severely uncontrolled asthma, which may result in maternal and/or fetal death.[28,146]

Information on the safety of leukotriene receptor antagonists (LTRAs) for asthma during pregnancy is limited.[136,150] In one study of 96 women using LTRAs, no increased risk for preterm delivery, gestational diabetes, preeclampsia, or pregnancy loss was found, compared with 122 women with asthma who used SABA.[136] However, there was a small decrease in birth weight among users of LTRAs, and an increase in the prevalence of major structural anomalies compared with a nonasthmatic group, albeit among a small sample size.[136] Sarkar and colleagues[150] also found a decrease in mean birth weight among users of LTRAs. Current guidelines do not specifically recommend the use of LTRAs during pregnancy, due to the limited data available, unless the woman's asthma was previously well controlled on these medications before pregnancy.[28]

How Should Exacerbations be Treated in Pregnancy?

Women with asthma should receive vigorous treatment of an exacerbation during pregnancy to reduce the risk of readmission and to improve outcomes for the fetus.[28] At least one study has found that pregnant women were significantly less likely to be prescribed oral steroids, either in the emergency department or on discharge from hospital, compared with nonpregnant women.[133] Following discharge from hospital, the pregnant women were 3 times more likely to report an ongoing asthma exacerbation than the nonpregnant women.[133] Another study found that hospitalizations were more common during pregnancy than before pregnancy, and emergency department presentations and oral steroid courses were less likely during pregnancy than before pregnancy,[19] suggesting either that treatment approaches differ in pregnancy or there are changes in the frequency or severity of exacerbations during pregnancy.[19] A severe asthma attack presents more of a risk to the fetus than the use of asthma medications because of the potential for fetal hypoxia, so therapy should be maximized during any asthma exacerbation which occurs.[28] Management of an asthma emergency during pregnancy should involve cooperation between the respiratory specialist and obstetrician, to achieve close monitoring of lung function and fetal activity as well as maintenance of oxygen saturation above 95%.[28]

Two randomized controlled trials of asthma therapy during pregnancy have addressed treatment of exacerbations as well as treatment to prevent exacerbations. Wendel and colleagues[151] studied 84 women with 105 exacerbations during pregnancy, who were randomized to receive methylprednisolone with intravenous aminophylline or methylprednisolone alone at the time of admission to hospital. Although women receiving aminophylline reported more side effects, there was no difference in length of hospital stay between treatments.[151] The women were further randomized on discharge to receive inhaled β_2-agonist with either oral steroid taper alone or ICS (beclomethasone) plus oral steroid taper. The readmission rate was reduced by 55% with the inclusion of ICS on discharge.[151]

The second trial compared the use of inhaled beclomethasone and oral theophylline for the prevention of asthma exacerbations during pregnancy in women with moderate asthma.[152] There was no difference in the rate of severe exacerbation between groups nor in perinatal outcomes.[152] Inhaled beclomethasone was a suitable alternative to theophylline for asthma treatment during pregnancy, but did not reduce the exacerbation rate. Other studies have described a reduction in exacerbations with the use of ICS medication,[21,32] emphasizing the importance of women using appropriate preventive medication for asthma control during pregnancy.

How Should Asthma Management be Approached in Pregnancy?

While most women with asthma have disease of mild severity,[91] changes in disease status are to be expected during pregnancy. The NAEPP report indicates that individual treatment plans are required to address specific circumstances and patient needs, and that self-management of asthma is an important component of overall management.[28] It is important that changes in lung function and asthma control are detected early. Women should receive education about the use of regular peak flow monitoring at home and they should be provided with a written asthma action plan outlining how to respond to changes in their asthma and when to seek medical advice.[28,153]

An Australian study found that pregnant women with asthma have poor asthma skills and knowledge.[141] At the beginning of pregnancy 40% of women self-reported nonadherence to ICS medication, 16% had inadequate inhaler technique, and 42% had inadequate knowledge about their asthma medications.[141] Regular peak flow monitoring was performed by 3%, and 15% had a written action plan.[141] Asthma self management education during pregnancy was subsequently provided in an antenatal clinic

---

Table 4
Structured clinical assessment of asthma during pregnancy

1. Asthma control	Symptoms	Type (dyspnea, wheeze, cough, chest tightness)
		Pattern (response to triggers and treatment, intensity, frequency)
		Timing (nocturnal, on waking, with exercise)
	Lung function	Airflow limitation
2. Exacerbations	Frequency	
	Severity	
3. Asthma skills	Inhalation device selection and technique	
	Asthma knowledge	
	Self-monitoring	
	Adherence	
	Written action plan	
4. Asthma treatment	Compare with recommendations	
	Optimize ICS dose	
	Step up treatment category according to guidelines	
5. Asthma triggers and comorbidities	Identify	Comorbidities (rhinitis, gastroesophageal reflux, obesity)
	Avoidance strategies	

setting, contributing to an improvement in skills among pregnant women. During the 30- to 60-minute session with an asthma educator, women received education about asthma control and assessment of management skills, including trigger avoidance, smoking cessation, inhaler technique, and medication adherence. Women assessed as unstable and requiring medical review were referred to their primary care physician or to a respiratory physician for review. An individualized written action plan was provided. Asthma education during pregnancy was associated with significant improvements in all aspects of self-management as well as a significant increase in ICS use in women with moderate and severe asthma.[141] Women with severe asthma also reported fewer nighttime asthma symptoms and less use of reliever medications after receiving education.[141]

Pregnant women with asthma have a need for further education, information, and self-management skills.[128] An outline of a structured clinical assessment of asthma during pregnancy is given in **Table 4**. Few women report discussing their concerns about medications with their physician.[131] A multidisciplinary approach to prenatal and asthma care may benefit pregnant women, and is recommended.[28] Chambers[131] found that 40% of women would continue using ICS medication solely on the recommendation of their obstetrician. Recent studies have proposed that nurses and midwives have key roles to play in educating pregnant women with asthma, in culturally sensitive ways, which will empower them to alter their behavior and make lifestyle changes that control asthma symptoms.[104,154] Significant deficiencies in asthma knowledge and self-management skills among pregnant women might be greatly improved by asthma education, potentially leading to better asthma control and improved fetal outcomes.

SUMMARY

Asthma is a highly prevalent medical problem during pregnancy. Exacerbations of asthma or poorly controlled disease can increase the risk of adverse perinatal outcomes, which may influence future health. Well-controlled asthma during pregnancy is not considered to be a significant risk to the baby, and regular monitoring of maternal asthma throughout pregnancy is recommended. By controlling asthma and preventing severe exacerbation, ICS may provide protection against adverse outcomes. Improvements in asthma management that address health behavior issues such as maternal smoking, poor

self-management skills, and nonadherence to medication will be important in improving perinatal outcomes for women with asthma.

REFERENCES

1. Berg CL, Mackay AP, Qin C, et al. Overview of maternal morbidity during hospitalization for labor and delivery in the United States: 1993–1997 and 2001–2005. Obstet Gynecol 2009;113:1075.
2. Kwon HL, Belanger K, Bracken MB. Asthma prevalence among pregnant and childbearing-aged women in the United States: estimates from national health surveys. Ann Epidemiol 2003;13:317.
3. Kukla L, Bouchalova M, Shkiriak-Nyzhnyk Z, et al. Chronic morbidity in women, namely in pregnancy (comparative study between West, Central and East European countries). Lik Sprava 2008;1–2:43.
4. Clark JM, Hulme E, Devendrakumar V, et al. Effect of maternal asthma on birthweight and neonatal outcome in a British inner-city population. Paediatr Perinat Epidemiol 2007;21:154.
5. Clifton VL, Engel P, Smith R, et al. Maternal and neonatal outcomes of pregnancies complicated by asthma in an Australian population. Aust N Z J Obstet Gynaecol 2009;49:619.
6. Gluck JC, Gluck PA. The effects of pregnancy on asthma: a prospective study. Ann Allergy 1976; 37:164.
7. Schatz M, Harden K, Forsythe A, et al. The course of asthma during pregnancy, post partum, and with successive pregnancies: a prospective analysis. J Allergy Clin Immunol 1988;81:509.
8. Kircher S, Schatz M, Long L. Variables affecting asthma course during pregnancy. Ann Allergy Asthma Immunol 2002;89:463.
9. Juniper EF, Daniel EE, Roberts RS, et al. Improvement in airway responsiveness and asthma severity during pregnancy. A prospective study. Am Rev Respir Dis 1989;140:924.
10. Kwon HL, Belanger K, Bracken MB. Effect of pregnancy and stage of pregnancy on asthma severity: a systematic review. Am J Obstet Gynecol 2004; 190:1201.
11. Sims CD, Chamberlain GV, de Swiet M. Lung function tests in bronchial asthma during and after pregnancy. Br J Obstet Gynaecol 1976;83:434.
12. Juniper EF, Daniel EE, Roberts RS, et al. Effect of pregnancy on airway responsiveness and asthma severity. Relationship to serum progesterone. Am Rev Respir Dis 1991;143:S78.
13. Beckmann CA. Peak flow values by gestation in women with asthma. Clin Nurs Res 2008;17:174.
14. Belanger K, Hellenbrand ME, Holford TR, et al. Effect of pregnancy on maternal asthma symptoms and medication use. Obstet Gynecol 2010;115: 559.

15. Tamasi L, Bohacs A, Bikov A, et al. Exhaled nitric oxide in pregnant healthy and asthmatic women. J Asthma 2009;46:786.

16. Murphy VE, Clifton VL, Gibson PG. Asthma exacerbations during pregnancy: incidence and association with adverse pregnancy outcomes. Thorax 2006;61:169.

17. Enriquez R, Griffen MR, Carroll KN, et al. Effect of maternal asthma and asthma control during pregnancy and perinatal outcomes. J Allergy Clin Immunol 2007;120:625.

18. Schatz M, Dombrowski MP, Wise R, et al. Asthma morbidity during pregnancy can be predicted by severity classification. J Allergy Clin Immunol 2003;112:283.

19. Murphy VE, Gibson P, Talbot PI, et al. Severe asthma exacerbations during pregnancy. Obstet Gynecol 2005;106:1046.

20. Apter AJ, Greenberger PA, Patterson R. Outcomes of pregnancy in adolescents with severe asthma. Arch Intern Med 1989;149:2571.

21. Stenius-Aarniala BS, Hedman J, Teramo KA. Acute asthma during pregnancy. Thorax 1996;51:411.

22. Baibergenova A, Thabane L, Akhtar-Danesh N, et al. Is fetal gender associated with emergency department visits for asthma during pregnancy? J Asthma 2006;43:293.

23. Jana N, Vasishta K, Saha SC, et al. Effect of bronchial asthma on the course of pregnancy, labour and perinatal outcome. J Obstet Gynaecol 1995;21:227.

24. Mabie WC, Barton JR, Wasserstrum N, et al. Clinical observations on asthma and pregnancy. J Matern Fetal Med 1992;1:45.

25. Stenius-Aarniala B, Piirila P, Teramo K. Asthma and pregnancy: a prospective study of 198 pregnancies. Thorax 1988;43:12.

26. Bakhireva LN, Jones KL, Schatz M, et al. Asthma medication use in pregnancy and fetal growth. J Allergy Clin Immunol 2005;116:503.

27. Schatz M, Dombrowski MP, Wise R, et al. The relationship of asthma-specific quality of life during pregnancy to subsequent asthma and perinatal morbidity. J Asthma 2010;47:46.

28. National Heart, Lung, and Blood Institute, National Asthma Education and Prevention Program Asthma and Pregnancy Working Group. NAEPP expert panel report. Managing asthma during pregnancy: recommendations for pharmacologic treatment—2004 update. J Allergy Clin Immunol 2005;115:34.

29. Carroll KN, Griffin MR, Gebretsadik T, et al. Racial differences in asthma morbidity during pregnancy. Obstet Gynecol 2005;106:66.

30. Chung KD, Demissie K, Rhoads GG. Asthma in pregnancy—its relationship with race, insurance, maternal education, and prenatal care utilization. J Natl Med Assoc 2004;96:1414.

31. Hendler I, Schatz M, Momirova V, et al. Association of obesity with pulmonary and nonpulmonary complications of pregnancy in asthmatic women. Obstet Gynecol 2006;108:77.

32. Schatz M, Leibman C. Inhaled corticosteroid use and outcomes in pregnancy. Ann Allergy Asthma Immunol 2005;95:234.

33. Hartert TV, Neuzil KM, Shintani AK, et al. Maternal morbidity and perinatal outcomes among pregnant women with respiratory hospitalizations during influenza season. Am J Obstet Gynecol 2003;189:1705.

34. Williams DA. Asthma and pregnancy. Acta Allergol 1967;22:311.

35. Douwes J, Gibson P, Pekkanen J, et al. Non-eosinophilic asthma: importance and possible mechanisms. Thorax 2002;57:643.

36. Jain S, Kaminoto L, Bramley AM, et al. Hospitalized patients with 2009 H1N1 influenza in the United States, April–June 2009. N Engl J Med 2009;361:1935.

37. Scriven J, Mcewen R, Mistry S, et al. Swine flu: a Birmingham experience. Clin Med 2009;9:534.

38. Minerbi-Codish I, Fraser D, Avnun L, et al. Influence of asthma in pregnancy on labor and the newborn. Respiration 1998;65:130.

39. Rastogi D, Wang C, Lendor C, et al. T-helper type 2 polarization among asthmatics during and following pregnancy. Clin Exp Allergy 2006;36:892.

40. Nelson-Piercy C. Asthma in pregnancy. Thorax 2001;56:325.

41. Lyons HA, Antonio R. The sensitivity of the respiratory center in pregnancy and after the administration of progesterone. Trans Assoc Am Physicians 1959;72:173.

42. Lye SJ, Porter DG. Demonstration that progesterone 'blocks' uterine activity in the ewe in vivo by a direct action on the myometrium. J Reprod Fertil 1978;52:87.

43. Tan KS, Thomson NC. Asthma in pregnancy. Am J Med 2000;109:727.

44. Rubio Ravelo L, Gago Rodriguez B, Almirall Collazo JJ, et al. Comparative study of progesterone, estradiol and cortisol concentrations in asthmatic and non-asthmatic women. Allergol Immunopathol (Madr) 1988;16:263.

45. Molvarec A, Tamasi L, Losonczy G, et al. Circulating heat shock protein 70 (HSPA1A) in normal and pathological pregnancies. Cell Stress Chaperones 2010;15:237.

46. Tamasi L, Bohacs A, Tamasi V, et al. Increased circulating heat shock protein 70 levels in pregnant asthmatics. Cell Stress Chaperones 2010;15:295.

47. Chaouat G, Ledee-Bataille N, Dubanchet S, et al. Reproductive immunology 2003: reassessing the Th1/Th2 paradigm? Immunol Lett 2004;92:207.

48. Clifton VL, Murphy VE. Maternal asthma as a model for examining fetal sex-specific effects on maternal

physiology and placental mechanisms that regulate human fetal growth. Placenta 2004;25 (Suppl A):S45.

49. Tamasi L, Bohacs A, Pallinger E, et al. Increased interferon-gamma- and interleukin-4-synthesizing subsets of circulating T lymphocytes in pregnant asthmatics. Clin Exp Allergy 2005;35:1197.

50. Bohacs A, Pallinger E, Tamasi L, et al. Surface markers of lymphocyte activation in pregnant asthmatics. Inflamm Res 2010;59:63.

51. Osei-Kumah A, Smith R, Clifton VL. Maternal and cord plasma cytokine and chemokine profile in pregnancies complicated by asthma. Cytokine 2008;43:187.

52. Osei-Kumah A, Wark PA, Smith R, et al. Asthma during pregnancy alters immune cell profile and airway epithelial chemokine release. Inflamm Res 2010;59:349.

53. Beecroft N, Cochrane GM, Milburn HJ. Effect of sex of fetus on asthma during pregnancy: blind prospective study. BMJ 1998;317:856.

54. Dodds L, Armson BA, Alexander S. Use of asthma drugs is less among women pregnant with boys rather than girls. BMJ 1999;318:1011.

55. Kwon HL, Belanger K, Holford TR, et al. Effect of fetal sex on airway lability in pregnant women with asthma. Am J Epidemiol 2005;163:217.

56. Murphy VE, Gibson PG, Giles WB, et al. Maternal asthma is associated with reduced female fetal growth. Am J Respir Crit Care Med 2003;168:1317.

57. Bakhireva LN, Schatz M, Lyons Jones K, et al. Fetal sex and maternal asthma control in pregnancy. J Asthma 2008;45:403.

58. Firoozi F, Ducharme FM, Lemiere C, et al. Effect of fetal gender on maternal asthma exacerbations in pregnant asthmatic women. Respir Med 2009;103:144.

59. Acs N, Puho E, Banhidy F, et al. Association between bronchial asthma in pregnancy and shorter gestational age in a population-based study. J Matern Fetal Med 2005;18:107.

60. Bahna SL, Bjerkedal T. The course and outcome of pregnancy in women with bronchial asthma. Acta Allergol 1972;27:397.

61. Demissie K, Breckenridge MB, Rhoads GG. Infant and maternal outcomes in the pregnancies of asthmatic women. Am J Respir Crit Care Med 1998;158:1091.

62. Kallen B, Otterblad Olausson P. Use of anti-asthmatic drugs during pregnancy. 1. Maternal characteristics, pregnancy and delivery complications. Eur J Clin Pharmacol 2007;63:363.

63. Lehrer S, Stone J, Lapinski R, et al. Association between pregnancy-induced hypertension and asthma during pregnancy. Am J Obstet Gynecol 1993;168:1463.

64. Liu S, Wen SW, Demissie K, et al. Maternal asthma and pregnancy outcomes: a retrospective cohort study. Am J Obstet Gynecol 2001;184:90.

65. MacMullen NJ, Shen JJ, Tymkow C. Adverse maternal outcomes in women with asthma versus women without asthma. Appl Nurs Res 2010;23(1):e9–13.

66. Mihrshahi S, Belousova E, Marks GB, et al. Pregnancy and birth outcomes in families with asthma. J Asthma 2003;40:181.

67. Sobande AA, Archibong EI, Akinola SE. Pregnancy outcome in asthmatic patients from high altitudes. Int J Gynaecol Obstet 2002;77:117.

68. Triche EW, Saftlas AF, Belanger K, et al. Association of asthma diagnosis, severity, symptoms, and treatment with risk of preeclampsia. Obstet Gynecol 2004;104:585.

69. Wen SW, Demissie K, Liu S. Adverse outcomes in pregnancies of asthmatic women: results from a Canadian population. Ann Epidemiol 2001;11:7.

70. Martel MJ, Rey E, Beauchesne MF, et al. Use of inhaled corticosteroids during pregnancy and risk of pregnancy induced hypertension: nested case-control study. BMJ 2005;330:230.

71. Schatz M, Dombrowski M, Wise R, et al. Spirometry is related to perinatal outcomes in pregnant women with asthma. Am J Obstet Gynecol 2006;194:120.

72. Dombrowski MP, Schatz M, Wise R, et al. Asthma during pregnancy. Obstet Gynecol 2004;103:5.

73. Schatz M, Zeiger RS, Hoffman CP, et al. Perinatal outcomes in the pregnancies of asthmatic women: a prospective controlled analysis. Am J Respir Crit Care Med 1995;151:1170.

74. Tata LJ, Lewis SA, McKeever TM, et al. A comprehensive analysis of adverse obstetric and pediatric complications in women with asthma. Am J Respir Crit Care Med 2007;175:991.

75. Alexander S, Dodds L, Armson BA. Perinatal outcomes in women with asthma during pregnancy. Obstet Gynecol 1998;92:435.

76. Perlow JH, Montgomery D, Morgan MA, et al. Severity of asthma and perinatal outcome. Am J Obstet Gynecol 1992;167:963.

77. Martel MJ, Rey E, Beauchesne MF, et al. Use of short-acting beta2-agonists during pregnancy and the risk of pregnancy-induced hypertension. J Allergy Clin Immunol 2007;119:576.

78. Siddiqui S, Goodman N, McKenna S, et al. Pre-eclampsia is associated with airway hyperresponsiveness. BJOG 2008;115:520.

79. Clifton VL, Giles WB, Smith R, et al. Alterations of placental vascular function in asthmatic pregnancies. Am J Respir Crit Care Med 2001;164:546.

80. Read MA, Leitch IM, Giles WB, et al. U46619-mediated vasoconstriction of the fetal placental vasculature in vitro in normal and hypertensive pregnancies. J Hypertens 1999;17:389.

81. Lao TT, Huengsburg M. Labour and delivery in mothers with asthma. Eur J Obstet Gynecol Reprod Biol 1990;35:183.

82. Norjavaara E, de Verdier MG. Normal pregnancy outcomes in a population-based study including 2,968 pregnant women exposed to budesonide. J Allergy Clin Immunol 2003;111:736.

83. Sheiner E, Mazor M, Levy A, et al. Pregnancy outcome of asthmatic patients: a population-based study. J Matern Fetal Med 2005;18:237.

84. Getahun D, Ananth CV, Peltier MR, et al. Acute and chronic respiratory diseases in pregnancy: association with placental abruption. Am J Obstet Gynecol 2006;195:1180.

85. Olesen C, Thrane N, Nielsen GL, et al. A population-based prescription study of asthma drugs during pregnancy: changing the intensity of asthma therapy and perinatal outcomes. Respiration 2001;68:256.

86. Bracken MB, Triche EW, Belanger K, et al. Asthma symptoms, severity, and drug therapy: a prospective study of effects on 2205 pregnancies. Obstet Gynecol 2003;102:739.

87. Doucette JT, Bracken MB. Possible role of asthma in the risk of preterm labor and delivery. Epidemiology 1993;4:143.

88. Gordon M, Niswander KR, Berendes H, et al. Fetal morbidity following potentially anoxigenic obstetric conditions. VII. Bronchial asthma. Am J Obstet Gynecol 1970;106:421.

89. Murphy VE, Gibson PG, Smith R, et al. Asthma during pregnancy: mechanisms and treatment implications. Eur Respir J 2005;25:731.

90. Greenberger PA, Patterson R. The outcome of pregnancy complicated by severe asthma. Allergy Proc 1988;9:539.

91. Firoozi F, Lemiere C, Ducharme FM, et al. Effect of maternal moderate to severe asthma on perinatal outcomes. Respir Med 2010;104(9):1278–87.

92. Hammoud AO, Bujold E, Sorokin Y, et al. Smoking in pregnancy revisited: findings from a large population-based study. Am J Obstet Gynecol 2005;192:1856.

93. Clifton VL, Rennie N, Murphy VE. Effect of inhaled glucocorticoid treatment on placental 11beta-hydroxysteroid dehydrogenase type 2 activity and neonatal birthweight in pregnancies complicated by asthma. Aust N Z J Obstet Gynaecol 2006;46:136.

94. Clifton VL, Vanderlelie J, Perkins AV. Increased anti-oxidant enzyme activity and biological oxidation in placentae of pregnancies complicated by asthma. Placenta 2005;26:773.

95. Mayhew TM, Jenkins H, Todd B, et al. Maternal asthma and placental morphology: effects of severity, treatment and fetal sex. Placenta 2008;29:366.

96. Murphy VE, Johnson RF, Wang YC, et al. The effect of maternal asthma on placental and cord blood protein profiles. J Soc Gynecol Investig 2005;12(5):349–55.

97. Murphy VE, Zakar T, Smith R, et al. Reduced 11beta-hydroxysteroid dehydrogenase type 2 activity is associated with decreased birth weight centile in pregnancies complicated by asthma. J Clin Endocrinol Metab 2002;87:1660.

98. Syed RZ, Zubairi AB, Zafar MA, et al. Perinatal outcomes in pregnancy with asthma. J Pak Med Assoc 2008;58:525.

99. Schatz M, Dombrowski MP, Wise R, et al. The relationship of asthma medication use to perinatal outcomes. J Allergy Clin Immunol 2004;113:1040.

100. Bakhireva LN, Schatz M, Lyons Jones K, et al. Asthma control during pregnancy and the risk of preterm delivery or impaired fetal growth. Ann Allergy Asthma Immunol 2008;101:137.

101. Bowden AP, Barrett JH, Fallow W, et al. Women with inflammatory polyarthritis have babies of lower birth weight. J Rheumatol 2001;28:355.

102. Fonager K, Sorensen HT, Olsen J, et al. Pregnancy outcome for women with Crohn's disease: a follow up study based on linkage between national registries. Am J Gastroenterol 1998;93:2426.

103. Skomsvoll JF, Ostensen M, Irgens LM, et al. Obstetrical and neonatal outcome in pregnant patients with rheumatic disease. Scand J Rheumatol Suppl 1998;107:109.

104. MacMullen NJ, Tymkow C, Shen JJ. Adverse maternal outcomes in women with asthma: differences by race. MCN Am J Matern Child Nurs 2006;31:263.

105. Bertrand JM, Riley SP, Popkin J, et al. The long term pulmonary sequelae of prematurity: the role of familial airway hyperreactivity and the respiratory distress syndrome. N Engl J Med 1985;312:742.

106. Kramer MS, Coates AL, Michoud MC, et al. Maternal asthma and idiopathic preterm labor. Am J Epidemiol 1995;142:1078.

107. Chan KN, Noble-Jamieson CM, Elliman A, et al. Airway responsiveness in low birthweight children and their mothers. Arch Dis Child 1988;63:905.

108. Breton M-C, Beauchesne M-F, Lemiere C, et al. Risk of perinatal mortality associated with asthma during pregnancy. Thorax 2009;64:101.

109. Blais L, Kettani F, Elftouh N, et al. Effect of maternal asthma on the risk of specific congenital malformations: a population-based cohort study. Birth Defects Res A Clin Mol Teratol 2010;88:216.

110. Kallen B, Otterblad Olausson P. Use of anti-asthmatic drugs during pregnancy. 3. Congenital malformations in the infants. Eur J Clin Pharmacol 2007;63:383.

111. Tata LJ, Lewis SA, McKeever TM, et al. Effect of maternal asthma, exacerbations and asthma

medication use on congenital malformations in offspring: a UK population-based study. Thorax 2008;63:981.

112. Blais L, Beauchesne MF, Rey E, et al. Use of inhaled corticosteroids during the first trimester of pregnancy and the risk of congenital malformations among women with asthma. Thorax 2007;62:320.

113. Blais L, Beauchesne M, Lemiere C, et al. High doses of inhaled corticosteroids during the first trimester of pregnancy and congenital malformations. J Allergy Clin Immunol 2009;124:1229.

114. Blais L, Forget A. Asthma exacerbations during the first trimester of pregnancy and the risk of congenital malformations among asthmatic women. J Allergy Clin Immunol 2008;121:1379.

115. Lin S, Munsie JW, Herdt-Losavio ML, et al. Maternal asthma medication use and the risk of gastroschisis. Am J Epidemiol 2008;168:73.

116. Lin S, Herdt-Losavio M, Gensburg L, et al. Maternal asthma, asthma medication use, and the risk of congenital heart defects. Birth Defects Res A Clin Mol Teratol 2009;85:161.

117. Park-Wyllie L, Mazzotta P, Pastuszak A, et al. Birth defects after maternal exposure to corticosteroids: prospective cohort study and meta-analysis of epidemiological studies. Teratology 2000;62:385.

118. Rodriguez-Pinilla E, Martinez-Frias ML. Corticosteroids during pregnancy and oral clefts: a case-control study. Teratology 1998;58:2.

119. Kallen B, Rydhstroem H, Aberg A. Congenital malformations after the use of inhaled budesonide in early pregnancy. Obstet Gynecol 1999;93:392.

120. Silverman M, Sheffer A, Diaz PV, et al. Outcome of pregnancy in a randomized controlled study of patients with asthma exposed to budesonide. Ann Allergy Asthma Immunol 2005;95:566.

121. Schatz M, Zeiger RS, Hoffman CP, et al. Increased transient tachypnea of the newborn in infants of asthmatic mothers. Am J Dis Child 1991;145:156.

122. Kelly YJ, Brabin BJ, Milligan P, et al. Maternal asthma, premature birth, and the risk of respiratory morbidity in schoolchildren in Merseyside. Thorax 1995;50:525.

123. Weinstein RE, Gurvitz M, Greenberg D, et al. Altered cerebral dominance in atopy and in children of asthmatic mothers. Ann N Y Acad Sci 1992;650:25.

124. Leonard H, De Klerk N, Bourke J, et al. Maternal health in pregnancy and intellectual disability in the offspring: a population-based study. Ann Epidemiol 2005;16:448.

125. Schatz M, Harden K, Kagnoff M, et al. Developmental follow-up in 15-month-old infants of asthmatic vs. control mothers. Pediatr Allergy Immunol 2001;12:149.

126. Martel M, Rey E, Beauchesne M, et al. Control and severity of asthma during pregnancy are associated with asthma incidence in offspring: two-stage case-control study. Eur Respir J 2009; 34:579.

127. Martel M, Beauchesne M, Malo J, et al. Maternal asthma, its control and severity in pregnancy, and the incidence of atopic dermatitis and allergic rhinitis in the offspring. J Pediatr 2009;155:707.

128. Beckmann CA. A descriptive study of women's perceptions of their asthma during pregnancy. MCN Am J Matern Child Nurs 2002;27:98.

129. Burdon JG, Goss G. Asthma and pregnancy. Aust N Z J Med 1994;24:3.

130. Lipson A. Asthma and pregnancy—misleading and incorrect recommendation on the effect of medication on the foetus—and a remedy. Aust N Z J Med 1994;24:407.

131. Chambers K. Asthma education and outcomes for women of childbearing age. Case Manager 2003; 14:58.

132. Enriquez R, Wu P, Griffin MR, et al. Cessation of asthma medication in early pregnancy. Am J Obstet Gynecol 2006;195:149.

133. Cydulka RK, Emerman CL, Schreiber D, et al. Acute asthma among pregnant women presenting to the emergency department. Am J Respir Crit Care Med 1999;160:887.

134. Dombrowski MP, Bottoms SF, Boike GM, et al. Incidence of preeclampsia among asthmatic patients lower with theophylline. Am J Obstet Gynecol 1986;155:265.

135. Kurinczuk JJ, Parsons DE, Dawes V, et al. The relationship between asthma and smoking during pregnancy. Women Health 1999;29:31.

136. Bakhireva LN, Jones KL, Schatz M, et al. Safety of leukotriene receptor antagonists in pregnancy. J Allergy Clin Immunol 2007;119:618.

137. Hensley Alford SM, Lappin RE, Peterson L, et al. Pregnancy associated smoking behavior and six year postpartum recall. Matern Child Health J 2009;865:2009.

138. Roelands J, Jamison MG, Lyerly AD, et al. Consequences of smoking during pregnancy on maternal health. J Womens Health (Larchmt) 2009;18:867.

139. Newman RB, Momirova V, Dombrowski MP, et al. The effect of active and passive household cigarette smoke exposure on pregnant women with asthma. Chest 2010;137:601.

140. Murphy VE, Clifton VL, Gibson PG. The effect of cigarette smoking on asthma control during exacerbations in pregnant women. Thorax 2010;65(8): 739–44.

141. Murphy VE, Gibson PG, Talbot PI, et al. Asthma self-management skills and the use of asthma education during pregnancy. Eur Respir J 2005; 26:435.

142. Liu LY, Coe CL, Swenson CA, et al. School examinations enhance airway inflammation to antigen

challenge. Am J Respir Crit Care Med 2002;165: 1062.

143. Nickel C, Lahmann C, Muehlbacher M, et al. Pregnant women with bronchial asthma benefit from progressive muscle relaxation: a randomised, prospective, controlled trial. Psychother Psychosom 2006;75:237.

144. Schatz M, Zeiger RS, Harden KM, et al. The safety of inhaled beta-agonist bronchodilators during pregnancy. J Allergy Clin Immunol 1988; 82:686.

145. Mann RD, Kubota K, Pearce G, et al. Salmeterol: a study by prescription-event monitoring in a UK cohort of 15,407 patients. J Clin Epidemiol 1996; 49:247.

146. Schatz M. Breathing for two: Now we can all breathe a little easier. J Allergy Clin Immunol 2005;115:31.

147. Breton M, Martel M, Vilain A, et al. Inhaled corticosteroids during pregnancy: a review of methodologic issues. Respir Med 2008;102:862.

148. Rahimi R, Nikfar S, Abdollahi M. Meta-analysis finds use of inhaled corticosteroids during pregnancy safe: a systematic meta-analysis review. Hum Exp Toxicol 2006;25:447.

149. Schatz M, Zeiger RS, Harden K, et al. The safety of asthma and allergy medications during pregnancy. J Allergy Clin Immunol 1997;100:301.

150. Sarkar M, Koren G, Kalra S, et al. Montelukast use during pregnancy: a multicentre, prospective comparative study of infant outcomes. Eur J Clin Pharmacol 2009;65:1259.

151. Wendel PJ, Ramin SM, Barnett-Hamm C, et al. Asthma treatment in pregnancy: a randomized controlled study. Am J Obstet Gynecol 1996;175:150.

152. Dombrowski MP, Schatz M, Wise R, et al. Randomized trial of inhaled beclomethasone dipropionate versus theophylline for moderate asthma during pregnancy. Am J Obstet Gynecol 2004;190:737.

153. McDonald CF, Burdon JG. Asthma in pregnancy and lactation. A position paper for the Thoracic Society of Australia and New Zealand. Med J Aust 1996;165:485.

154. Henley-Einion A. Midwifery basics: caring for women with medical conditions (2). Respiratory disorders in pregnancy. Pract Midwife 2008;11:48.

Pregnancy in Cystic Fibrosis

John R. McArdle, MD

KEYWORDS

- Cystic fibrosis • Pregnancy • Birth outcomes
- Genetic screening

Cystic fibrosis (CF) is a life-shortening genetic disorder that is inherited in an autosomal recessive fashion. CF affects roughly 1 individual per 3000 live births among Caucasians, with lesser gene frequency among different races.[1] The disease is characterized by alterations in the presence or function of the Cystic Fibrosis Transmembrane Conductance Regulator (CFTR) on the membrane of epithelial cells. CFTR functions as a transport channel, and also serves to regulate the function of other membrane channels, helping to control the composition and volume of epithelial secretions.[2] Alterations in airway mucus lead to recurrent sinopulmonary infections, bronchiectasis, and progressive lung disease in many patients, with respiratory failure the most common cause of death among CF patients. CF patients also frequently suffer from pancreatic exocrine insufficiency, leading to malabsorption and malnutrition. As patients with CF age, CF-related diabetes mellitus (CFRD) is an increasing complication, which may further complicate their level of nutrition and pulmonary function.[3] Lung and/or liver transplantation may be performed in those with advanced disease.

Advances in the care of patients with CF have led to significant prolongation in survival, with median survival increasing from 18 years in 1980 to 37.4 years in 2008.[4] The improved health and longevity of CF women naturally leads to a larger number who may become or desire to become pregnant. The presence of dysfunction in the lungs, pancreas, reproductive tract, and other organs can pose significant challenges to the CF pregnancy (**Table 1**).

FERTILITY

Men

Men with CF usually manifest impaired fertility, with more than 95% of men infertile without assisted reproductive techniques.[5] Congenital bilateral absence of the vas deferens (CBAVD) is commonly present, and is thought to result from in utero involution due to obstruction by desiccated secretions.[6] The absence of the vas deferens is generally identifiable by palpation. The epididymis and seminal vesicles may also be atrophic.[7] Semen from men with CF has been found to be of low volume, with low pH and low fructose levels.[4,7] Testicular spermatogenesis is generally, though not universally, preserved.

Men with CF wishing to father children should undergo semen analysis to assess for azospermia.[8] Assisted reproductive techniques, including microsurgical epididymal sperm aspiration (MESA), percutaneous epididymal sperm aspiration (PESA) or testicular sperm harvesting, either through testicular aspiration or biopsy. MESA provides larger amounts of sperm than PESA, often allowing enough sperm to attempt fertilization across multiple cycles. PESA may require repetition if pregnancy is not achieved in the first cycle. Intracytoplasmic sperm injection may be used over conventional in vitro fertilization because of the relatively low number of sperm harvested.[8] Meniru and colleagues[9] were able to successfully harvest sperm by either aspiration or testicular biopsy in 100% of 62 patients with CBAVD. Uniform success was also noted by Hubert and colleagues[10] in 25 men with CBAVD.

Section of Pulmonary & Critical Care Medicine, Yale University School of Medicine, 333 Cedar Street, PO Box 208057, New Haven, CT 06520-8057, USA
E-mail address: j.mcardle@cox.net

Clin Chest Med 32 (2011) 111–120
doi:10.1016/j.ccm.2010.10.005
0272-5231/11/$ — see front matter © 2011 Elsevier Inc. All rights reserved.

Table 1
Selected series of pregnancies in women with cystic fibrosis published since 2000

Author/Year	Location	Number	Maternal Outcome	Fetal Outcome	Predictors of Outcome
Edenborough et al,[29] 2000	UK	72	65% with intravenous antibiotics during pregnancy Median survival following birth 11.9 y	70% live births 46% preterm	Maternal FEV$_1$ below 60% associated with prematurity
Gilljam et al,[32] 2000	Canada	92	80% live births 19% maternal mortality at mean follow up of 11 y	8% preterm	FEV$_1$ <50% *Burkholderia cepacia* colonization Pancreatic insufficiency associated with maternal mortality, though outcome no worse than for CF population at large
Boyd et al,[33] 2004	UK	84	74% live births Women who became pregnant were healthier than those who did not	17% preterm	
Gillet et al,[30] 2002	France	75	85% live births Mean weight gain 5.5 kg 3 deaths in year after pregnancy	18% preterm 29.8% low weight	FEV$_1$ <50% associated with maternal mortality
Barak et al,[31] 2005	Israel	11	8/11 with spontaneous vaginal deliveries	25% preterm 1 infant with esophageal atresia	
McMullen et al,[25] 2006	USA	216	More use of intravenous antibiotics and hospitalization during pregnancy 20.6% treated for DM during pregnancy	Not reported	Improved 10-y survival rates in those who became pregnant compared with matched controls
Goss et al,[34] 2006	USA	680	67% live births 77% 10-y survival		No lung function cutoff in which pregnancy found to be harmful
Ødegaard et al,[35] 2002	Norway/Sweden	33	Half needed supplementary nutrition	24% preterm	FEV$_1$ <60%, diabetes, liver disease, lower weight gain associated with preterm delivery
Cheng et al,[36] 2006	USA (single center)	43	84% live births TPN use common Postpartum length of stay longer than normal	36% preterm	FEV$_1$ <50% associated with lower infant weight

Abbreviations: DM, diabetes mellitus; FEV$_1$, forced expiratory volume in 1 second; TPN, total parenteral nutrition.

Women

CF is associated with impaired growth, and delays in puberty and menarche, traditionally attributed to pancreatic insufficiency and the nutritional effects of maldigestion and malabsorption in combination with chronic illness.[11] Delays in menarche relative to non-CF controls has been noted even in those who are well nourished with excellent pulmonary health, raising the question of whether CFTR mutations might have a more direct relationship with reproductive function.[12] For those who have reached menarche, anovulatory cycles have been an important cause of impaired fertility in CF women, again frequently, but not exclusively, due to impaired nutrition and poor overall health. The isolation of CFTR protein in the hypothalamus may suggest central dysregulation of ovulation as a possible mechanism for delays in sexual maturation and abnormalities in ovulation.[13]

CFTR is present in the endometrium, cervical mucosa, and Fallopian tubes. The cervical mucus of women with CF is often thicker and more tenacious than normal, leading to obstruction of the cervical os[14]; this may result in mechanical obstruction to sperm penetration, reducing the likelihood of fertilization. CFTR may also lead to altered ion content of uterine secretions. These secretions are usually rich in bicarbonate ions, and this milieu may play a role in capacitation of sperm (the process by which sperm become capable of fertilization).[15] Bicarbonate ions are secreted by CFTR, and alterations in CFTR presence or function leads to reduced bicarbonate in uterine secretions, potentially impairing the process of sperm capacitation.

Despite these possible impairments to fertility, many women with CF are able to conceive normally. Misperceptions about fertility may lead to poor advice regarding contraception by health care providers.[16] Women with CF should be assumed to be capable of conception when they become sexually active, and advised accordingly regarding contraception.

GENETIC SCREENING

For women with CF desiring pregnancy, determination of her CF genotype should be performed if unknown, and carrier screening for her partner should be offered.[17] There are currently more than 1400 gene defects described that can lead to CF.[17] The genetic testing currently available is less than 100% sensitive, with significant variations in sensitivity given the different gene frequencies among different ethnic groups. Given a gene frequency of roughly 1:25 among Caucasians,

the likelihood of a woman with CF giving birth to a child with CF would be expected to be 1 in 50 if the father belonged to this ethnic group. Negative carrier screening has different implications depending on the sensitivity of the test used. Screening tests with 85%, 90%, or 95% sensitivity would be expected to reduce the risk of being a carrier from 1:25 to 1:165, 1:246, and 1:491, respectively if the partner tested negative.[18] While negative testing would be associated with a decreased risk of giving birth to an affected child, no test currently available provides 100% assurance against having a child with CF.

Psychosocial counseling is also advisable in women with CF who desire pregnancy. An open dialog, with free expression of reproductive desires and fears, is optimal. It should be recognized that the desire to have children may result in a decision not to follow the medical advice provided, and women should be confident of the support of their treatment team if their decision runs counter to the team's recommendations.[19] It is often necessary, particularly in those with advanced lung disease, to discuss challenging topics, including the rigors of pregnancy and its impact on women with impaired lung function, the need for frequent prenatal visits to assure optimization of the mother's health status, the demands of caring for an infant and toddler and the impact these may have on self care, and the very real possibility that the mother may die or require lung transplantation while the child is still young. It is important that these issues be handled delicately but openly, with the understanding that such topics may be very difficult for some women to face. Psychological support should be available for those in need, as depression, anxiety, anger, or grief may become more difficult to manage in the face of such reproductive challenges.

MEDICATION USE DURING PREGNANCY

The medical regimen for patients with CF is often complex, with the use of pancreatic enzyme supplements, inhaled, oral or intravenous antibiotics, mucolytics, and anti-inflammatory medications and others commonly employed to combat manifestations of this illness. Considerations during pregnancy include timing of exposure, with certain medications manifesting teratogenicity during organogenesis in the first trimester and others posing risks to organ function, growth, and viability later in pregnancy.[17] It is uncommon for drugs to be tested during pregnancy unless they are intended specifically for use during pregnancy. Extrapolations about safety include results of animal studies, clinical experience during pregnancy in humans, and knowledge about how the mechanism of action would be expected to affect pregnancy. The health and well-being of the mother should be primary in making decisions about medication use in CF pregnancies, particularly in the setting of infectious exacerbations, which are an important cause of morbidity and declining lung function in CF patients.

Antibiotics

Oral antibiotics are commonly employed both for periods of exacerbation and as chronic therapy in patients with CF. Azithromycin, when used 3 times weekly as maintenance therapy, has been demonstrated to improve lung function and decrease the frequency of infectious exacerbations in patients with CF who are chronically colonized with Pseudomonas aeruginosa.[20] Available human data suggest there is probably no risk from this agent during pregnancy, though the long-term use in CF differs from the more commonly used short-course therapy in which this experience is derived. Quinolones are frequently used to treat infectious exacerbations in nonpregnant patients but are usually avoided during pregnancy. Animal data during pregnancy reveal an association with cartilage dyscrasias, though similar problems have not been seen with human use.[21] Penicillins and cephalosporin use during pregnancy appears to be safe based on available experience.[17] Trimethoprim-sulfamethoxazole use is generally avoided during the first and third trimesters of pregnancy, with trimethoprim associated with neural defects during the first trimester and sulfonamides associated with icterus of the newborn with third-trimester use. Tetracyclines should be avoided during the second and third trimesters because of tooth and bone discoloration in the fetus. Rifamycins should also be avoided during pregnancy, as first-trimester use is associated with fetal damage in animals and third-trimester use may increase bleeding risks for mother and neonate.[17]

Among intravenous antibiotics, imipenem has demonstrated fetal damage in animals, and carbapenems should be avoided during pregnancy.[17] Aminoglycosides such as gentamicin and tobramycin can be associated with nephrotoxicity and damage to the eighth cranial nerve. However, they have been used safely in CF and other patients during pregnancy, and may be used during pregnancy with close attention to drug levels, with once-daily dosing preferable.[22] There are few data on the use of vancomycin during pregnancy, and though there is no evidence of harm, it should be used with caution.

Inhalational use of antibiotics is frequently employed in patients with CF to reduce the frequency of infectious exacerbations or improve lung function. Commonly used antibiotics for inhalation include tobramycin, colistimethate, and aztreonam. The systemic absorption of these agents is low, and while concerns exist about fetal harm with aminoglycoside and colistimethate use during pregnancy, these low levels of absorption suggest that use during pregnancy is likely safe.[11,23]

Mucolytics

Recombinant human DNase (dornase alpha) is a useful mucolytic in patients with CF, owing to the high concentration of extracellular DNA in CF sputum.[24] There are few data on the use of dornase in pregnancy. Most series describing CF pregnancies make no mention of the frequency of dornase use during these pregnancies. McMullen and colleagues[25] examined data from the Epidemiologic Study of Cystic Fibrosis (ESCF), a longitudinal database of 24,000 individuals with CF living in the United States and Canada. The investigators reported on 216 pregnancies and noted that 39.4% of women received dornase during pregnancy. However, this study was intended to evaluate the impact of pregnancy on women with CF, and no comparison of birth outcomes between the groups was undertaken. Hypertonic saline use is associated with a decrease in infectious exacerbations in CF patients, and is unlikely to pose any risk to mother or fetus.[26]

Others

Pancreatic enzyme replacement therapy is required in a large majority of CF patients because of the maldigestion associated with pancreatic insufficiency. These agents appear to pose no significant risk during pregnancy. Acid suppressive therapy is frequently used with pancreatic enzyme replacement, and proton pump inhibitors are considered safe for use in pregnancy.[17] Fat soluble vitamins, including vitamins A, D, E, and K, are frequently supplemented in CF patients. These agents are considered safe at prophylactic doses. Vitamin A doses should be less than 10,000 IU daily, as higher doses used early in pregnancy are associated with neural crest defects.[14] Among glucose-lowering drugs, insulins are not associated with teratogenesis. Sulfonylureas are not felt to be associated with teratogenic risks but pose a risk for neonatal hypoglycemia, and therefore insulin is the preferred agent. Thiazolidinediones such as pioglitazone manifest fetal toxicity in animals, and should be avoided.[17]

IMPACT ON MATERNAL LUNG FUNCTION AND MORTALITY

The first report of a "successful" pregnancy by a CF female, published in 1960, included the sobering fact that the mother succumbed to her illness 6 weeks after delivery.[27] Concern for the impact of pregnancy on maternal lung function and mortality was further raised by the publication by Edenborough and colleagues[28] of the results of 22 pregnancies between 1982 and 1992 in 20 women with CF seen at 3 centers in England. In their series, mothers lost an average of 13% of their forced expiratory volume in 1 second (FEV_1) and 11% of their forced vital capacity (FVC) during pregnancy, though function returned to prepregnancy baseline in the majority after delivery. Eighteen of the pregnancies resulted in live births, with 6 of the 18 births occurring after preterm cesarean section precipitated by declining pulmonary health in the mother. Four of the 6 mothers with a baseline FEV_1 under 60% predicted died within 3.2 years of giving birth. All mothers with FEV_1 greater than 60% remained alive during follow-up. There was one tension pneumothorax during the third trimester of pregnancy, which was successfully treated.[28] Edenborough and colleagues[29] published a second series reporting on 72 pregnancies in 55 CF women between 1977 and 1996 from 11 CF centers in the United Kingdom (this series included the 22 pregnancies in the previously mentioned series). The investigators noted that 65% of pregnancies required intravenous antibiotics for respiratory symptoms. Ten of these patients underwent premature caesarean delivery for reasons of infection and decreasing lung function, 2 of whom suffered from pneumothorax. Mothers with lower FEV_1 (<60% predicted) at baseline were more likely to deliver prematurely and demonstrate decreased weight gain than those with higher lung function at baseline. Twelve of the mothers, accounting for 17 pregnancies and 13 live births, died in follow-up, with 7 of the children younger than 5 years and 10 younger than 10 years at the time of the mother's death.[29]

Gillet and colleagues[30] performed a retrospective study of the French CF Registry, and reported on 90 pregnancies in 80 women between 1980 and 1999. This study matched these patients to a group of nonpregnant CF patients with the same genotype followed in the same care center network. During pregnancy, 77.5% of women received intravenous antibiotics as compared with 59.1% before pregnancy, suggesting either increased exacerbation frequency or lowered threshold to administer intravenous therapy in this group. Declines in lung function from before to after pregnancy did not significantly differ between the pregnant patients and controls. One death occurred during pregnancy, in a woman with prepregnancy FEV_1 of 61%, with death related to *Pseudomonas* sepsis. Three women died within 1 year of giving birth, all of whom had FEV_1 under 50% predicted at baseline. All told, maternal mortality within 1 year of birth was 15% for those with baseline FEV_1 under 50% predicted and 3% in those with FEV_1 above 50% predicted.[30]

Subsequent series have demonstrated less ominous results. Barak and colleagues[31] reported on 8 CF women with 11 pregnancies. Four of these 11 women had baseline FEV_1 under 50% predicted, only 1 of whom experienced a significant decline in lung function during pregnancy. In all, 10 of the 11 pregnancies were associated with stable pulmonary function. Gilljam and colleagues[32] analyzed data from the Toronto CF database from 1961 to 1998 and identified 92 pregnancies in 54 women. Pregnancy was not associated with greater declines in lung function than in the general CF population. In a mean follow-up time of 11 years, 19% of the women had died, with prepregnancy FEV_1 less than 50%, colonization with *Burkholderia cepacia*, and pancreatic insufficiency associated with decreased survival. Mortality in this cohort was not altered by pregnancy when compared with the entire adult female cohort.[32] Boyd and colleagues[33] reported a population-based cohort from the United Kingdom gleaned from the UK CF Database. These investigators found that CF women who became pregnant had an earlier age at diagnosis, were less likely to have an FEV_1 below 50%, and were less commonly homozygous for the deltaF508 mutation, suggesting that those achieving pregnancy were healthier than the CF population at large.[33] McMullen and colleagues[25] examined data from 1995 to 2003 in the Epidemiologic Study of Cystic Fibrosis (ESCF), a longitudinal observational study in the United States and Canada. A total of 216 women with at least one pregnancy were compared with a matched group of never-pregnant women at prepregnancy, intrapregnancy, and postpregnancy time periods. Declines in FEV_1 were seen in both groups from the baseline to follow-up period, with no significant difference between the pregnant and nonpregnant groups. The patients who became pregnant had an increased frequency of hospitalization and treatment of exacerbation during the period of pregnancy, despite similar rates in the year before pregnancy.[25] Again it remains unclear whether the pregnant cohort became ill more frequently, or was more likely to report symptoms or have the symptoms addressed more aggressively during pregnancy. Goss and colleagues[34] conducted a parallel cohort study on all women older than 12 years enrolled in the US CF Foundation National Patient Registry from 1985 to 1997. The study found that women who reported pregnancy had higher lung function at baseline than those who did not, as well as higher body weight, suggesting that better overall health was associated with a desire or ability to become pregnant. Women who became pregnant had improved 10-year survival (77% vs 58%). These results held true for those with an FEV_1 of less than 40% before pregnancy as well as in those with diabetes mellitus (DM).[34] Pregnancy did not appear to increase mortality in this population as compared with nonpregnant controls. Ødegaard and colleagues[35] reported on 23 women with 33 pregnancies followed at CF centers in Sweden and Norway, and found that women with lower baseline lung function were more likely to deliver prematurely. The group as a whole, however, did not manifest a decline in lung function during pregnancy, but did receive more intravenous antibiotics during pregnancy than in the year before or following pregnancy. Women with low lung function were more likely to deliver preterm, but did not have accelerated decline in lung function compared with those with FEV_1 greater than 60% predicted.[35] Lastly, a single-center study from the University of Washington reported outcomes of 43 pregnancies among 25 CF women.[36] Twenty-four of these women delivered live infants, of whom 16 had their obstetric care at the University of Washington Medical Center. Seven of the 16 women had FEV_1 under 50% predicted. A lower FEV_1 at the beginning of pregnancy was associated with lower birth weight, more days of hospitalization, and intravenous antibiotics, though gestational age at delivery was similar to those with higher lung function at baseline. Eleven of the patients had their vaginal deliveries induced, 9 of these owing to nutritional or pulmonary decompensation on the part of the mother. One maternal death occurred 28 days postpartum in a woman with prepregnancy FEV_1 of 37% predicted. A very aggressive nutritional management strategy was used in this cohort, with 6 of 16 women receiving total parenteral nutrition during their pregnancy.[36]

On balance, there appears to be evidence for increased use of antibiotics and hospitalization during pregnancy in women with CF, but no clear FEV_1 cutoff predictive of poor maternal outcome. There is no convincing evidence that pregnancy itself is associated with increased maternal mortality or accelerated loss of lung function.

NUTRITION AND DIABETES MELLITUS DURING PREGNANCY

Women with CF are frequently affected by pancreatic insufficiency and malabsorption, in conjunction with increased resting energy expenditure, which makes low body weight and malnutrition important concerns in CF women even in the absence of pregnancy. The increase in resting energy expenditure during pregnancy can make weight gain during pregnancy challenging. Patients with CF also develop increasing rates of glucose intolerance with age, due to decreased insulin production, impaired insulin sensitivity, and increased hepatic glucose production. The rates of CFRD may be greater than 50% in patients older than 30 years when rigorous screening is employed.[37]

Gestational diabetes is caused by impaired tissue insulin sensitivity related to secretion of leptin, prolactin, cortisol, and placental lactogen as well as pregnancy-induced weight gain, caloric intake, and decreased physical activity.[38] Pregnancies complicated by gestational diabetes have increased rates of several complications, including macrosomia, polyhydramnios, preeclampsia, and metabolic abnormalities in the neonate among others.[39–41] Gilljam and colleagues[3] noted the development of gestational diabetes in 14% of 54 women who developed pregnancy between 1961 and 1998 in addition to 3 women who had CFRD before pregnancy, suggesting rates of gestational DM higher than seen in the general population. Hardin and colleagues[42] evaluated the metabolic impact of pregnancy in 8 pregnant women with CF and compared them with 8 CF women who were not pregnant and 9 pregnant women without CF. Of the 8 pregnant women with CF, 7 developed gestational diabetes as screened by oral glucose tolerance test (OGTT) by the end of the second trimester. The CF women, pregnant or nonpregnant, manifested a higher resting energy expenditure compared with the pregnant women without CF. Hepatic glucose production (HGP) was higher in CF subjects with impaired suppression of HGP by insulin as compared with pregnant women without CF. Rates of protein turnover were significantly higher in both groups of CF patients. Insulin resistance and HGP increased in both CF pregnancies and non-CF pregnancies, though women with CF had baseline impairments in each, leading to greater incidence of gestational DM.[42] Women with CF who are considering pregnancy should be screened with an OGTT to detect occult CFRD prior to pregnancy as well as during pregnancy to detect gestational DM.[17] The preferred treatment for CFRD is insulin, with too few data existing on the use of oral agents to routinely recommend their use.[3]

Pregnancy poses significant energy cost, with estimates of 80,000 kilocalories required for a 60-kg woman through pregnancy.[43] Weight gain of at least 11 kg is recommended,[44] with higher levels advocated for those with a prepregnancy body mass index (BMI; calculated as body weight divided by height squared) of less than 19.8 kg/m^2. Pancreatic insufficiency leads to malabsorption of fats, and chronic lung disease can increase energy expenditure in patients with CF, making weight gain challenging for the CF pregnancy. Low BMI in pregnancy is associated with both premature delivery and low birth weight.[45] In addition to the increased caloric needs and energy expenditure, reflux symptoms, common in both CF and pregnancy, may limit the ability to use nutritional supplements or nasogastric feeding in CF pregnancies. Cheng and colleagues,[36] in reporting pregnancy outcomes at their center at the University of Washington, achieved a median weight gain of 10.9 kg for their pregnant population as a whole and used total parenteral nutrition (TPN) for support of patients with poor weight gain. These patients had demonstrated lower weight gain and higher rates of prematurity than those not requiring TPN, though infant weight was appropriate for gestational age in each group. While the optimal nutritional strategy remains incompletely defined, the use of nasogastric, gastrostomy, or parenteral routes of nutritional support may be helpful in optimizing weight gain for the CF patient failing to gain weight or losing weight during pregnancy.

BIRTH OUTCOMES OF CF PREGNANCIES

Several different series have provided data for birth outcomes of CF pregnancies. There does not appear to be evidence that pregnancy in patients with CF is associated with an increased risk of fetal demise or birth defects. The majority of CF pregnancies result in live births, ranging from 67% to 85% in series from the United States, United Kingdom, Canada, and France.[29,30,32–34] These results do not differ from pregnancy outcomes in women without CF. The most common complication of CF pregnancies is preterm delivery, with attendant risks of prematurity to the newborn. Barak and colleagues[31] reported a 25% preterm delivery rate in their Israeli cohort, with prematurity associated with low prepregnancy lung function. The series by Ødegaard and colleagues[35] of 33 pregnancies from Norway and Sweden reported a preterm delivery rate of 24%, noting an association between low maternal weight gain and lower lung function with prematurity. Of their 6 women with prepregnancy FEV$_1$ below 60%, 4 delivered prematurely (67%) as opposed to 15% in those with an FEV$_1$ above 60%. Gillet and colleagues[30] reported an 18% preterm delivery rate and 29.8% of infants with low birth weight in their review of 90 pregnancies reported to the French CF Registry. In their series, low baseline FVC was associated with preterm labor. Edenborough and colleagues[29] reported a 46% prematurity rate among 48 live births in their cohort from the United Kingdom. The group who delivered prematurely had a mean FEV$_1$ of 60% as opposed to 80% in those who delivered at term. DM was also more common among those delivering prematurely. The Toronto CF database reported a low rate of prematurity, with only 6 of 74 deliveries occurring prematurely, with no differences in prematurity in those with FEV$_1$ above and below 50% predicted.[32] Most available data would suggest an increased risk for prematurity in pregnancy involving women with CF, with a suggestion that pregnancies occur in women with lower prepregnancy lung function and that diabetes is more likely to deliver preterm.

OBSTETRIC AND POSTPARTUM CONSIDERATIONS

An obstetrician with experience in high-risk pregnancies is a crucial part of the treatment team, along with a physician with expertise in the care of CF, a nutritionist, and an anesthesiologist.[43] Antenatal visits should occur every 4 weeks through the second trimester, every 2 weeks thereafter, and weekly close to term, with careful attention to weight gain, glucose tolerance, and respiratory status in addition to usual obstetric care.[17] During delivery, implantable venous access devices should not be relied on as the sole means of intravenous access, as they do not have the capability of supporting large volume fluid infusions should they be necessary. Vaginal delivery is the norm in CF pregnancies, with guidelines recommending cesarean section for maternal compromise such as deteriorating lung function or for fetal indications similar to non-CF pregnancies.[17] Epidural analgesia can serve to reduce the respiratory and cardiovascular work of labor, and is recommended in recently published pregnancy guidelines. Forceps or ventouse assistance may be used in women with compromised respiratory status to shorten the second stage of labor.[43]

In cases where cesarean section is necessary, spinal epidural or pure epidural anesthesia offers the possibility of optimizing postpartum pain control to allow more effective chest physiotherapy in the immediate postpartum period. In cases where general anesthesia is necessary, the involvement of an intensivist for assistance with ventilatory management may be warranted.[17]

Breast feeding results in an increased maternal caloric intake, and may not be appropriate for women with severe nutritional failure. Cheng and colleagues[36] noted that all mothers in their single-center series had a return to prepregnancy weight within 2 months of delivery, reflecting a weight loss in CF mothers that is more rapid than in the general population. Ongoing attention to nutrition and continued adherence to medications and chest physiotherapy is important in the postpartum period, as the demands of caring for an infant with attendant sleep deprivation may compromise the mother's ability to perform self care. It may be helpful to actively engage the woman's partner or other family members to allow adequate time for the woman to complete her routine daily CF regimen. Breast feeding should not deter the physician from aggressive treatment of respiratory exacerbations, though care should be taken to assess all medications for safety in women who are breast feeding.

PREGNANCY FOLLOWING LUNG TRANSPLANTATION

Lung transplantation offers improved quality of life to patients with CF and advanced lung disease.[46] Successful pregnancies following transplant of other solid organs such as heart, liver, and kidneys have been reported, with no significant risk of increased congenital anomalies or neonatal infections. Chronic rejection remains a significant challenge after lung transplantation. Outcomes for lung transplant recipients remain inferior to those seen with other solid organs.[47] The International Society for Heart and Lung Transplantation reports 5-year survival rates of 51% and 10-year survival rates of 28%, though a large study from the United Kingdom reported 10-year survival rates of 51%.[47,48]

Gyi and colleagues[49] reported the outcomes of 4 pregnancies in CF transplant recipients and combined results for 6 prior pregnancies found in the literature. In these 10 pregnancies, 9 resulted in live births and 1 pregnancy was terminated. Of the 9 births, 5 were premature and with low birth weight, but no fetal anomalies were reported.

Among the mothers, prepregnancy evidence for chronic rejection was present and an additional 3 developed rejection during pregnancy; this was associated with progressive decline in lung function postpartum. The National Lung Transplantation Pregnancy Registry, established in 1991, reported results on 14 lung transplant pregnancies, not confined to CF patients, and noted a 63% rate of prematurity, 53% risk of hypertension during pregnancy, and 27% incidence of a rejection episode during pregnancy. Fifty-three percent of the pregnancies ended in a live birth, with 33% terminated and 13% resulting in spontaneous abortions.[50]

A physician experienced in the management of transplant recipients and CF is essential. Careful follow-up of calcineurin inhibitor use during pregnancy is warranted, as dose increases may be required.[46] Although abundant data are lacking, therapy is likely with common immunosuppressants including prednisone, azathioprine, tacrolimus, and cyclosporine A.[46] Based on case series, it is considered unlikely that azathioprine increases the risk of congenital anomalies, although a recent report of 476 pregnancies with azathioprine exposure for the treatment of mostly inflammatory bowel disease and systemic lupus erythematosis[51] showed an association between medication exposure and atrial or ventricular septal defect based on 7 affected exposed children (adjusted odds ratio 3.18, 95% confidence interval 1.45–6.04). The odds ratio decreased a small amount when corrected to concomitant drug exposure, and it is possible that this finding may have been due to chance, the underlying disease, and potentially an ascertainment bias whereby the diagnosis of these defects is dependent on the extent that fetal or neonatal echocardiography is performed. Based on experimental animal studies and human case reports, tacrolimus is not expected to increase the risk of congenital anomalies. However, the existing data do not establish its safety. Experimental animal studies do not predict an increase in congenital anomalies after pregnancy exposure to cyclosporin. A small number of human cases are also reassuring. Women should be screened frequently for viremia due to herpes simplex virus and cytomegalovirus, with therapy initiated accordingly. Women should be screened for hypertension, renal dysfunction, and preeclampsia frequently, and should undergo regular assessment of graft function because of the risk of rejection. Current recommendations are to wait a period of at least 2 years after transplantation prior to pregnancy, such that graft function and the presence of obliterative bronchiolitis can be assessed.[46]

SUMMARY

As women with CF enter adulthood with improved health, the desire to bear and raise children is not infrequent. Careful assessment of health, including nutrition, lung function, and glucose tolerance status should be undertaken for women with CF considering pregnancy. Although pregnancy poses considerable physiologic stress, there is no clear evidence that the outcome of women with CF who become pregnant is any worse than for the population of CF women at large. The pregnancies may require intensive use of medical resources and more frequent hospitalizations to optimize maternal and fetal outcome. However, the shortened survival conferred by CF does lead to high rates of maternal death before the child's tenth birthday.

Genetic counseling and prenatal screening of the partner can be informative regarding the possibility of giving birth to a child with CF. Pregnancies in women with CF are not associated with an increased risk of fetal anomalies, but do carry a significant risk of prematurity and low birth weight, complications that seem to be more likely in those with poor weight gain and poor prepregnancy lung function. Careful attention to the possibility of gestational diabetes and aggressive nutritional management, potentially including tube feeding or parenteral feeding, are recommended to optimize outcome for both mother and child. Lung transplantation poses its own unique challenges, and careful assessment of drug levels, screening for infection, and graft dysfunction are recommended.

REFERENCES

1. Hamosh A, FitzSimmons SC, Macek M, et al. Comparison of the clinical manifestations of cystic fibrosis in black and white patients. J Pediatr 1998; 132(2):255–9.

2. Riordan JR, Rommens JM, Kerem B, et al. Identification of the cystic fibrosis gene: cloning and characterization of complementary DNA. Science 1989; 245(4922):1066–73.

3. Curran DR, McArdle JR, Talwalkar JS. Diabetes mellitus and bone disease in cystic fibrosis. Semin Respir Crit Care Med 2009;30(5):514–30.

4. Cystic Fibrosis Foundation Patient Registry: Annual Data Report 2008. 2009. Available at: http://www. cff.org/UploadedFiles/research/ClinicalResearch/ 2008-Patient-Registry-Report.pdf. Accessed May 19, 2010.

5. Kaplan E, Shwachman H, Perlmutter AD, et al. Reproductive failure in males with cystic fibrosis. N Engl J Med 1968;279(2):65–9.

6. Anguiano A, Oates RD, Amos JA, et al. Congenital bilateral absence of the vas deferens. A primarily genital form of cystic fibrosis. JAMA 1992;267(13): 1794–7.

7. Holsclaw DS. Cystic fibrosis and fertility. Br Med J 1969;3(5666):356.

8. Popli K, Stewart J. Infertility and its management in men with cystic fibrosis: review of literature and clinical practices in the UK. Hum Fertil (Camb) 2007; 10(4):217–21.

9. Meniru GI, Forman RG, Craft IL. Utility of percutaneous epididymal sperm aspiration in situations of unexpected obstructive azoospermia. Hum Reprod 1997;12(5):1013–4.

10. Hubert D, Patrat C, Guibert J, et al. Results of assisted reproductive technique in men with cystic fibrosis. Hum Reprod 2006;21(5):1232–6.

11. Sueblinvong V, Whittaker LA. Fertility and pregnancy: common concerns of the aging cystic fibrosis population. Clin Chest Med 2007;28(2): 433–43.

12. Johannesson M, Landgren BM, Csemiczky G, et al. Female patients with cystic fibrosis suffer from reproductive endocrinological disorders despite good clinical status. Hum Reprod 1998;13(8): 2092–7.

13. Johannesson M, Bogdanovic N, Nordqvist AC, et al. Cystic fibrosis mRNA expression in rat brain: cerebral cortex and medial preoptic area. Neuroreport 1997;8(2):535–9.

14. Oppenheimer EA, Case AL, Esterly JR, et al. Cervical mucus in cystic fibrosis: a possible cause of infertility. Am J Obstet Gynecol 1970;108(4): 673–4.

15. Sutton KA, Jungnickel MK, Florman HM. Of fertility, cystic fibrosis and the bicarbonate ion. Nat Cell Biol 2003;5(10):857–9.

16. Edenborough FP. Pregnancy in women with cystic fibrosis. Acta Obstet Gynecol Scand 2002;81(8): 689–92.

17. Edenborough FP, Borgo G, Knoop C, et al. Guidelines for the management of pregnancy in women with cystic fibrosis. J Cyst Fibros 2008;7(Suppl 1): S2–32.

18. Lemna WK, Feldman GL, Kerem B, et al. Mutation analysis for heterozygote detection and the prenatal diagnosis of cystic fibrosis. N Engl J Med 1990; 322(5):291–6.

19. Simcox AM, Hewison J, Duff AJ, et al. Decision-making about pregnancy for women with cystic fibrosis. Br J Health Psychol 2009;14(Pt 2):323–42.

20. Saiman L, Marshall BC, Mayer-Hamblett N, et al. Azithromycin in patients with cystic fibrosis chronically infected with *Pseudomonas aeruginosa*: a randomized controlled trial. JAMA 2003;290(13):1749–56.

21. Loebstein R, Addis A, Ho E, et al. Pregnancy outcome following gestational exposure to fluoroquinolones: a

multicenter prospective controlled study. Antimicrob Agents Chemother 1998;42(6):1336–9.

22. Czeizel AE, Rockenbauer M, Olsen J, et al. A teratological study of aminoglycoside antibiotic treatment during pregnancy. Scand J Infect Dis 2000;32(3):309–13.

23. Geller DE, Pitlick WH, Nardella PA, et al. Pharmaco-kinetics and bioavailability of aerosolized tobramy-cin in cystic fibrosis. Chest 2002;122(1):219–26.

24. Fuchs HJ, Borowitz DS, Christiansen DH, et al. Effect of aerosolized recombinant human DNase on exacerbations of respiratory symptoms and on pulmonary function in patients with cystic fibrosis. The Pulmozyme Study Group. N Engl J Med 1994; 331(10):637–42.

25. McMullen AH, Pasta DJ, Frederick PD, et al. Impact of pregnancy on women with cystic fibrosis. Chest 2006;129(3):706–11.

26. Elkins MR, Robinson M, Rose BR, et al. A controlled trial of long-term inhaled hypertonic saline in patients with cystic fibrosis. N Engl J Med 2006; 354(3):229–40.

27. Siegel B, Siegel S. Pregnancy and delivery in a patient with cystic fibrosis of the pancreas. Obstet Gynecol 1960;16:438–40.

28. Edenborough FP, Stableforth DE, Webb AK, et al. Outcome of pregnancy in women with cystic fibrosis. Thorax 1995;50(2):170–4.

29. Edenborough FP, Mackenzie WE, Stableforth DE. The outcome of 72 pregnancies in 55 women with cystic fibrosis in the United Kingdom 1977–1996. BJOG 2000;107(2):254–61.

30. Gillet D, de Braekeleer M, Bellis G, et al. Cystic fibrosis and pregnancy. Report from French data (1980–1999). BJOG 2002;109(8):912–8.

31. Barak A, Dulitzki M, Efrati O, et al. Pregnancies and outcome in women with cystic fibrosis. Isr Med Assoc J 2005;7(2):95–8.

32. Gilljam M, Antoniou M, Shin J, et al. Pregnancy in cystic fibrosis. Fetal and maternal outcome. Chest 2000;118(1):85–91.

33. Boyd JM, Mehta A, Murphy DJ. Fertility and preg-nancy outcomes in men and women with cystic fibrosis in the United Kingdom. Hum Reprod 2004; 19(10):2238–43.

34. Goss CH, Rubenfeld GD, Otto K, et al. The effect of pregnancy on survival in women with cystic fibrosis. Chest 2003;124(4):1460–8.

35. Ødegaard I, Stray-Pedersen B, Hallberg K, et al. Maternal and fetal morbidity in pregnancies of Norwegian and Swedish women with cystic fibrosis. Acta Obstet Gynecol Scand 2002;81(8):698–705.

36. Cheng EY, Goss CH, McKone EF, et al. Aggressiv prenatal care results in successful fetal outcome in CF women. J Cyst Fibros 2006;5(2):85–91.

37. Moran A, Hardin D, Rodman D, et al. Diagnosi screening and management of cystic fibrosis relate diabetes mellitus: a consensus conference repor Diabetes Res Clin Pract 1999;45(1):61–73.

38. Kapoor N, Sankaran S, Hyer S, et al. Diabetes pregnancy: a review of current evidence. Cu Opin Obstet Gynecol 2007;19(6):586–90.

39. Metzger BE, Lowe LP, Dyer AR, et al. Hyperglycem and adverse pregnancy outcomes. N Engl J Me 2008;358(19):1991–2002.

40. Dodd JM, Crowther CA, Antoniou G, et al. Screenin for gestational diabetes: the effect of varying bloo glucose definitions in the prediction of advers maternal and infant health outcomes. Aust N Z Obstet Gynaecol 2007;47(4):307–12.

41. Crowther CA, Hiller JE, Moss JR, et al. Effect of trea ment of gestational diabetes mellitus on pregnanc outcomes. N Engl J Med 2005;352(24):2477–86.

42. Hardin DS, Rice J, Cohen RC, et al. The metabol effects of pregnancy in cystic fibrosis. Obstet Gyne col 2005;106(2):367–75.

43. Thorpe-Beeston JG. Contraception and pregnanc in cystic fibrosis. J R Soc Med 2009;102(Suppl 1 3–10.

44. Hilman BC, Aitken ML, Constantinescu M. Preg nancy in patients with cystic fibrosis. Clin Obste Gynecol 1996;39(1):70–86.

45. Kotloff RM, FitzSimmons SC, Fiel SB. Fertility an pregnancy in patients with cystic fibrosis. Clin Ches Med 1992;13(4):623–35.

46. Budev MM, Arroliga AC, Emery S. Exacerbation o underlying pulmonary disease in pregnancy. Cr Care Med 2005;33(Suppl 10):S313–8.

47. Morton J, Glanville AR. Lung transplantation i patients with cystic fibrosis. Semin Respir Crit Car Med 2009;30(5):559–68.

48. Meachery G, De Soyza A, Nicholson A, et a Outcomes of lung transplantation for cystic fibros in a large UK cohort. Thorax 2008;63(8):725–31.

49. Gyi KM, Hodson ME, Yacoub MY. Pregnancy i cystic fibrosis lung transplant recipients: case serie and review. J Cyst Fibros 2006;5(3):171–5.

50. Armenti VT, Radomski JS, Moritz M, et al. Repo from the National Transplantation Pregnanc Registry (NTPR): outcomes of pregnancy after trans plantation. Clin Transpl 2004;103–14.

51. Cleary BJ, Källén B. Early pregnancy azathioprin use and pregnancy outcome. Birth Defects Res Clin Mol Teratol 2009;85:647–54.

Pneumonia Complicating Pregnancy

Veronica Brito, MD[a], Michael S. Niederman, MD[b,c],*

KEYWORDS
- Pregnancy • Pneumonia • Cesarean section • Aspiration

Community-acquired pneumonia (CAP) is a common illness that can be serious, particularly in pregnant patients. Pneumonia is the most common cause of fatal nonobstetric infection in pregnant patients.[1–3] Pneumonia is a cause of respiratory failure in pregnant patients, but newer data suggest that not all pneumonias are more common or more serious in pregnant women than in other populations in contrast to older studies. However, because pneumonia can affect both mother and fetus, it may lead to an increased likelihood of complicated preterm delivery compared with pregnancies in which infection is absent.

The reported incidence of pneumonia in pregnant women varies, probably because of the differences in the populations studied and the timing of the studies. A summary of studies that report the incidence of pneumonia in pregnancy is seen in **Table 1**.[4–8] Incidence of pneumonia of 6 in 1000 deliveries was reported before the seventies, declining in the seventies and eighties; more recent studies showed an increase, which may reflect women with chronic illnesses being able to become pregnant; prevalence of immune deficiencies (such as human immunodeficiency virus [HIV] infection), and rising illicit drug use in pregnant women. Although the incidence of pneumonia in pregnancy has declined, rates may be higher in large urban hospitals than in community settings, because of the pattern of the different populations at risk. Also, the available data generally come from those who are seen in a hospital and may not reflect milder forms of illness seen in a physician's office.

Pneumonia can also present in the postpartum period. Postpartum hospital admissions are generally related to infectious processes. Among the nonobstetric infections, gallbladder disease is the leading cause of postpartum admissions, followed by pneumonia. The odds of being admitted with pneumonia in the postpartum period are more than twice as high for patients who underwent cesarean deliveries compared with vaginal deliveries.[9] This higher prevalence may be due to more abdominal discomfort and splinting after cesarean deliveries. Other potential mechanisms may include comorbidities in patients necessitating cesarean deliveries, which may predispose patients to infections.

There are very few formally collected data sets about nosocomial pneumonia in the pregnant or postpartum patient, but in this category, one form is aspiration pneumonia complicating labor and delivery. Mendelson originally described gastric acid aspiration in obstetric patients undergoing labor and delivery,[10,11] and in the past, as many as 2% of all maternal deaths were due to aspiration.[11] The pregnant woman is physiologically predisposed to aspiration, because of the elevation of the intragastric pressure due to the gravid uterus, a relaxed gastroesophageal sphincter due to the circulating progesterone, and the delayed gastric emptying that accompanies pregnancy. These factors, the sedation and analgesia given during labor, and the vigorous

[a] Pulmonary and Critical Care Medicine, Winthrop-University Hospital, Mineola, NY, USA
[b] Department of Medicine, Winthrop University Hospital, 222 Station Plaza North, Suite 509, Mineola, NY, 11501, USA
[c] Department of Medicine, SUNY at Stony Brook, NY, USA
* Corresponding author. Department of Medicine, Winthrop University Hospital, 222 Station Plaza North, Suite 509, Mineola, NY, 11501.
E-mail address: mniederman@winthrop.org

Clin Chest Med 32 (2011) 121–132
doi:10.1016/j.ccm.2010.10.004
0272-5231/11/$ – see front matter © 2011 Elsevier Inc. All rights reserved.

Table 1
Reported incidence of pneumonia occurring in pregnancy

Study	Year of Publication	Setting	Results
Benedetti et al[4]	1982	89,219 deliveries in a university hospital	0.4 per 1000
Madinger et al[5]	1989	32,179 at a community hospital	0.78 per 1000
Berkowitz and LaSalsa[6]	1990	1120 case records at a large city hospital	2.72 per 1000
Munn et al[7]	1999	Comparison study to identify risk factors associated with antepartum pneumonia (59 cases vs 118 controls)	0.78–2.7 per 1000
Jin et al[8]	2003	Incidence of pneumonia in live births in the province of Alberta, Canada	1.47 per 1000

abdominal palpation during examinations all increase the threat of aspiration. Spinal anesthesia for cesarean section delivery could suppress cough reflex for at least 4 hours after delivery, possibly increasing the risk of aspiration during and after delivery.[12] The incidence of this complication has declined over time, with an increased awareness of the problem and with efforts directed toward prevention. In Mendelson's original series, the incidence was 1 in 667 deliveries,[11,13] but in the 1970s, the rate was as low as 1 in 6000 vaginal deliveries but 1 in 430 cesarean sections. More recent studies of cesarean section patients report a rate of 1 in 1431 to 1 in 1547.[11] Current strategies for raising gastric pH may be especially valuable for the cesarean section patient. Mortality from this complication has been very low in recent years, with 1 death in 9200 pregnancies.[11]

The impacts of pregnancy on pneumonia risk are listed (**Box 1**). Alterations in maternal cellular immunity have been described during pregnancy, especially in the second and third trimester, generally to protect the fetus from rejection by the mother. These include decreased lymphocyte proliferative response, especially in the second and third trimesters; decreased natural killer cell activity; changes in T-cell populations with a decrease in circulating helper T cells; reduced lymphocyte cytotoxic activity; and production of substances by the trophoblast that block maternal recognition of fetal major histocompatibility antigens.[2,14] Hormonal changes during pregnancy, including elevation of progesterone, human gonadotropin, α-fetoprotein, and cortisol, may also inhibit cell-mediated immune function.[14] These changes can predispose to infection with specific pathogens, such as viruses, fungi, and tuberculosis. Catanzaro[15] have shown that the hormonal changes lead to an increase in 17-estradiols, which can enhance the in vitro growth of *Coccidioides immitis*.[15]

Some of the physiologic changes of pregnancy may also predispose pregnant women to a severe pneumonia course, including elevation of the diaphragm by up to 4 cm, decrease in functional residual capacity, increase in oxygen consumption, and increase in lung water.[2,16,17] These alterations may decrease the ability of the pregnant woman to clear respiratory secretions and potentially aggravate airway obstruction associated with pulmonary infections. The elevation of the diaphragm, the associated decrease in functional residual capacity, and the increase in oxygen consumption during pregnancy make the pregnant woman less able to tolerate even brief periods of hypoxia, particularly in the third trimester.

ETIOLOGY OF PNEUMONIA IN PREGNANCY

The available data on infectious agents causing pneumonia in pregnancy show similar results to the pathogens that can cause lung infection in nonpregnant adults. These data are derived mainly from observational, and often retrospective, studies in which only routine microbiological investigations have been used. Sputum and blood cultures were the main methods of diagnosis (**Box 2**).[2,17] Hopwood[18] identified a cause in only 9 of 23 cases, with a mixture of gram-positive bacteria, gram-negative bacteria, and influenza A virus. Benedetti and colleagues[4] found a bacterial pathogen in 21 of 39 patients, with pneumococcus being the predominant pathogen accounting for 13 cases and *Hemophilus influenzae*, the next most common pathogen. Madinger and colleagues[5] also found *Streptococcus pneumoniae* (pneumococcus) to be the most common and *H influenzae*, the second-most common pathogen isolated. In these studies, serologic testing was rarely performed to search for atypical pathogens, such as *Mycoplasma* or *Chlamydophila*. Berkowitz and

Box 1
Alterations in pregnancy leading to an increased incidence and risk of complications from pneumonia

Immunologic changes

    Reduced lymphocyte proliferative response

    Diminished cell-mediated cytotoxicity

    Reduced number of helper T cells

    Reduced lymphokine response to alloantigens

Maternal physiologic changes

    Increase in oxygen consumption

    Increase in lung water

    Elevation of diaphragm

    Aspiration more likely in labor and delivery

Coexisting illnesses/habits

    Smoking

    Anemia

    Asthma

    Cystic fibrosis

    Illicit drug use

    HIV infection

    Recent viral respiratory infection of influenza

    Immunosuppressive illness and therapy

    Placental abruption

Labor and delivery

    Increases risk of aspiration pneumonia (can be modified)

Data from Khan S, Niederman MS. Pneumonia in the pregnant patient. In: Rosene-Montela K, Bourjeily G, editors. Pulmonary problems in pregnancy. New York (NY): Humana Press; 2009. p. 177—96.

Box 2
Bacteriology of pneumonia in pregnancy (in decreasing order of frequency)

Streptococcus pneumoniae (including drug-resistant streptococcus pneumonia)

Hemophilus influenzae

No pathogens identified

Atypical pneumonia agents:

    Legionella species (more common in severe pneumonia)

    Mycoplasma pneumoniae

    Chlamydophila pneumoniae

Viral agents

    Influenza A

    Varicella

Staphylococcus aureus (including methicillin-resistant strains)

Pseudomonas aeruginosa (with bronchiectasis, cystic fibrosis)

Aspiration

Fungi

    Coccidioidomycosis

Pneumocystis jiroveci (with HIV infection)

Data from Khan S, Niederman MS. Pneumonia in the pregnant patient. In: Rosene-Montela K, Bourjeily G, editors. Pulmonary problems in pregnancy. New York (NY): Humana Press; 2009. p. 177—96.

LaSala[6] also found pneumococcus and *H influenzae* to be the most common pathogens.

These studies are limited by a lack of comprehensive diagnostic testing, but even today, routine diagnostic testing is not recommended,[19] and even when performed, the yield is affected by type of material analyzed (sputum, bronchial washing, blood cultures), whether the patient was receiving antibiotics at the time of study, and whether serologies and antigen detection are performed. Atypical pathogens are not identified by routine cultures of sputum, yet are common causes of pneumonia in the nonpregnant patient. As described in numerous case reports and selected limited series, CAP in pregnancy may be caused by mumps, infectious mononucleosis, swine influenza, influenza A, including the novel H1N1 virus, *Staphylococcus aureus* (including methicillin-resistant forms), legionella, varicella, *Chlamydophila pneumoniae*, coccidioidomycosis, and other fungal pneumonias.[3,15,20–26] Whether infection with any of these agents is more common in pregnancy than in the nonpregnant state is unknown, but certain pathogens represent a greater hazard to the pregnant woman, because of her physiologic defects in cell-mediated immunity.

During pregnancy, varicella has been reported in 1 to 5 per 10,000 births, and the complications present a challenge for clinicians, mother, and fetus. With varicella, pneumonia usually complicates primary infection in 0.3% to 1.8% of all cases, but as many as 9% of primary cases during pregnancy can be complicated by pneumonia.[27] Influenza A is a common infection in pregnant women during epidemics and carries a higher mortality than in the nonpregnant patient,[25] with the maternal mortality rates being as high as 30% to 50% in the 1918 epidemic.[2,3,17,28] In the

Asian flu epidemic of 1957 to 1958, 10% of all deaths occurred in pregnant women, and almost 50% of women of childbearing age who died were pregnant.[25,29] This increased mortality was especially noted in the third trimester. During the 2009 to 2010 H1N1 influenza epidemic, severe illness caused by influenza was seen in pregnant women, increasing their morbidity and mortality and impacting the health of mother and fetus. Pregnant patients with H1N1 who were hospitalized showed an increased risk of obstetric complications, including premature and emergency cesarean delivery, and an increased risk of fetal complications, such as fetal distress and fetal death. Antivirals given early in the presentation of the disease seemed to improve outcomes in these patients.[30]

Another viral infection documented in pregnancy was severe acute respiratory syndrome (SARS) infection caused by a coronavirus. One series[31] described 12 patients with SARS during pregnancy, with 7 in the first trimester, and 5 in the second and third. Overall mortality was 25%, with half being admitted to the intensive care unit (ICU) and one-third requiring mechanical ventilation. Fetal complications were common, with 4 of the 7 infections that occurred in the first trimester leading to spontaneous abortion and most of the others leading to preterm labor and babies that were small for gestational age.

Other current microbiologic considerations should be recognized in patients with CAP. Up to 40% of S pneumoniae may be antibiotic-resistant (drug-resistant streptococcus pneumonia [DRSP]). In vitro resistance of S pneumoniae is fairly low level in many cases; however, the impact of such resistance on outcomes when usual therapies are administered is difficult to document.[19] If the patient has received any antibiotic in the 3 months preceding CAP and the pneumonia is due to pneumococcus, the organism is more likely to be resistant to an agent that was recently used.[32] In addition to recent antibiotic therapy, another risk of DRSP is exposure to a child in day care, a potentially common risk for women who are pregnant.[19] Community-acquired strains of methicillin—resistant S aureus (CA-MRSA) are not being reported commonly but may cause serious forms of CAP after influenza infection.[33] The organism can lead to a severe, bilateral necrotizing infection, because of the production of various toxins, including the Panton-Valentine leukocidin. Although this organism most commonly leads to skin and soft tissue infection, there is a case report of a severe necrotizing pneumonia due to CA-MRSA, which seeded the lung 9 days postpartum from septic pelvic thrombophlebitis because of an infected episiotomy site.[34] Two other recent case reports[35,36] of CA-MRSA in the fourteenth week of pregnancy in a 21-year-old woman and in a woman in her thirty-second week of pregnancy described successful treatment with a combination of linezolid and rifampin. In the second case, clindamycin, an agent that can reduce bacterial toxin production and serve as an antibacterial agent was also added. Aspiration is a form of pneumonia that can be a postpartum or obstetric complication, causing a chemical pneumonitis or a bacterial infection involving the pathogens found in the oropharynx and gastric contents, primarily anaerobes and gram-negative enteric organisms.

CLINICAL FEATURES AND MANAGEMENT OF BACTERIAL/ATYPICAL PATHOGEN PNEUMONIA
Clinical Findings

The clinical presentations of pneumonia during pregnancy has not been found to differ substantially from the findings in nonpregnant adults and include fever, cough, pleuritic chest pain, rigors, chills, sputum production, and dyspnea.[37–39] A report by Ramsey and Ramin[39] found that 9.3% of pregnant pneumonia patients reported a productive cough; 32.2%, shortness of breath; and 27.1%, pleuritic chest pain.

Disease Severity

Although most women do not have multilobar illness,[4] in one series, the presence of this finding was correlated with a greater risk of a complicated course of illness, a finding also seen in nonpregnant patients.[40] Many different methods are used to define severity of illness in patients with CAP, but the Pneumonia Severity Index (PSI), which incorporates historical data, laboratory information, and physical findings, developed in the United States, can help to define the need for inpatient and ICU care.[41] The PSI uses a complex scoring system assessment of patient age, comorbidity, and laboratory and clinical data to define a patient's risk of death. The calculated score is used to place the patient into one of 5 groups, each with increasing mortality risk. In its original derivation, pregnant patients were omitted, but Shariatzadeh and Marrie[38] have observed that all pregnant patients evaluated by them fell into the low-risk classes I and II, similar to age-matched controls. However, twice as many pregnant patients were hospitalized as age-matched controls with similar PSI scores yet with a shorter length of stay. Thus, the PSI may underestimate the need for inpatient care in pregnancy, or physicians were being more cautious with admitting pregnant women even in there was a fairly low predicted mortality risk. Similarly, Yost and colleagues[40] found that a PSI-based recommendation would have meant that two–thirds of admitted pregnant CAP patients could have been sent home, but if this had been done, 10 of 79 would probably have required readmission because of a complicated course.

Although guidelines suggest criteria for ICU admission in the CAP patient, these recommendations should probably be liberalized for the pregnant patient, because of a reduced physiologic ability to tolerate hypoxemia. Also, if certain infections are present, such as varicella-zoster or other viruses, the potential for rapid progression in pregnancy is high enough that expectant ICU observation may be justified. In the H1N1 epidemic, the hospitalization rate in pregnant women was 4 times higher than in the general population and was associated with a high risk of death and ICU admission.[42] Also, death from H1N1 in pregnant women was more common than for seasonal influenza.[43] Criteria for severe CAP used in the new American Thoracic Society/Infectious Diseases Society of America (ATS/IDSA) guidelines but not specific to pregnant women include the presence of at least one major criterion, such as the need for mechanical ventilation or septic shock requiring vasopressors, or the presence of 3 minor criteria.[19] The minor criteria include respiratory rate of at least 30 breaths per minute, PaO_2/FiO_2 ratio less than or equal to 250 mm Hg, multilobar infiltrates, confusion or disorientation, blood urea nitrogen greater than or equal to 20 mg/dL, white blood cell count less than 400 per mm^3, platelet count less than 100,000 per mm^3, hypotension requiring aggressive fluid resuscitation, and hypothermia. The guideline also suggested that criteria such as hypoglycemia, hyponatremia, asplenia (as in sickle cell disease), and unexplained acidosis be considered in deciding the need for ICU admission.[19]

Diagnostic Testing

Hopwood[18] recommended that all women with persistent upper respiratory distress have a chest radiograph to avoid delays in recognizing the presence of CAP. In one series, 98% of patients with antepartum pneumonia had positive findings on their chest radiographs at admission or on repeat examination, including infiltrates, atelectasis, pleural effusion, pneumonitis, or pulmonary edema.[7] In another series[4] of pneumonia in pregnancy, 28 of 39 patients had an infiltrate confined to a single lobe, whereas the remainder had multilobar pneumonia, and only 1 had a pleural effusion. Madinger and colleagues[5] reported that although all 25 pregnant patients who had pneumonia did have signs and symptoms

of lung infection, the diagnosis was initially overlooked in 5 patients. This may explain why respiratory failure, empyema, and other serious complications adding to morbidity complicated diagnosis in half of those with pneumonia.

The ATS/IDSA guidelines for the management of adults with CAP also recommended that all patients with suspected CAP should have a chest radiograph (with an abdominal shield during pregnancy).[19] All admitted patients should also have an assessment of gas exchange (oximetry or arterial blood gas), routine blood chemistry, and blood counts. Blood cultures can give false-positive results and are only recommended in patients with severe illness, especially if there has been no prior therapy with antibiotics; for these patients, 2 sets of blood cultures are recommended. Sputum culture and Gram stain should be obtained if a drug-resistant pathogen or an organism not covered by usual empiric antibiotic therapy is suspected. Routine serologic testing is not recommended for any population with CAP. However, for patients with severe CAP, Legionella urinary antigen and pneumococcal urinary antigen tests are recommended, and aggressive efforts at establishing an etiologic diagnosis should be made, including consideration of bronchoscopy.

Antimicrobial Therapy

Initial therapy is empiric, based on the expected organisms, and should be directed in all patients at S pneumoniae (including DRSP in patients with recent antibiotic therapy or underlying chronic heart or lung disease and those with exposure to a child in daycare); H influenzae (especially in cigarette smokers); and atypical pathogens, such as C pneumoniae, Mycoplasma pneumoniae, and, in the setting of severe CAP, Legionella pneumophila. In choosing an antibiotic for bacterial pneumonia, the agent's safety in pregnancy and efficacy must be considered. Penicillins, cephalosporins, and erythromycin are all safe and potentially effective antimicrobials for CAP.[44] The penicillins are only 50% protein-bound and can cross the placenta to achieve fetal concentrations that are 50% of maternal levels. Clindamycin is probably also safe, but there is limited clinical experience with this agent.[45] The fluoroquinolones are commonly used to treat CAP in nonpregnant patients but are usually avoided during pregnancy, because of the risk of fetal arthropathy and malformations in animal studies and because they can be mutagens and carcinogens. However, sporadic reports of safe use in pregnancy have appeared, suggesting that they can be used if absolutely necessary.[46] Other drugs to be avoided in pregnancy include tetracyclines (the mother is at risk of fulminant hepatitis, and these agents can stain and deform fetal teeth and cause bony deformities); chloramphenicol (which can cause bone marrow suppression in fetus, and if given near term, can cause "gray baby syndrome" with gray facies, flaccidity, and cardiovascular collapse); and sulfa compounds (can cause fetal kernicterus).[47] Aminoglycosides should be used only if there is a clinical indication of serious gram-negative infection, because there is significant risk of ototoxicity to the fetus. Vancomycin poses serious risk to the fetus, causing fetal nephrotoxicity and ototoxicity, and similarly, should only be used if absolutely necessary. Linezolid is a protein synthesis inhibitor. Linezolid has no safety data available in human pregnancies. A few case reports describe use of this drug in MRSA pneumonia.[35,36]

Current guidelines for CAP recommend that patients should not receive empiric therapy with a β-lactam (penicillin or cephalosporin) alone and that all patients be treated for atypical pathogens and pneumococcus. For an outpatient with mild CAP and no risks of DRSP, therapy should be with an oral macrolide such as azithromycin, which is better tolerated than erythromycin. Clarithromycin is not recommended for use in pregnancy, because of adverse embryonic and fetal outcomes in animal studies. If an outpatient with mild illness is at risk of DRSP, therapy should be given with a macrolide combined with high-dose amoxicillin (3 g/d), cefpodoxime, or cefuroxime (500 mg twice daily).

If the patient is admitted to hospital, therapy should be initially given intravenously with azithromycin or erythromycin if the patient has no risks of DRSP and intravenous macrolide and ceftriaxone or cefotaxime rather than cefuroxime[19] in patients at risk of DRSP. Yost and colleagues[40] studied 119 women with CAP who were hospitalized, and 83% received erythromycin monotherapy, with only one having a poor clinical response but with 5 requiring discontinuation because of intestinal symptoms. Azithromycin may be better tolerated as an intravenous macrolide than erythromycin.

In the ICU-admitted patient with severe CAP, no patient should get monotherapy, and combination therapy should be with cefotaxime or ceftriaxone plus a macrolide (azithromycin or erythromycin) if pseudomonal risks are not present. Pseudomonal risks include bronchiectasis, prolonged corticosteroid therapy, and cystic fibrosis, and if present, should be treated with an antipseudomonal β-lactam (imipenem, meropenem, cefepime, or piperacillin-tazobactam), an aminoglycoside (amikacin, gentamicin, tobramycin), and a macrolide. CA-MRSA should be considered in patients with severe CAP after influenza. However, although the safety of vancomycin and linezolid in pregnancy is not established, benefits of these drugs in patients with severe pneumonia probably outweigh the risks of the drugs, and patients should be counseled accordingly.

Supportive Care

Supportive therapy of the pregnant patient with pneumonia is similar to the nongravid state; hydration, antipyretic therapy, and supplemental oxygen remain key. The goal of oxygen therapy is to maintain the arterial oxygen tension at greater than 70 mm Hg, because hypoxemia is less well tolerated in pregnant women. Respiratory alkalosis leads to reduction in uterine blood flow, and thus, work of breathing should be decreased whenever possible in the pregnant pneumonia patient; adequate oxygenation may require the use of noninvasive ventilation. Respiratory failure mandating mechanical ventilation has occurred in pregnancy and requires close monitoring of mother and fetus. Preterm labor is a known complication of systemic infections, which should be suspected and addressed based on gestational age, fetal maturity, and maternal and fetal wellbeing.

Prevention of Aspiration

Pregnancy can increase the risk of aspiration, particularly in the peripartum period.[10] Patients can aspirate bacteria from the oropharynx (enteric gram-negatives or anaerobes), solid particulate matter from the stomach, or liquid stomach contents, including gastric acid. The aspiration of bacteria leads to a pneumonia that usually begins at least 24 hours after the event. When particulate matter is aspirated, it can lead to immediate bronchospasm, cough, and possibly cyanosis. Aspiration of gastric contents leads to symptoms that begin 6 to 8 hours after the event, at which time the patient usually presents with tachypnea, bronchospasm, pulmonary edema, or hypotention.[10] The risk of pneumonitis is substantially increased if the aspirated fluid has a pH of less than 2.4.[48]

The major thrust of management is prevention. Regional anesthesia is preferred over general anesthesia. In the latter scenario, airway protection with cricoid pressure and rapid sequence induction at the time of endotracheal intubation can reduce the risk of aspiration.[11] Raising gastric acid pH pharmacologically may also help avoid some of the complications of aspiration, but no data document a clear benefit or preference for antacids over histamine type-2 blockers and proton pump inhibitors.[49]

VIRAL PNEUMONIA EVALUATION AND MANAGEMENT

Influenza Virus

The influenza viruses are myxoviruses of 3 antigenically different types, A, B, and C, that can cause disease in humans, but most epidemics in humans are due to type A, as was the case with the novel H1N1 virus. First identified in 1933, influenza remains a significant cause of morbidity and mortality from febrile respiratory illness worldwide.[28,50] Pregnant women are at increased risk of acquiring influenza and developing complications of infection. In one study by Neuzil and colleagues,[28] pregnant women were affected more often than nonpregnant women. Influenza also led to hospitalization for acute cardiopulmonary illness more often in older women during the third trimester and in those with underlying medical conditions, such as asthma.[28,51] Historically, influenza in pregnancy has been associated with a high rate of morbidity and mortality, and epidemic infection may lead to more complications than sporadic infection.[52] The course of influenza was first reported during the epidemic of 1918 when 1350 cases in pregnant women who had an influenza-like illness were evaluated, and pneumonia was a complication in 585(43%) of these. In 52% of these patients, pregnancy was interrupted, and there were 308 (23%) maternal deaths. The mortality was highest in the last 3 months of pregnancy, especially when complicated by pneumonia.[50] Overall, in the 1918 epidemic, influenza during pregnancy had a 30% maternal mortality, increasing to 50% in the presence of pneumonia.[53] Mortality rose in parallel with gestational age to a maximum of 61% when influenza was contracted after 36 weeks of gestation. In the 1957 epidemic, 50% of women of childbearing age who died were pregnant and 10% of all the influenza deaths were among pregnant women.

However, since 1958, pregnancy has not been associated with an enhanced morbidity and mortality from influenza until the H1N1 infections in 2009 to 2010. Influenza pneumonia occurred in 12% of 102 pregnant patients with influenza in the 2003-to-2004 season and led to complications, such as respiratory failure, meningitis, and myocarditis.[3] In April of 2009, the first cases of influenza A H1N1 were registered in Mexico and were associated with an unexpected number of deaths. Data from the surveillance system of the Mexican health authorities[54] showed a death rate of about 1% of all confirmed 6945 cases, and the highest risk group was in the 10- to 39-year-old age group. Out of the 63 deaths in the period from April to July, 2009 in Mexico, 4 were in pregnant women. All pregnant workers were taken out of work during the period of the pandemic in Mexico. Surveillance data from the US Centers for Disease Control (CDC)[30] collected between August 21 and December 31, 2009 showed that 5% of 509 hospitalized pregnant women died, and those with delayed antiviral therapy (more than 4 days after onset of symptoms) were more likely to be admitted to an ICU (relative risk 6.0) and have worse outcomes, such as death. The most common comorbid conditions found in these patients were asthma and obesity. In that subset, it seemed that patients with advanced pregnancy (second and third trimester) were at a higher risk of death, with four of the 56 deaths having occurred in the first trimester (7.1%), 15 in the second (26.8%), and 36 in the third (64.5%). Previous reports from the US CDC database collected in the first 2 months of the pandemic[55] showed a high mortality in pregnant women. Six deaths occurred in pregnant women in the initial months of the epidemic, all in women who had developed pneumonia and subsequent acute respiratory distress syndrome requiring mechanical ventilation. A case-series from the state of Victoria in Australia[56] identified 43 pregnant patients admitted to the hospital with H1N1, 8 of whom were in the ICU. Again, asthma, obesity, and diabetes were conditions commonly present in these patients, but about half had no comorbidities and the only identified risk factor of influenza was pregnancy. Pneumonia was a common complication found in 11 of the 43 pregnant patients. Only one patient died and there were 2 fetal deaths and one neonatal death, pointing to the importance of worse outcomes for mother and fetus. Influenza was associated with preterm delivery, and 36% of patients delivered while admitted to the hospital for influenza.

The clinical symptoms of influenza do not seem to be altered by pregnancy, even if it is a more severe illness than in the nonpregnant patient. The incubation period is 1 to 4 days, and symptoms include cough, fever, malaise, coryza, headache, and myalgias.[57] In an uncomplicated case, influenza may resolve in 3 days or less. If symptoms persist for more than 5 days, especially in a pregnant patient, complications, such as pneumonia, should be considered. Pneumonia, either a viral or a secondary bacterial infection, is a well-recognized complication of influenza.

When pneumonia complicates influenza in pregnancy, antibiotics should be started and should be directed at the likely pathogens that can cause secondary infection, including pneumococcus, *H influenzae,* and *S aureus* including MRSA. Therapy for these organisms has been discussed earlier, but antiviral agents should be started if a viral pneumonia is likely, especially early in the course of illness.[2] Antiviral agents, such as amantadine and rimantadine, can prevent illness in exposed patients and reduce the duration of symptoms if given within 48 hours of its onset. Amantadine is effective against Influenza A, whereas oseltamivir and zanamivir are active against influenza A and B; all can be used for prophylaxis in high-risk pregnant women or for therapy in complicated cases.[2] Animal reports of teratogenicity with the use of Amantadine seem to be species-specific. Although many reports describe various congenital malformations associated with the use of amantadine and oseltamivir, none provide sufficient information for a conclusion on the developmental toxicity of these drugs to be reached. Despite these concerns, pregnancy is certainly not a contraindication for the use of antivirals, because during the 2009 H1N1 epidemics, the use of antiviral therapy with oseltamivir, zanamivir, and amantadine, alone or in combination, was associated with better outcomes if initiated earlier at onset of the symptoms (before day 2).[30] The CDC recommends that for pregnant patients, antiviral drugs should be started as soon as possible after the onset of influenza symptoms. Oseltamivir and zanamivir are found in breast milk; however, the concentrations of oseltamivir in breast milk is about 1% of serum levels, and no adverse effects of lactation exposure to zanamivir was found in rats.

Although antivirals can be prophylactic after exposure, the primary method of influenza prevention is vaccination. The recommendation of the Advisory Committee on Immunization Practices is that all women who will be pregnant during the influenza season receive the vaccine. The same principle applies to the novel H1N1 virus vaccine. Vaccination can also be performed safely in any trimester of pregnancy but should be avoided in the first trimester, if possible, unless the timing of the influenza season necessitates immunization at that time.[58,59] The inactivated form of the vaccine (not the nasal vaccine) is used for pregnant women and other high-risk groups. Breast-feeding is not a contraindication to vaccination.[59]

Varicella Pneumonia

Varicella is a particular problem that can complicate pregnancy, having a higher incidence and severity than in nonpregnant patients and with the potential to complicate the course of pregnancy and lead to congenital defects. Pneumonia is the most serious complication of varicella, but when varicella is present in the pregnant patient, it carries a high mortality, between 35% and 40%.[3,27] Haake and colleagues[27] reviewed 34 cases of varicella pneumonia in pregnancy and found a 35% mortality. Although only 5% to 10% of cases occur in adults, this population accounts for 25% to 55% of fatal cases. A recent series from Spain indicated that among the 46 patients studied with varicella pneumonia, 24% were treated in the ICU but none of them died, including 2 females who were pregnant.[60] Varicella-zoster (VZ) is a DNA virus that usually causes a benign, self-limited illness in children (chickenpox), but up to 10% of the adult population is susceptible to primary infection.[17] Studies show that the infection rate in pregnant women is as high as 4% to 6.8%, but after a close exposure, the risk of infection may be as high as 70%.[61] Pregnancy may also increase the rate of pneumonia as a complication of primary infection, and smoking may also be a risk factor of developing this complication, with infected smokers having a higher rate of pneumonia than infected nonsmokers.[62]

Pregnancy also enhances the virulence of the VZ virus as a consequence of functional T-cell abnormalities and of the higher levels of circulating corticosteroids, along with circulatory overload and altered respiratory reserve. Most reports have shown that when varicella pneumonia complicates pregnancy, it is usually in the third trimester and that infection occurring at this time is more severe and complicated than if it occurs earlier.[20,63] The incidence of pulmonary involvement in primary varicella infection is approximately 16%.[3]

The varicella virus can have a period of incubation of 10 days to 3 weeks.[3] In the mother, the virus is in the blood for 24 to 48 hours before the exanthem, and during this period, 24% of fetuses develop transplacental infection,[64] which can lead to congenital malformations in 1.2% of exposed fetuses. Clinically, varicella pneumonia presents 2 to 5 days after the onset of fever, vesicular rash (chickenpox), and malaise and is heralded by the onset of pulmonary symptoms,[2,20] including cough, dyspnea, pleuritic chest pain, and even hemoptysis. In one series, all patients with VZ pneumonia had oral mucosal ulcerations. Severity of illness may range from asymptomatic radiographic infiltrates to fulminant respiratory failure and acute lung injury.[20] Typically, chest radiographs reveal interstitial, diffuse miliary or nodular infiltrates that resolve by 14 days unless complicated by acute lung injury and respiratory failure.[64] The severity of infiltrates has been described to peak with the height of the skin eruption. One of the late radiographic sequelae of varicella pneumonia is diffuse pulmonary calcification.[65]

All patients with VZ pneumonia require antiviral agents (acyclovir) and early hospitalization. Mechanical ventilation may be needed in up to half of all pregnant women, and this group has a mortality rate of at least 25%. Registry and other data on acyclovir, a DNA polymerase inhibitor in the pregnant patient, have shown no increase in birth defects following in utero exposure to this drug.[66–68] In a study of 312 pregnancies in which acyclovir was used, no increase in the number or pattern of birth defects was seen.[67] However, there is no evidence of the efficacy of acyclovir for improving outcome, although some studies have suggested that this therapy can reduce the risk of developing respiratory failure and mortality for mother and fetus. Haake and colleagues[27] reviewed the early initiation of therapy within 36 hours of admission and found that those receiving early therapy had an improved hospital course after the fifth hospital day, lower mean temperature, less tachypnea, and improved oxygenation compared with those who were not treated. The recommended dose is 7.5 mg/kg every 8 hours intravenously, although doses of 3 to 18 mg/kg have been used. Treatment is recommended for 7 days. Some small series have suggested a benefit from adjunctive corticosteroid therapy.[3]

The effects of varicella on the fetus include intrauterine infection in 10% to 20%. Traditionally, fetal involvement has occurred in 3 patterns: "varicella embryopathy" stemming from maternal disease developing before 20 weeks' gestation, congenital varicella from 20 weeks' gestation until term but more commonly close to term, and neonatal disease occurring when the pregnant patient has active lesions at the time of delivery.[69] Varicella embryopathy was first described in 1947 and has since been redefined by several authors, but it includes limb hypoplasia, skin scarring, central nervous system involvement, and other skeletal lesions. This embryopathy has been reported with infection occurring as late as 26 weeks.[69]

The largest series of congenital varicella reported 1373 pregnancies complicated by VZ from 1980 to 1993. Fetal abnormalities occurred most commonly in the children of women infected between 13 and 20 weeks of gestation than at any other time in pregnancy.[70] Fetal anomalies varied from skin lesions to lethal multiorgan system involvement. Because of concern about fetal effects, the use of prophylactic immune globulin is recommended within 96 hours of exposure to prevent maternal illness in women without prior varicella infection (negative Ig G titers) or immunization. Although the use of VZ immune globulin in a pregnant woman may not eliminate the incidence of embryopathy, if given before maternal infection develops, it may decrease or attenuate fetal disease.[70] Immunoprophylaxis with zoster immune globulin should be given early after close exposure of a seronegative pregnant women, with the aim of preventing disease in the mother but not in the fetus. Although expensive, one analysis suggested that the use of this approach is likely to be cost-effective.[22] The varicella vaccine, however, is contraindicated in pregnancy because it is a live- attenuated vaccine.

Other Viruses

Pneumonia may complicate up to 50% of adult measles cases, and bacterial superinfection is common. In one report of 3 cases of rubeola during pregnancy, all patients had bacterial superinfection and 2 had preterm labor.[26]

SARS is caused by a coronavirus, which can affect pregnant women, leading to symptoms that are the same as in nonpregnant women and include fever, chills, rigors, malaise, and myalgias.[71] Patients are most infectious in the second week of illness. Laboratory findings include marked lymphopenia and thrombocytopenia, and chest radiographs show patchy to generalized interstitial infiltrates.[71] The case fatality was 25% in 12 cases that were reported in pregnancy, and other complications included first-trimester spontaneous abortions, preterm births, and intrauterine growth restriction. Treatment includes broad-spectrum antibiotics to cover superimposed bacterial infections, high-dose corticosteroids, and, possibly, ribavirin, which has been teratogenic in animals.[31]

FUNGAL PNEUMONIA

Fungal pathogens can cause pneumonia in pregnancy, including *Cryptococcus neoformans, Histoplasma capsulatum, Sporothrix schenkii, Blastomyces dermatitidis, and Coccidioides immitis.*[39] Fungal pneumonia in pregnancy is rare and usually resolves without treatment in healthy women. However, disseminated disease carries a more serious prognosis and can complicate pregnancy, particularly with infection in the third trimester and in those with HIV infection.[15,21]

Coccidioidomycosis generally occurs in the Southwestern United States and symptoms include fever, cough, headache, malaise, weight loss, and erythema nodosum. Although most patients have pulmonary involvement (including an infiltrate, pleural effusion, miliary infiltrates, or cavitation), disseminated disease involves the central nervous system, skin, and bones. Those with erythema nodosum have a lower rate of disseminated disease and a higher rate of recovery.[21]

For disseminated disease or severe pneumonia, treatment with intravenous amphotericin B is recommended, followed by oral fluconazole postpartum.[21,72] Earlier series used ketoconazole and itraconazole, but fluconazole is preferred as a more effective, more bioavailable agent.[21] Fluconazole has been associated in case reports with congenital anomalies similar to Antley-Bixler syndrome, mainly with high-dose and prolonged use of the drug, such as doses used to treat systemic fungal infections. Although case reports do not establish teratogenicity, it is unlikely that occurrence of an unusual genetic abnormality with high-dose fluconazole would occur by chance alone. Animal reports on reproductive effects of amphotericin B are incomplete. Although the lack of birth defects in infants exposed in utero to the drug does not establish its safety, the use of amphotericin in severe fungal pneumonia should not be delayed. The severity of fungal infections and the potential for morbidity and mortality may justify the use of drugs such as fluconazole. Proper patient counseling should happen in those cases. Other fungal infections have been reported in pregnancy but are uncommon, and the impact of pregnancy on these infections and the bearing of these infections on the outcome of pregnancy is uncertain.[2]

PNEUMONIA COMPLICATING HIV INFECTION

Pregnancy can theoretically accelerate the progression of underlying HIV infection-related immune suppression, and respiratory infection can be the AIDS-defining illness for some pregnant patients, leading to an increased risk of maternal and fetal mortality.[73] Also, vertical transmission of HIV infection to the newborn is a serious concern. Antiretroviral therapy may improve CD4+ count and reduce the risk of respiratory infection, but if this therapy is stopped in pregnancy, the risk of respiratory infection rises.

Bacterial respiratory infections are the most common respiratory complication of HIV infection, but a low CD4+ count (<200 cells per μL) predisposes to bacterial pneumonia and to pneumonia with *Pneumocystis jiroveci* (PCP), which can be a serious infection risk for both mother and fetus. In one review of 22 patients with PCP in pregnancy, 59% with respiratory failure necessitating mechanical ventilation, 50% mortality for the mothers, 5 intrauterine deaths, and 4 neonatal deaths were reported.[74] Women with PCP infection should receive therapy with trimethoprim-sulfa (TMP-SMX), along with corticosteroids if hypoxemia is present. These patients should be monitored for preterm labor and at the time of delivery, and women receiving TMP-SMX or dapsone should have their newborns monitored closely for hyperbilirubinemia and kernicterus. Immune reconstitution inflammatory syndrome may occur in the postpartum period. For HIV-infected women without active PCP, prophylaxis is best done when the CD4+ cell count falls to less than 200 cells per μL using TMP-SMX, but because of teratogenic risk with this medication in the first trimester, consideration should be given to the use of aerosolized pentamidine because of its lack of systemic absorption.

SUMMARY

Pneumonia in pregnancy is associated with a higher morbidity and mortality than in the nonpregnant population. Several physiologic and immunologic changes that occur in pregnancy may predispose to infection and impair the ability of pregnant patients to respond to respiratory pathogens. The early recognition and treatment of the diverse etiologic agents of pneumonia can improve outcomes for fetus and mother. Antibiotics should be selected with fetal safety in mind. Pneumonia can be prevented by avoidance of aspiration, use of influenza vaccination, and treatment with appropriate prophylaxis of known HIV-positive patients with a CD4 cell count of less than 200 cells per mL or those with a previous earlier history of pneumonia.

REFERENCES

1. Kaunitz AM, Hughes JM, Grimes DA, et al. Causes of maternal mortality in the United States. Obstet Gynecol 1985;65:605–12.
2. Rodrigues JM, Niederman MS. Pneumonia complicating pregnancy. Clin Chest Med 1992;13:679–91.
3. Goodnight WH, Soper DE. Pneumonia in pregnancy. Crit Care Med 2005;33:S390–7.
4. Benedetti TJ, Valle R, Ledger WJ. Antepartum pneumonia in pregnancy. Am J Obstet Gynecol 1982; 144:413–7.
5. Madinger NE, Greenspoon JS, Elrodt AG. Pneumonia during pregnancy: has modern technology improved maternal and fetal outcome? Am J Obstet Gynecol 1989;161:657–62.
6. Berkowitz K, LaSala A. Risk factors associated with increasing prevalence of pneumonia during pregnancy. Am J Obstet Gynecol 1990;163:981–5.
7. Munn MB, Groome LJ, Atterbury JL, et al. Pneumonia as a complication of pregnancy. J Matern Fetal Med 1999;8:151–4.
8. Jin Y, Carriere KC, Marrie TJ, et al. The effects of community acquired pneumonia during pregnancy

ending in a live birth. Am J Obstet Gynecol 2003;18: 800–6.

9. Belfort MA, Clark SL, Saade GR, et al. Hospital readmission after delivery: evidence for an increased incidence of nonurogenital infection in the immediate postpartum period. Am J Obstet Gynecol 2010;35:e1–7.

10. Baggish MS, Hooper S. Aspiration as a cause of maternal death. Obstet Gynecol 1974;43:327–36.

11. Engelhardt T, Webster NR. Pulmonary aspiration of gastric contents in anaesthesia. Br J Anaesth 1999;83:453–60.

12. Gayat E, Lecarpentier E, Retout S, et al. Cough reflex sensitivity after elective caesarean section under spinal anaesthesia and after vaginal delivery. Br J Anaesth 2007;99:694–8.

13. Dines DE, Baker WG, Scantland WA. Aspiration pneumonitis—Mendelson's syndrome. JAMA 1961; 176:229–31.

14. Lederman MM. Cell-mediated immunity and pregnancy. Chest 1984;86:6S–9S.

15. Catanzaro A. Pulmonary mycosis in pregnant women. Chest 1984;86:14S–9S.

16. Rigby FB, Pastorek JG II. Pneumonia during pregnancy. Clin Obstet Gynecol 1996;39:107–19.

17. Khan S, Niederman MS. Pneumonia in the pregnant patient. In: Rosene-Montela K, Bourjeily G, editors. Pulmonary problems in pregnancy. New York (NY): Humana Press; 2009. p. 177–96.

18. Hopwood HG. Pneumonia in pregnancy. Obstet Gynecol 1965;25:875–9.

19. Mandell LA, Wunderink RG, Anzueto A, et al. Infectious diseases society of America/American thoracic society consensus guidelines on the management of community-acquired pneumonia in adults. Clin Infect Dis 2007;44:S27–72.

20. Harris RE, Rhoades ER. Varicella pneumonia complicating pregnancy: report of a case and review of the literature. Obstet Gynecol 1965;25:734–40.

21. Spinello I, Johnson R, Baqui S. Coccidioidomycosis and pregnancy. Ann N Y Acad Sci 2007;1111:358–64.

22. McKendrik MW, Lau J, Alston S, et al. VZV infection in pregnancy: a retrospective review over 5 years in Sheffield and discussion on the potential utilisation of varicella vaccine in prevention. J Infect 2007;55:64–7.

23. Biem J, Roy L, Halik J, et al. Infectious mononucleosis complicated by necrotizing epiglottitis, dysphagia, and pneumonia. Chest 1989;96:204–5.

24. Gherman RB, Leventis LL, Miller RC. Chlamydial psittacosis during pregnancy: a case report. Obstet Gynecol 1995;86:648–50.

25. McKinney WP, Volkert P, Kaufman J. Fatal swine influenza pneumonia during late pregnancy. Arch Intern Med 1990;150:213–5.

26. Stein SJ, Greenspoon JS. Rubeola during pregnancy. Obstet Gynecol 1991;78:925–9.

27. Haake DA, Zakowski PC, Haake DL, et al. Early treatment with acyclovir for varicella pneumonia in otherwise healthy adults: retrospective controlled study and review. Rev Infect Dis 1990;12:788–98.

28. Neuzil KM, Reed GW, Mitchel EF, et al. Impact of influenza on acute cardiopulmonary hospitalizations in pregnant women. Am J Epidemiol 1998;148: 1094–102.

29. Winterbauer RH, Ludwig WR, Hammar SP. Clinical course, management and long-term sequelae of respiratory failure due to influenza viral pneumonia. Johns Hopkins Med J 1977;141:148–55.

30. Siston AM, Rasmussen SA, Honein MA, et al. Pandemic 2009 influenza A(H1N1) virus illness among pregnant women in the United States. JAMA 2010;303: 1517–25.

31. Wong SF, Chow KM, Leung TN, et al. Pregnancy and perinatal outcomes of women with SARS. Am J Obstet Gynecol 2004;191:292–7.

32. Vanderkooi OG, Low DE, Green K, et al. Predicting antimicrobial resistance in invasive pneumococcal infections. Clin Infect Dis 2005;40:1288–97.

33. Micek ST, Dunne M, Kollef MH. Pleuropulmonary complications of Panton-Valentine leukocidin-positive community-acquired methicillin-resistant Staphylococcus aureus: importance of treatment with antimicrobials inhibiting exotoxin production. Chest 2005;128:2732–8.

34. Rotas M, McCalla S, Liu C, et al. Methicillin-resistant staphylococcus aureus necrotizing pneumonia arising from an infected episiotomy site. Obstet Gynecol 2007;109:533–6.

35. Mercieri M, Di Rosa R, Pantosti A, et al. Critical pneumonia complicating early -stage pregnancy. Anesth Analg 2010;110:852–4.

36. Broadfield E, Doshi N, Alexander PD, et al. Cunning and community-acquired pneumonia. Lancet 2009; 373:270.

37. Finland M, Dublin TD. Pneumococcal pneumonias complicating the pregnancy and puerperium. JAMA 1939;250:1027–32.

38. Shariatzadeh MR, Marrie TJ. Pneumonia during pregnancy. Am J Med 2006;119:872–6.

39. Ramsey PS, Ramin KD. Pneumonia in pregnancy: medical complications of pregnancy. Obstet Gynecol Clin North Am 2001;28:553–69.

40. Yost NP, Bloom SL, Richey SD, et al. An appraisal of treatment guidelines for antepartum community acquired pneumonia. Am J Obstet Gynecol 2000;183:131–5.

41. Fine MJ, Auble TE, Yealy DM, et al. A prediction rule to identify low-risk patients with community- acquired pneumonia. N Engl J Med 1997;336:243–50.

42. Louie JK, Acosta M, Jamieson DJ, et al. Severe 2009 H1N1 influenza in pregnant and postpartum women in california. N Engl J Med 2010;362:27–35.

43. Callaghan WM, Chu SY, Jamieson DJ. Deaths from seasonal influenza among pregnant women in the

United States, 1998–2005. Obstet Gynecol 2010; 115:919–23.

44. Hollingsworth H. Pneumonia in pregnancy. Obstet Gynecol 1985;65:605–12.

45. Maccato ML. Respiratory insufficiency due to pneumonia in pregnancy. Obstet Gynecol Clin North Am 1991;18:289–99.

46. Loebstein R, Addis A, Ho E, et al. Pregnancy outcome following gestational exposure to fluoroquinolones: a multicenter prospective controlled study. Antimicrob Agents Chemother 1998;42:1336–9.

47. Levin S, Jupa JE. Principles of antibiotic use in obstetrics and gynecology. Obstet Gynecol Annu 1976;5:293–313.

48. Hollingsworth HM, Pratter MR, Irwin RS. Acute respiratory failure in pregnancy. J Intensive Care Med 1989;4:11–34.

49. Paranjothy S, Griffiths JD, Broughton HK, et al. Interventions at caesarean section for reducing the risk of aspiration pneumonitis. Cochrane Database Syst Rev 2010;1:CD004943.

50. Harris JW. Influenza occurring in pregnant women. JAMA 1919;72:978–80.

51. Hartert TV, Neuzil KM, Shintani AK, et al. Maternal morbidity and perinatal outcomes among pregnant women with respiratory hospitalizations during influenza season. Am J Obstet Gynecol 2003;2:145–55.

52. Laibl VR, Sheffield JS. Influenza and pneumonia in pregnancy. Clin Perinatol 2005;32:727–38.

53. Larsen JW. Influenza and pregnancy. Clin Obstet Gynecol 1982;25:599–603.

54. Echevarría-Zuno S, Mejía-Aranguré JM, Mar-Obeso AJ, et al. Infection and death from influenza A H1N1 virus in Mexico: a retrospective analysis. Lancet 2009;374:2072–9.

55. Jamieson DJ, Honein MA, Rasmussen SA, et al. Pandemic 2009 influenza A(H1N1) virus illness among pregnant women in the United States. Lancet 2009;374:451–8.

56. Hewagama S, Walker SP, Stuart RL, et al. 2009 H1N1 influenza A and pregnancy outcomes in Victoria, Australia. Clin Infect Dis 2010;50:686–90.

57. Cox NJ, Subbarao K. Influenza. Lancet 1999;354: 1277–82.

58. Deinard AS, Ogburn P. Influenza vaccination program effects on maternal health and pregnancy outcome. Am J Obstet Gynecol 1981;140:240–5.

59. Harper SA, Fukuda K, Uyeki TM, et al. Prevention and control of influenza. Recommendations of the advisory committee on immunization practices. MMWR Recomm Rep 2004;53:1–40.

60. Chiner E, Ballester I, Betlloch I, et al. Varicella-zoster virus pneumonia in an adult population: ha mortality decreased? Scand J Infect Dis 2010;42 215–21.

61. Sauerbrei A, Sonntag S, Wutzler P. [Prevalence c varicella zoster in pregnant patients]. Zentralbl Gy nakol 1990;112:223–6 [in German].

62. Ellis M, Neal K, Webb A. Is smoking a risk factor fo pneumonia in adults with chickenpox? BMJ 1986 294:1002.

63. Zambrano MA, Martinez A, Minguez JA, et al. Vari cella pneumonia complicating pregnancy. Acta Ob stet Gynecol Scand 1995;74:318–20.

64. Cox SM, Cunningham FG, Luby J. Management c varicella pneumonia complicating pregnancy. Am . Perinatol 1990;7:300–1.

65. Eder SE, Apuzzio JJ, Weiss G. Varicella pneumoni during pregnancy: treatment of two cases with acyclovir. Am J Perinatol 1988;5:16–8.

66. Centers for Disease Control. Pregnancy outcome following systemic prenatal acyclovir exposure June 1, 1984–June 30, 1993. MMWR 1993;42 806–9.

67. Andrews EB, Yankasas BC, Cordero JF, et al Acyclovir in pregnancy registry: six years experi ence. Obstet Gynecol 1992;79:7–13.

68. Stone KM, Reiff-Eldridge R, White AD, et al. Preg nancy outcomes following systemic prenata acyclovir exposure: conclusions from the interna tional acyclovir pregnancy registry, 1984–1999 Birth Defects Res A Clin Mol Teratol 2004;7C 201–7.

69. Katz VL, Kuller JA, McMahon MJ, et al. Varicella during pregnancy: maternal and fetal effects. Wes J Med 1995;163:446–50.

70. Enders G, Miller E, Cradock-Watson J, et al. Conse quences of varicella and herpes zoster in preg nancy: prospective study of 1739 cases. Lance 1994;343:1548–51.

71. Peiris JS, Yuen KY, Osterhaus AS, et al. The severe acute respiratory syndrome. N Engl J Med 2003 349:2431–41.

72. Ely EW, Peacock JE, Haponik EE, et al. Crypto coccus pneumonia complicating pregnancy. Medi cine 1998;77:153–67.

73. Kumar RM, Uduman SA, Khurrana AK. Impact o pregnancy on maternal AIDS. J Reprod Med 1997 42:429–34.

74. Ahmad H, Mehta NJ, Manikal VM, et al. Pneumocys tis carinii pneumonia in pregnancy. Chest 2001;120 666–71.

Infiltrative Lung Diseases in Pregnancy

N. Freymond, MD[a,b], V. Cottin, MD, PhD[a,b], J.F. Cordier, MD[a,b],*

KEYWORDS

- Infiltrative lung disease • Pregnancy • Women • Gender
- Connective tissue disease • Systemic vasculitis
- Sarcoidosis • Lymphangioleiomyomatosis

Most infiltrative lung diseases (ILDs) are not commonly associated with pregnancy because only a minority of them occur in women of child-bearing age. However, ILDs may arise de novo in pregnancy or a previous known ILD may be exacerbated during pregnancy. Pregnancy may affect the diagnosis, management, and outcome of ILD. Conversely, ILD may affect pregnancy. ILD may occur as a result of drugs administered commonly or specifically during pregnancy. On the other hand, some conditions, such as lymphangioleiomyomatosis (LAM) have long been considered as contraindications to pregnancy. Conversely, sarcoidosis or rheumatoid arthritis (RA) with ILD have not been considered to alter the management of pregnancy, labor, or delivery. The respiratory risk induced by pregnancy also depends on the severity of respiratory impairment, whatever its cause (with forced vital capacity [FVC] <50% of predicted values and/or forced expiratory volume in 1 second <30% of predicted values are usually poorly tolerated during pregnancy).

RESPIRATORY MECHANICS AND PHYSIOLOGY IN PREGNANCY

The gravid uterus affects respiratory mechanics, altering diaphragm position and thoracic cage configuration; however, diaphragmatic motion is not impaired. Lung volume decreases by the second half of pregnancy, including expiratory reserve volume and residual volume, resulting in a 9.5% to 25% reduction of functional residual capacity.[1] The reduction in functional residual capacity is counterbalanced by an increase in inspiratory capacity, leading to a minimal change in total lung capacity.[2] Increased progesterone levels stimulate central respiratory drive, leading to hyperventilation, dyspnea,[3] and increased tidal volume. Alveolar-capillary diffusion is normal or even improved as a consequence of chronic hyperventilation. These changes in respiratory physiology must be taken into account when interpreting lung function tests in pregnant women suffering from ILD. Decrease in lung volumes resulting from ILD should thus be interpreted taking into account these physiologic changes, whereas decrease in alveolar-capillary diffusion capacity if present cannot be attributed to pregnancy.

IATROGENIC ILD AND CONCEPTION

ILD could be a consequence of drugs administered to induce pregnancy. Ovarian hyperstimulation syndrome may complicate the therapeutic induction of ovulation with an incidence of 0.1% to 0.2% of treatment cycles.[4] Several grades of severity have been described.[5] Severe forms occurring in 0.5% to 5% of all cases of hyperstimulation are characterized by manifestations related to intra-abdominal or pleural fluid accumulation, especially with pleural effusion. Acute respiratory distress syndrome has been reported in 2.4% of cases, especially after massive hydration. Scattered pulmonary infiltrates are also common, often in association with diaphragm elevation, pleural effusion, and atelectasis.[4]

[a] Department of Respiratory Medicine, Reference Centre for Rare Pulmonary Diseases, Hospices Civils de Lyon, Louis Pradel Hospital, Lyon, France
[b] University of Lyon I, UMR754 INRA, IFR 128, Lyon, France
* Corresponding author. Hôpital Louis Pradel, 28 Avenue Doyen Lepine, 69677 Lyon (Bron) Cedex, France.
E-mail address: jean-francois.cordier@chu-lyon.fr

Clin Chest Med 32 (2011) 133–146
doi:10.1016/j.ccm.2010.11.006
0272-5231/11/$ – see front matter © 2011 Published by Elsevier Inc.

Two cases of acute eosinophilic pneumonia developed after the intramuscular injection of progesterone given as luteal phase support after in vitro fertilization.[6] Both patients developed respiratory symptoms 3 weeks after the first injection, and evolved to acute respiratory distress, with 1 requiring mechanical ventilation. The symptoms improved as treatment was shifted to vaginal progesterone administration together with corticosteroids. Sesame oil (as excipient) and benzyl alcohol (as preservative) were both incriminated in the development of the hypersensitivity reaction. Three further cases have been reported.[7–9] Patients with ovarian hyperstimulation are also at an increased risk for venous thromboembolism, with deep venous thrombosis having a special predilection for upper extremities. The reasons for this predilection relate to estradiol-rich ascitic fluid being drained by the thoracic duct into upper extremity veins. The higher concentration of estradiol in this fluid is believed to lead to increase local thrombin generation by decreasing thrombomodulin activity.

CONNECTIVE TISSUE DISEASE–ASSOCIATED ILD

Connective tissue diseases are generally more common in women than in men, and predominate between the ages of 20 and 40 years. Possible explanations for this female predilection include endogenous hormonal changes related to menstruation and pregnancy history, exogenous hormonal treatments, especially oral contraceptives, gender differences in lifestyle factors, genetic differences, and the suspected role of noninherited genetic factors such as noninherited maternal antigens (maternal-fetal genotype incompatibility) and microchimerism.[10] Microchimerism, that is, the persistence of fetal cells in women after pregnancy and of maternal cells in her offspring, might predispose to autoimmune disorders and influence their pattern through a process analogous to graft-versus-host disease. Specifically, the persistence of fetal cells in the mother after pregnancy could either improve or worsen the manifestations of autoimmune disease.[11] Some evidence for a role of microchimerism has been found in systemic sclerosis (SSc), systemic lupus erythematosus (SLE), and RA.[10]

Rheumatoid Arthritis

ILD, occurring in at least 10% of patients with RA,[12,13] usually develops within the first 5 years after the diagnosis of rheumatic disease, and most commonly corresponds to a histopathologic pattern of usual interstitial pneumonia. An imaging pattern indicative of usual interstitial pneumonia is associated with a poor outcome.[14,15] In contrast to the female predominance of RA, ILD has a male predominance in RA with a male/female ratio of about 3:1.

It has long been appreciated that clinical improvement in RA occurs in more than 70% of patients during the second and third trimesters.[16] During the last months of pregnancy, regulatory T-cell lymphocytes are upregulated, with overexpression of interleukin-4 and interleukin-10 that might reduce disease activity. However, RA flares up in the first 3 to 4 months postpartum in most cases (~90%)[17]; the evolution of ILD does not parallel that of rheumatic disease, and pregnancy generally has little effect on RA-related ILD. Several studies have reported that pregnancy in patients with RA does not carry any particular fetal risk.[18,19] However, others suggest that RA could contribute to reduced birth weight[20] or to an increased risk of preeclampsia and the need for cesarean section.[21,22]

Evaluation of RA and of associated ILD through preconception counseling is recommended to best inform patients of the potential risks associated with pregnancy and to avoid exposing pregnant women to potentially teratogenic medications. Corticosteroids such as prednisone are metabolized in large part by the placenta but may still be associated with a risk of hypertension, diabetes, and premature rupture of membranes. Their use is certainly justifiable in severe illnesses such as ILD but should be done with proper counseling. Nonsteroidal antiinflammatory agents are not commonly used during pregnancy. Use of these drugs in early pregnancy has been shown in some but not all epidemiologic studies to increase the risk of cardiac defects and gastroschisis. Use in late pregnancy is avoided because of concerns with premature ductal closure. Methotrexate is teratogenic in animals and seems to increase the incidence of congenital abnormalities in humans as well. This drug is avoided in pregnancy. Among 101 pregnancies in women with RA exposed to methotrexate during the first trimester (at doses of 5–25 mg/wk), 66% were uneventful, 23% had miscarriages, and 5% had newborns with minor neonatal malformations (metatarsus varus, eyelid angioma).[23] The rate of induced abortions was 18%. Leflunomide is highly teratogenic and interferes with embryo development and viability in experimental animals and a washout period of at least 3.5 months after its discontinuation is necessary before conception.

Published experience with tumor necrosis factor-alpha (TNF-α) inhibitors in pregnancy is limited to some case reports and an ongoing registry. TNF-α inhibitors are classified by the

United States Food and Drug Administration as pregnancy risk category B, indicating that no adverse effects on pregnancy have been observed in animal studies, but that additional investigations are needed in humans. Nevertheless, TNF-α inhibitors have recently been implicated in cases of VATER syndrome (5 areas in which a child may incur abnormalities, ie, vertebrae, anus, trachea, esophagus, and renal; there may also be cardiac and limb conditions, which changes the acronym to VACTERL). The incidence of congenital abnormalities is considered to be much less than 3% of pregnant women who received TNF-α inhibitors.[24] Overall, TNF-α inhibitors should be avoided during pregnancy, and their withdrawal is advised once pregnancy is recognized.

Data on the safety of abatacept (an inhibitor of T-cell costimulation through interaction between B7 and CTLA-4 molecules) and rituximab (anti-CD20 chimeric monoclonal antibody with B-cell inhibitory activity) during pregnancy are insufficient. Therefore a decision to weigh the advantage of discontinuing the drug before conception or at the onset of pregnancy against the risk of untreated or uncontrolled disease on the mother and fetus should be discussed with every patient. Antimalarial agents, hydroxychloroquine, and sulfasalazine are justifiable in pregnancy as no significant associations with congenital abnormalities have been reported. These drugs may be administered until birth (**Table 1**).[25] Cyclosporine A may be given with caution. The risk of azathioprine during pregnancy is generally considered as being low.[25] Bisphosphonates are unlikely to lead to significant adverse pregnancy outcomes based on experimental animal studies; however, human data are limited.

SLE

SLE predominantly affects women of childbearing age and pleural disease is the most common pulmonary manifestation. It may rarely involve lung parenchyma, leading especially to acute lupus pneumonitis and alveolar hemorrhage.

Prospective studies indicate that pregnancy may confer a modestly increased risk of SLE exacerbation,[26] especially in patients with a history of renal involvement. Lupus activity may increase during pregnancy,[26,27] resulting in moderate to severe lupus flares in 15% to 30% of cases, and a higher risk in patients with active disease in the prior 6 months (58% worsening in pregnancy during high disease activity vs 8% in quiescent disease).[28] The more active the disease is before conception, the more likely exacerbation occurs during pregnancy or in puerperium.[29] Therefore, whenever possible, pregnancy should be delayed until the disease has been stable for at least 6 months. Lupus flares during pregnancy are generally not severe, with mainly skin and joint involvement, usually controlled by low or moderate doses of corticosteroids. Corticosteroids, hydrochloroxychloroquine, and azathioprine may be continued during pregnancy if necessary in patients with SLE.[30]

The postpartum period carries a particularly high risk of lupus pneumonitis.[31] Acute lupus pneumonitis occurring in 1% to 4% of patients[32] typically develops in those with established SLE, but may be the initial manifestation of the disease. Its presentation is coupled with acute dyspnea, fever, hypoxemia, and alveolar opacities on pulmonary imaging. Corticosteroids are generally beneficial, but the course of acute lupus pneumonitis may be fatal. Alveolar hemorrhage, which

Table 1
Administration of drugs and biological agents during pregnancy

Use Justifiable in Rare Circumstances	Use Justifiable When Indicated	Use Almost Never Justifiable
Anti-TNF (infliximab, etanercept, adalimumab; very limited data) Cyclosporine A (not teratogenic in animals; growth retardation, but limited data)	Corticosteroids (caution required at high doses) Azathoprine (caution at high doses) Hydroxychloroquine Sulfasalazine (folic acid supplementation required) Intravenous polyvalent immunoglobulins	Methotrexate Cyclophosphamide Mycophenolate mofetil Rituximab Leflunomide D-Penicillamine

In-depth review of medication safety in pregnancy can be found at www.Reprotox.org, distributed in Micromedix, Inc's TOMES Reprorisk module.
Data from Refs.[26,138–140]

occurs in less than 2% of patients with SLE, especially in young women,[31] is a severe complication often associated with nephritis, with mortality estimated to be 50% to 90%.[32] High-dose corticosteroids with or without immunosuppressive agents are the treatment of choice. Two cases of alveolar hemorrhage during pregnancy have been reported in SLE, with recovery after the termination of pregnancy in one case,[33] and favorable outcome for both the mother and child in the other case.[34]

Complications of pregnancy that are more frequent in women with SLE than in healthy women comprise spontaneous abortion,[35] preterm birth (20%–54%),[36–39] premature rupture of membranes, HELLP (hemolysis, elevated liver enzyme, low platelet count) syndrome, intrauterine fetal death with antiphospholipid antibodies, intrauterine fetal growth restriction (20%–30%),[40] and preeclampsia (13%–35%).[40–42] In a prospective study of 267 pregnancies, 85.8% were successful.[28] High disease activity increased the number of fetal deaths with a relative risk approaching 3. The highest risk of SLE on pregnancy derives from immunoglobulin G antiprothrombin antibodies.[43] Antiphospholipid antibodies are linked with thrombotic events and adverse pregnancy and fetal outcomes including miscarriage and fetal demise, and the combination of low-molecular-weight heparin with aspirin is recommended. However, unfractionated heparin in combination with acetylsalicylic acid may be preferable, according to a Cochrane review.[44]

SSc

SSc is characterized by the excessive synthesis and deposition of extracellular matrix as well as microvascular obliteration in various organs. ILD and pulmonary arterial hypertension are the 2 most common respiratory manifestations in SSc in 40% to 80% and 12% to 50% of cases, respectively, and are the most predominant causes of death.[45] The skin, peripheral vasculature, kidneys, myocardium, and esophagus may also be involved. High-resolution computed tomography (HRCT) of the chest can identify early ILD. Treatment options for ILD in SSc are limited to cyclophosphamide and lung transplantation in patients less than 60 to 65 years of age with end-stage pulmonary fibrosis.

SSc occurs 3 to 5 times more frequently in women than in men, and with an increased risk in women with lower parity.[10] SSc has long been considered a strict contraindication to pregnancy, with patients being informed about the high risk of poor fetal and maternal outcome, including maternal death.[46] There are few reports on the onset of scleroderma symptoms during pregnancy or worsening after pregnancy. Women with SSc currently have a high likelihood of successful pregnancy if it is carefully planned once the disease is stable, and close monitoring and appropriate management are achieved.[47] Retrospective studies have found an increased frequency of preterm births and of small full-term infants, but the incidence of miscarriage and the neonatal survival rate did not differ from healthy controls.[48] The main risk in pregnant women with SSc is renal crisis with acute-onset severe hypertension that may be life threatening for both mother and child. The disease is stable in 61% to 88% of cases and is exacerbated in 7% to 20% of pregnancies.[48,49] Some symptoms common in pregnancy, such as peripheral edema, gastroesophageal reflux, arthralgias, and dyspnea, may especially occur. Classically, Raynaud phenomenon is improved as a result of increased cardiac output in the second half of pregnancy.[49]

A prospective study reported 17 pregnancies in patients with severe SSc, including 5 with ILD. Three patients with FVC less than 65% of predicted values had preterm births, but all the children survived. Another patient required therapeutic abortion, and died of acute respiratory failure. One patient with ILD and FVC less than 55% required interruption of pregnancy during the first trimester.[49]

Hydroxychloroquine and low-dose corticosteroids may be safe in renal crisis, even during pregnancy. Given their unmistakable advantage compared with any other antihypertensives in this case, angiotensin-converting enzyme inhibitors are recommended despite the risk of teratogenicity and kidney dysfunction at birth. D-Penicillamine, cyclophosphamide, and methotrexate need to be avoided during pregnancy and breast-feeding, but azathioprine may be used. A single case report related a successful pregnancy in a patient receiving low-dose cyclosporine A.[50]

Polymyositis and Dermatomyositis

Polymyositis and dermatomyositis are characterized by chronic striated-muscle inflammation and possible characteristic skin features in dermatomyositis. Polymyositis and dermatomyositis are twice as frequent in women than in men, with a bimodal age distribution peaking between 10 to 25 years and 30 to 60 years.[51] Lung involvement includes ILD, respiratory muscle involvement, aspiration pneumonia, and rarely pulmonary hypertension.

Dermatomyositis or polymyositis may develop before, during, or after pregnancy.[52,53] Substantial fetal mortality and morbidity seem to parallel maternal disease activity.[54] The outcome of pregnancy is especially poor when the disease occurs or flares early in gestation compared with exacerbations in the second or third trimester when the fetal prognosis is usually good.[55] In a parturient with polymyositis, general anesthesia should be avoided because of various risks, including delayed recovery from muscle relaxation, aspiration pneumonitis, arrhythmias, and cardiac failure. Regional anesthesia for cesarean section is likely a safer option.[56]

Muscle involvement and disease activity seem to be the main determinants of pregnancy outcome in patients with polymyositis or dermatomyositis, with 30% of healthy infants and 40% of abortions or fetal deaths in cases of active systemic disease versus 57% and 21.5%, respectively, in cases of inactive myositis.[54] As dermatomyositis usually responds to corticosteroids, the treatment may be continued during pregnancy. Patients with corticosteroid-resistant disease may be treated with immunosuppressive drugs, preferably azathioprine, or polyvalent intravenous immunoglobulin therapy. Nozaki and colleagues[57] reported a case of severe dermatomyositis developing during pregnancy; the patient showed no response to corticosteroids and received intravenous immunoglobulin therapy because of CO_2 narcosis during cesarean section with regional anesthesia. The patient could not be extubated until 2 months after the premature delivery of a healthy child. This case emphasizes the importance of multidisciplinary management around labor and delivery in patients with restrictive lung disease including those with respiratory muscle weakness. High levels of regional anesthesia may compromise respiratory muscles further, potentially leading to hypercapnic respiratory failure. The Trendelenburg position may also reduce functional residual capacity and further the restrictive physiology.

PULMONARY VASCULITIS
Anticytoplasmic Antibody-associated Granulomatosis Necrotizing Systemic Vasculitis

Anticytoplasmic antibody-associated granulomatous necrotizing systemic vasculitis (GSV) (formerly named Wegener granulomatosis) is a necrotizing granulomatous vasculitis of the small vessels involving the upper and lower respiratory tract, with or without glomerulonephritis. The incidence peaks in the fourth and fifth decades, and thus it is rarely encountered during pregnancy. However, GSV may have a more aggressive course in pregnant women and may thus require more active treatment.[58]

Out of 36 cases of active GSV in pregnant women reported in the literature between 1970 and 2008,[59] 11 were newly diagnosed in pregnancy, 21 were in remission, and 4 had active disease before conception. The worst scenario is related to active disease at the beginning of pregnancy or to the onset of vasculitis during pregnancy.[60,61] Even if the vasculitis is in remission at the time of conception, serious complications have been described during pregnancy, including preeclampsia, fetal macrosomia, or retroplacental hematoma.[60] Pregnancy in a patient with GSV should thus be considered at risk, and patients should be counseled to avoid pregnancy if the disease remains active. In patients with inactive disease, the risk of relapse of systemic vasculitis during pregnancy is unpredictable and does not correlate with initial disease severity.[60]

In most cases, treatment of GSV combines cyclophosphamide and corticosteroids. Patients given immunosuppressive drugs and corticosteroids conjointly have a more favorable pregnancy outcome than those treated with corticosteroids alone.[62,63] Conventional treatment with corticosteroids and cyclophosphamide seems to control disease activity in most cases, and the risk of fetal abnormality is significantly reduced after the first trimester. However, cyclophosphamide is known to cause fetal malformations, including facial and musculoskeletal deformities, especially during the first trimester. Cyclophosphamide may be safer during the second and third trimesters, although rare cases of fetal pancytopenia and impaired growth have been reported.[58] Azathioprine is less effective but safer than cyclophosphamide during pregnancy, although intrauterine growth retardation may be associated with it,[64] and maternal and fetal deaths have been encountered.[65] Given the systemic vasculitis, it is hard to decide whether the adverse outcomes described are associated with the disease itself or medications used to treat such disease. Methotrexate as maintenance therapy is contraindicated because of its teratogenicity. Overall, new onset of especially severe GSV should be treated with corticosteroids, but cyclophosphamide should be avoided if possible during the first trimester of pregnancy.

Churg-Strauss Syndrome

Churg-Strauss syndrome (CSS) is a rare necrotizing systemic vasculitis affecting small vessels and characterized by asthma, hypereosinophilia, and systemic manifestations with necrotizing granulomas. Lung infiltrates in CSS correspond to eosinophilic pneumonia and usually improve rapidly with corticosteroids. Disease severity is mainly a result of cardiac involvement in up to 60% of patients. Corticosteroids are the main treatment with immunosuppressive drugs needed in patients with poor prognostic factors including cardiac involvement.

A case report and review of the literature yielded 13 reports describing CSS in individuals who were either pregnant or near pregnancy.[66] The diagnosis was made during pregnancy in 6 patients, before conception in 4 patients, and after delivery in 3 patients. Sixty-seven percent of the reported pregnancies had a successful outcome; among them, 4 had received cyclophosphamide and/or azathioprine. Five fetal deaths occurred in patients who had not received immunosuppressive therapy, 3 from spontaneous abortions and 2 from elective terminations for unrelated reasons.[66] One pregnant woman died of extensive myocardial infarction; another died of cardiomyopathy 1 year after delivery; a third patient developed severe heart failure requiring heart transplantation after delivery; and 3 other pregnant women had cardiac involvement that remained stable with therapy throughout pregnancy. CSS may thus affect pregnant and peripartum women with variable effects on fetal and maternal health. Particular attention to patients with cardiac involvement is thus required.

Microscopic Polyangiitis

Microscopic polyangiitis is a rare, small-vessel, systemic vasculitis frequently associated with pauci-immune necrotizing glomerulonephritis and pulmonary capillaritis. Antineutrophil cytoplasmic antibodies with myeloperoxidase (MPO) specificity are found in more than 75% of patients.

Bansal and Tobin[67] were the first to report transplacental transfer of anti-MPO antineutrophil cytoplasmic antibodies resulting in neonatal pulmonary-renal syndrome, further indicating a pathogenetic role of antineutrophil cytoplasmic antibodies in vasculitis. A 32-year-old woman, who was not receiving immunosuppressive maintenance therapy for microscopic polyangiitis, had a relapse of vasculitis at week 33 of her second pregnancy; she required high-dose steroids and underwent urgent cesarean section because of severe preeclampsia. The neonate further developed vasculitis with alveolar hemorrhage and renal involvement (proteinuria and hematuria), and anti-MPO antibodies were detected in cord blood. He was treated with mechanical ventilation, high-dose corticosteroid therapy, and exchange transfusion, with clinical and biological recovery.

Another woman with microscopic polyangiitis remained in remission despite circulating anti-MPO antibodies during pregnancy with maintenance immunosuppressive therapy using azathioprine and prednisone; a healthy child born at 38 weeks had no clinical vasculitis, although the child's anti-MPO antibody blood titer was as high as that measured in the mother. Anti-MPO antibodies became undetectable in the child 4 months after birth.

Another woman with microscopic polyangiitis at 24 weeks of pregnancy who developed glomerulonephritis and alveolar hemorrhage was reported. She was treated with mechanical ventilation, cyclophosphamide, corticosteroids, and plasmapheresis, and delivered a healthy child at 35 weeks of gestation.[68]

SARCOIDOSIS

Sarcoidosis is a multisystem granulomatous disorder of unknown cause that typically occurs between the ages of 20 and 40 years. Sarcoidosis usually has a benign course, but other severe manifestations may result from cardiac, neurologic, ocular, kidney, or laryngeal involvement.

The frequency of pregnancy is estimated to be 0.02% to 0.05% of patients affected by sarcoidosis.[69,70] Sarcoidosis is unlikely to affect the outcome of pregnancy, but premature and low-birth-weight neonates have been reported.[71–73] If appropriately managed, pregnancy is likely to be well tolerated in patients with mild or well-controlled disease. An observational study over 14 years and published several decades ago noted mortality of 1.4% in 205 pregnant women with sarcoidosis,[71] and it is likely that mortality is now extremely low. In patients with stable or inactive sarcoidosis, pregnancy generally has no effect on the course of the disease, but postpartum exacerbation or development of new manifestations may occur 3 to 6 months after delivery.[72,74]

Sarcoidosis in pregnancy was first reported in a patient with thrombocytopenic purpura and spleen involvement who underwent splenectomy.[75] In a series of 16 pregnancies in 10 patients with sarcoidosis, lymphadenopathy, parenchymal lung involvement and hyper-gamma-globulinemia improved during pregnancy and relapsed after delivery; chronic uveitis was unchanged.[76] In another series of 35 pregnancies in 18 patients (including 6 with hypercalcemia), sarcoidosis remained unaltered during pregnancy.[77] However, respiratory failure is a rare but possible complication of sarcoidosis in pregnancy and may develop shortly after delivery, with efficacy of corticosteroids.[78]

Factors that indicate a poor prognosis of sarcoidosis in pregnancy include prominent parenchymal lesions on chest radiography, advanced radiographic staging, advanced maternal age, requirement for drugs other than corticosteroids, and the presence of extrapulmonary sarcoidosis.[79] Severe restrictive pulmonary disease also represents a serious risk.[80]

Corticosteroids are the main treatment of active sarcoidosis and suffice to control the disease in host cases.[81] Among the other drugs used, methotrexate is difficult to justify during pregnancy and breast-feeding and should be avoided. Azathioprine has been administered during pregnancy. Although rare adverse effects have been discussed in infants (thymic atrophy, leukopenia, chromosome aberrations, decreased birth weight, and increased risk of infection), azathioprine does not seem to be teratogenic in humans; the rate of malformations in children from treated women is comparable with that in the general population and the type of malformations is inconsistent. Hydroxychloroquine and cyclosporine A have been administered and do not seem to be major human teratogens[82]; however, human pregnancy data are limited, especially with cyclosporine A. Overall, the risk/benefit ratio of drugs other than corticosteroids (or rarely azathioprine) argues against their use as sarcoidosis therapy in pregnancy.

Vahid and colleagues[83] have proposed guidelines for the management of sarcoidosis during pregnancy. Patients should undergo baseline chest radiography and pulmonary function testing when they are planning for pregnancy; drug therapy should be avoided if possible; close follow-up after delivery is important because of possible exacerbation 3 to 6 months after delivery. Patients with advanced respiratory insufficiency, pulmonary hypertension, uncontrolled neurosarcoidosis, or myocardial sarcoidosis should be advised to avoid pregnancy.

LAM

Pulmonary LAM is a rare disease that usually occurs in women of child-bearing age. It can occur sporadically and further affects 30% to 40% of adult women with tuberous sclerosis complex. It is characterized by the nonneoplastic proliferation of abnormal smooth muscle cells with a peribronchial, perivascular, and perilymphatic distribution, leading to cystic lung lesions and eventual cystic destruction of lung structures.[84,85] Angiomyolipoma is present in up to 50% of patients with LAM.[86] The diagnosis is suspected in young women with progressive dyspnea, interstitial or cystic changes on chest radiography with normal or increased lung volumes, recurrent pneumothorax, or chylous effusion. Chest HRCT reveals multiple, small, diffusely distributed, thin-walled cysts (Fig. 1). Pulmonary function tests disclose an obstructive or mixed obstructive and restrictive pattern, and the diffusing capacity for carbon monoxide is commonly reduced. The diagnosis is made by lung biopsy, if required, or a combination of characteristic features, especially imaging.[87]

The role of sex hormones has been controversial in LAM, and there is no supportive evidence that

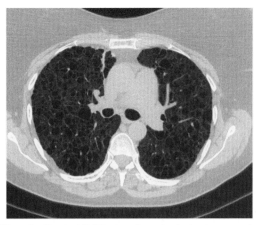

Fig. 1. Chest HRCT showing typical changes in a patient with LAM.

oral contraceptives are causally associated with the development or progression of pulmonary LAM.[87,88] LAM is believed to be accelerated by the administration of exogenous estrogens, and pregnancy may increase the rate of disease progression. Progesterone therapy has been used without evidence but is no longer recommended in LAM.[87] Controlled trials are currently being conducted for mTOR (mammalian target of rapamycin) inhibitors and metalloprotease inhibitors. However, very limited human pregnancy data exist with most of these products.

In 2 large series, the diagnosis of LAM was made during pregnancy in 20% of cases, and clear LAM exacerbation was observed in 14% of cases during pregnancy.[84,89] Many patients have an uneventful pregnancy, but women with LAM (especially with severely impaired lung function tests) must be warned before conception of the risk involved with pregnancy.[90] In addition, pregnancy in LAM is associated with an increased incidence of pneumothorax and chylous effusion[91,92]; and patients with poor baseline lung function are less likely to tolerate these complications. Several case reports have also described LAM presenting or worsening during pregnancy. Cohen and colleagues[93] surveyed 328 women with LAM: 15 women diagnosed with LAM during pregnancy had a high rate of pneumothorax (67%) and premature birth (47%). Moreover, women diagnosed with LAM before pregnancy had lower lung function after pregnancy than before pregnancy,[93] indicating that LAM diagnosed during pregnancy may be a marker of more aggressive disease.

The European Respiratory Society guidelines for the diagnosis and management of LAM[87] propose that all patients be informed of the risks of pneumothorax and chylous effusion, and pregnancy should be closely monitored. Ideally, information should be delivered to patients before pregnancy.

IDIOPATHIC INTERSTITIAL PNEUMONIAS
Idiopathic Pulmonary Fibrosis

Idiopathic pulmonary fibrosis is a nonneoplastic pulmonary disease characterized by the formation of scar tissue within the lungs in the absence of any known cause. Idiopathic pulmonary fibrosis affects more men than women, between the fifth and seventh decades of life, so it is extremely rare in pregnant women. Idiopathic ILD occurring before the age of 50 years should lead to the consideration of alternative diagnoses, such as nonspecific interstitial pneumonia, ILD related to connective tissue disease, pulmonary Langerhans cell histiocytosis (LCH), and so forth. However, a few cases of idiopathic pulmonary fibrosis in pregnant women have been reported, with different evolutions: 1 case with fatal outcome for the mother, 1 with termination of pregnancy by abortion, and 2 with successful pregnancy including 1 requiring mechanical ventilation of the mother[94–96]; no lung biopsy was performed to ascertain the diagnosis in these patients, making the diagnosis not certain.

Cryptogenic Organizing Pneumonia

Organizing pneumonia is a well-defined clinico-pathologic entity that may be cryptogenic or secondary to many causes, including infection, drug reaction, or connective tissue disease. It has only exceptionally been reported in pregnancy. A case of biopsy-proven cryptogenic organizing pneumonia was reported in a 27-year-old woman infected with human immunodeficiency virus, who used cocaine and who developed acute respiratory distress at 13 weeks of gestation; progressive improvement was achieved with corticosteroids, but premature rupture of membranes occurred at 34 weeks.[97] Another case of organizing pneumonia (with marked peripheral blood and alveolar eosinophilia) arose in a pregnant woman presenting with acute respiratory distress, in whom surgical lung biopsy demonstrated organizing pneumonia[98]; the response to steroids was poor, but death of the fetus was followed by rapid improvement of the pulmonary disease.

Respiratory Bronchiolitis-associated ILD

Respiratory bronchiolitis-associated ILD was present in a woman entering the third trimester of pregnancy.[99] She presented with worsening dyspnea and pulmonary infiltrates, but no infection was found. The diagnosis was made by video-assisted thoracoscopic lung biopsy. Treatment with steroids was successful.

EOSINOPHILIC PNEUMONIAS

A few cases of acute eosinophilic pneumonias in pregnancy have been reported in the literature. Treatment with corticosteroids was generally successful with no consequences on the outcome of pregnancy.[100–104] However, relapses may occur in the postpartum period.[105] Cesarean section at 34 weeks of gestation was required because of fetal distress in 1 critical case.[104]

DRUG-INDUCED LUNG DISEASE

Urinary tract infections and bacteriuria are common during pregnancy, and nitrofurantoin is 1 of the first-choice treatments.[106] Nitrofurantoin can evoke acute and chronic pulmonary manifestations with fever, cough, pleuritic chest pain, dyspnea (and, rarely, pleural effusion or pulmonary hemorrhage). Nitrofurantoin may cause acute hypersensitivity pneumonitis, acute permeability edema, subacute cellular interstitial pneumonia, nonspecific interstitial pneumonia, acute or chronic eosinophilic pneumonia, desquamative interstitial pneumonia, alveolar hemorrhage, and pulmonary fibrosis.[107,108] Acute-onset interstitial pneumonia related to nitrofurantoin has been observed in a woman at 16 weeks of gestation with improvement on methylprednisolone.[10] Other antibiotics commonly administered during pregnancy, including ampicillin, may provoke subacute, diffuse interstitial pneumonia or eosinophilic pneumonia.[110]

Carbamazepine may be given to treat epilepsy in pregnancy. Carbamazepine-induced interstitial pneumonia has been reported with different possible radiologic patterns.[111–114]

Drug-induced lung diseases in pregnancy are likely under-reported and underdiagnosed. In pregnant women developing ILD, a search should be systematically conducted for drug(s) causing iatrogenic pulmonary manifestations. Available databases on the Internet (especially www.pneumotox.com) are helpful when considering the diagnosis of drug-induced lung disease.

OTHER DISORDERS
Pulmonary Alveolar Lipoproteinosis

Pulmonary alveolar lipoproteinosis is a rare ILD characterized by the accumulation of abnormal lung surfactant in the alveoli and distal airways. It may be autoimmune (the most common form) with onset in adulthood, or secondary to various conditions including inhaled dusts and mycobacterial or cytomegalovirus infections. Autoimmune pulmonary alveolar proteinosis, 2 to 3 times more common in men than in women, is generally diagnosed in young to middle-aged adults.

Only 2 cases have been observed in pregnancy: a 23-year-old woman became pregnant in the setting of long-standing, severe alveolar proteinosis; 2 procedures involving whole-lung lavage were required during pregnancy because of respiratory deterioration, with favorable outcome for the mother and child.[115] Preterm labor occurred in a 19-year-old patient with familial alveolar proteinosis.[116]

Pulmonary LCH

LCH is characterized by the proliferation of and infiltration by Langerhans cells in several organ systems, especially the lungs, bones, skin, pituitary gland, liver, and lymph nodes. Pulmonary LCH affects adult smokers, predominantly between 20 and 40 years of age. The most common findings on chest HRCT are multiple nodular and/or cystic changes especially involving the middle and upper lobes, with progression of nodules to thick-walled, then thin-walled cysts.

Only a few cases of Langerhans cell granulomatosis in pregnancy have been recorded in the literature,[117–123] including 6 cases with pulmonary involvement. The disease was present before pregnancy and resulted in live births in all patients. A case of respiratory distress from bilateral pneumothorax and mediastinal emphysema has been reported[123]; cesarean section was performed under epidural anesthesia, without negative side effects on pulmonary function, and a low-weight-birth infant was delivered at the 28th week of gestation.

Pulmonary Lymphangitic Carcinomatosis

The influence of pregnancy on the occurrence and evolution of maternal tumors has long been debated. Lung involvement is frequent during the course of metastatic breast cancer, affecting 30% to 40% of patients, with 6% to 8% developing lymphangitic carcinomatosis.[124] Stomach and lung cancer may also cause pulmonary lymphangitic carcinomatosis.

Choriocarcinoma

Diffuse alveolar hemorrhage with diffuse ILD[125] and/or hemoptysis with multiple lung nodules[126] have been reported in malignant gestational trophoblastic disease (eg, choriocarcinoma) metastatic to the lungs.[127] Most patients have a history of molar pregnancy with lung metastasis usually diagnosed within 6 months after delivery. However,

the delay in appearance of lung metastasis may be longer, even as long as 37 years after delivery.[128]

Choriocarcinoma is a highly invasive, metastatic, and vascular germ-cell tumor of the uterus producing β-human chorionic gonadotrophin (β-hCG) and arising in any type of pregnancy. Very high levels of serum β-hCG allow the diagnosis without the need for biopsy. Choriocarcinoma after nonmolar pregnancies represents 17% of total gestational trophoblastic tumors requiring treatment.[129] Metastases of choriocarcinoma are evident at the time of diagnosis in up to 30% of patients, especially in the lungs, the most common site of metastasis[130]; metastatic disease was present in 31% of cases after live births and 43% after abortion in a series of choriocarcinomas after nonmolar pregnancy.[129] Metastatic pulmonary disease may present as infiltrative opacities and/or nodules, often asymptomatic, and with tumor embolism.[130] Diffuse pulmonary involvement may result in severe alveolar hemorrhage with respiratory failure and death.[125,131] However, the prognosis is usually good with chemotherapy.

Pulmonary Edema

Tocolytic pulmonary edema

Beta-adrenergic agonists, particularly ritodrine and terbutaline, used to inhibit uterine contractions and preterm labor, may elicit pulmonary edema during pregnancy in 0.25% to 5% of treated patients.[132,133] The mechanisms of pulmonary edema include prolonged exposure to catecholamines causing myocardial dysfunction, increased capillary permeability, and a large volume of intravenous fluid injected in response to maternal tachycardia. Corticosteroids administered in preterm labor can also contribute to fluid retention.

Drug-induced pulmonary edema usually resolves rapidly with the discontinuation of β-agonist therapy and diuretics. The possible side effects of β-agonists have led to the application of alternative tocolytic drugs, such as calcium channel blockers. However, pulmonary edema has also been reported after treatment with calcium channel blockers in pregnancy.[134–137] It is likely that pathologic conditions associated with spontaneous preterm labor (ie, multiple pregnancies, preeclampsia, chorioamnionitis, corticosteroid therapy) could increase water and sodium retention and predispose to pulmonary edema.[136] Additional risk factors for pulmonary edema in women with preterm delivery include tobacco use, cerclage placement, and erythrocyte transfusion.[137]

Preeclampsia and pulmonary edema

Preeclampsia, characterized by systemic hypertension, proteinuria, and peripheral edema, usually develops in the third trimester of pregnancy. Approximately 3% of all patients with preeclampsia develop pulmonary edema, frequently in the early postpartum period, and especially after abundant fluid replacement. Reduced serum albumin concentration and myocardial dysfunction contribute to edema formation. The standard therapeutic approach is to restrict fluid intake and to deliver nasal supplemental oxygen, diuretics, and inotropic vasodilators.

SUMMARY

ILDs are a heterogeneous group of disorders. Most of them rarely affect women of child-bearing age. They may occur in the context of connective tissue disease, and symptoms of the underlying disease may improve (as in RA), worsen (as in SLE), or remain unchanged during pregnancy. A multidisciplinary approach is necessary to provide information on the possible risks of pregnancy, to suggest the best timing for conception, and to provide adequate monitoring as well as supportive care. The possible increased risk of complications should be discussed before conception to allow informed decisions by patients. Ideally, the pulmonary disease must be stabilized before conception and immunosuppressive drugs contraindicated in pregnancy must be stopped for several months. Underlying pulmonary disease can be a significant challenge during pregnancy and the postpartum period, but pregnancies can now be managed in most cases despite coexisting ILD. Respiratory function and other evaluations should be performed before conception when possible as it is a major factor influencing maternal and neonatal outcome.

ACKNOWLEDGMENTS

The authors thank C. Silarakis and M.C. Thevenet for assistance in preparing the manuscript.

REFERENCES

1. Cugell DW, Frank NR, Gaensler EA, et al. Pulmonary function in pregnancy. I. Serial observations in normal women. Am Rev Tuberc 1953;67(5): 568–97.
2. Yannone ME, McCurdy JR, Goldfien A. Plasma progesterone levels in normal pregnancy, labor, and the puerperium. II. Clinical data. Am J Obstet Gynecol 1968;101(8):1058–61.
3. Weinberger SE, Weiss ST, Cohen WR, et al. Pregnancy and the lung. Am Rev Respir Dis 1980; 121(3):559–81.
4. Abramov Y, Elchalal U, Schenker JG. Pulmonary manifestations of severe ovarian hyperstimulation syndrome: a multicenter study. Fertil Steril 1999; 71(4):645–51.
5. Golan A, Ron-el R, Herman A, et al. Ovarian hyperstimulation syndrome: an update review. Obstet Gynecol Surv 1989;44(6):430–40.
6. Bouckaert Y, Robert F, Englert Y, et al. Acute eosinophilic pneumonia associated with intramuscular administration of progesterone as luteal phase support after IVF: case report. Hum Reprod 2004; 19(8):1806–10.
7. Khan AM, Jariwala S, Lieman HJ, et al. Acute eosinophilic pneumonia with intramuscular progesterone after in vitro fertilization. Fertil Steril 2008; 90(4):1200, e3–6.
8. Veysman B, Vlahos I, Oshva L. Pneumonitis and eosinophilia after in vitro fertilization treatment. Ann Emerg Med 2006;47(5):472–5.
9. Phy JL, Weiss WT, Weiler CR, et al. Hypersensitivity to progesterone-in-oil after in vitro fertilization and embryo transfer. Fertil Steril 2003;80(5):1272–5.
10. Olivier JE, Silman AJ. Why are women predisposed to autoimmune rheumatic diseases? Arthritis Res Ther 2009;11(5):252–60.
11. Waldorf KM, Nelson JL. Autoimmune disease during pregnancy and the microchimerism legacy of pregnancy. Immunol Invest 2008;37(5):631–44.
12. Olson AL, Swigris JJ, Sprunger DB, et al. Rheumatoid arthritis-interstitial lung disease-associated mortality. Am J Respir Crit Care Med 2010. [Epub ahead of print].
13. Tanaka N, Kim JS, Newell JD, et al. Rheumatoid arthritis-related lung diseases: CT findings. Radiology 2004;232(1):81–91.
14. Kim EJ, Elicker BM, Maldonado F, et al. Usual interstitial pneumonia in rheumatoid arthritis-associated interstitial lung disease. Eur Respir J 2010;35(6): 1322–8.
15. Cottin V. Pragmatic prognostic approach of rheumatoid arthritis-associated interstitial lung disease. Eur Respir J 2010;35(6):1206–8.
16. Nelson JL, Ostensen M. Pregnancy and rheumatoid arthritis. Rheum Dis Clin North Am 1997; 23(1):195–212.
17. Keeling SO, Oswald AE. Pregnancy and rheumatic disease: "by the book" or "by the doc". Clin Rheumatol 2009;28(1):1–9.
18. Neely NT, Persellin RH. Activity of rheumatoid arthritis during pregnancy. Tex Med 1977;73(8):59–63.
19. Spector TD, Silman AJ. Is poor pregnancy outcome a risk factor in rheumatoid arthritis? Ann Rheum Dis 1990;49(1):12–4.
20. Bowden AP, Barrett JH, Fallow W, et al. Women with inflammatory polyarthritis have babies of lower birth weight. J Rheumatol 2001;28(2):355–9.
21. Skomsvoll JF, Ostensen M, Irgens LM, et al. Pregnancy complications and delivery practice in women with connective tissue disease and inflammatory

rheumatic disease in Norway. Acta Obstet Gynecol Scand 2000;79(6):490–5.

22. Skomsvoll JF, Baste V, Irgens LM, et al. The recurrence risk of adverse outcome in the second pregnancy in women with rheumatic disease. Obstet Gynecol 2002;100(6):1196–202.

23. Martinez Lopez JA, Loza E, Carmona L. Systematic review on the safety of methotrexate in rheumatoid arthritis regarding the reproductive system (fertility, pregnancy, and breastfeeding). Clin Exp Rheumatol 2009;27(4):678–84.

24. Ali YM, Kuriya B, Orozco C, et al. Can tumor necrosis factor inhibitors be safely used in pregnancy? J Rheumatol 2010;37(1):9–17.

25. Ostensen M, Forger F. Management of RA medications in pregnant patients. Nat Rev Rheumatol 2009;5(7):382–90.

26. Petri M. Hopkins Lupus Pregnancy Center: 1987 to 1996. Rheum Dis Clin North Am 1997;23(1):1–13.

27. Carmona F, Font J, Cervera R, et al. Obstetrical outcome of pregnancy in patients with systemic lupus erythematosus. A study of 60 cases. Eur J Obstet Gynecol Reprod Biol 1999;83(2):137–42.

28. Clowse ME, Magder LS, Witter F, et al. The impact of increased lupus activity on obstetric outcomes. Arthritis Rheum 2005;52(2):514–21.

29. Ruiz-Irastorza G, Lima F, Alves J, et al. Increased rate of lupus flare during pregnancy and the puerperium: a prospective study of 78 pregnancies. Br J Rheumatol 1996;35(2):133–8.

30. Temprano KK, Bandlamudi R, Moore TL. Antirheumatic drugs in pregnancy and lactation. Semin Arthritis Rheum 2005;35(2):112–21.

31. Murin S, Wiedemann HP, Matthay RA. Pulmonary manifestations of systemic lupus erythematosus. Clin Chest Med 1998;19:641–65.

32. Keane MP, Lynch JP. Pleuropulmonary manifestations of systemic lupus erythematous. Thorax 2000;55(2):159–66.

33. Keane MP, Van De Ven CJ, Lynch JP 3rd, et al. Systemic lupus during pregnancy with refractory alveolar haemorrhage: recovery following termination of pregnancy. Lupus 1997;6(9):730–3.

34. Gaither K, Halstead K, Mason TC. Pulmonary alveolar hemorrhage in a pregnancy complicated by systemic lupus erythematosus. J Natl Med Assoc 2005;97(6):831–3.

35. Petri M, Allbritton J. Fetal outcome of lupus pregnancy: a retrospective case-control study of the Hopkins Lupus Cohort. J Rheumatol 1993;20(4):650–6.

36. Tincani A, Faden D, Tarantini M, et al. Systemic lupus erythematosus and pregnancy: a prospective study. Clin Exp Rheumatol 1992;10(5):439–46.

37. Cortes-Hernandez J, Ordi-Ros J, Paredes F, et al. Clinical predictors of fetal and maternal outcome in systemic lupus erythematosus: a prospective study of 103 pregnancies. Rheumatology (Oxford) 2002;41(6):643–50.

38. Clark CA, Spitzer KA, Nadler JN, et al. Preterm deliveries in women with systemic lupus erythematosus. J Rheumatol 2003;30(10):2127–32.

39. Yasmeen S, Wilkins EE, Field NT, et al. Pregnancy outcomes in women with systemic lupus erythematosus. J Matern Fetal Med 2001;10(2):91–6.

40. Johnson MJ, Petri M, Witter FR, et al. Evaluation of preterm delivery in a systemic lupus erythematosus pregnancy clinic. Obstet Gynecol 1995;86(3):396–9.

41. Moroni G, Ponticelli C. The risk of pregnancy in patients with lupus nephritis. J Nephrol 2003;16(2):161–7.

42. Chakravarty EF, Colon I, Langen ES, et al. Factors that predict prematurity and preeclampsia in pregnancies that are complicated by systemic lupus erythematosus. Am J Obstet Gynecol 2005;192(6):1897–904.

43. Bizzaro N, Tonutti E, Villalta D, et al. Prevalence and clinical correlation of anti-phospholipid-binding protein antibodies in anticardiolipin-negative patients with systemic lupus erythematosus and women with unexplained recurrent miscarriages. Arch Pathol Lab Med 2005;129(1):61–8.

44. Empson M, Lassere M, Craig J, et al. Prevention of recurrent miscarriage for women with antiphospholipid antibody or lupus anticoagulant. Cochrane Database Syst Rev 2005;2:CD002859.

45. Tyndall AJ, Bannert B, Vonk M, et al. Causes and risk factors for death in systemic sclerosis: a study from the EULAR Scleroderma Trials and Research (EUSTAR) database. Ann Rheum Dis 2010;69(10):1809–15.

46. Scarpinato L, Mackenzie AH. Pregnancy and progressive systemic sclerosis. Case report and review of the literature. Cleve Clin Q 1985;52(2):207–11.

47. Steen VD. Scleroderma and pregnancy. Rheum Dis Clin North Am 1997;23(1):133–47.

48. Steen VD, Conte C, Day N, et al. Pregnancy in women with systemic sclerosis. Arthritis Rheum 1989;32(2):151–7.

49. Steen VD, Medsger TA Jr. Fertility and pregnancy outcome in women with systemic sclerosis. Arthritis Rheum 1999;42(4):763–8.

50. Basso M, Ghio M, Filaci G, et al. A case of successful pregnancy in a woman with systemic sclerosis treated with cyclosporin. Rheumatology (Oxford) 2004;43(10):1310–1.

51. Saketkoo LA, Ascherman DP, Cottin V, et al. Interstitial lung disease in idiopathic inflammatory myopathy. Curr Rheumatol Rev 2010;6(2):108–19.

52. Park IW, Suh YJ, Han JH, et al. Dermatomyositis developing in the first trimester of pregnancy. Korean J Intern Med 2003;18(3):196–8.

53. Kanoh H, Izumi T, Seishima M, et al. A case of dermatomyositis that developed after delivery: the involvement of pregnancy in the induction of dermatomyositis. Br J Dermatol 1999;141(5):897–900.

54. Ishii N, Ono H, Kawaguchi T, et al. Dermatomyositis and pregnancy. Case report and review of the literature. Dermatologica 1991;183(2):146–9.

55. Pasrija S, Rana R, Sardana K, et al. A case of autoimmune myopathy in pregnancy. Indian J Med Sci 2005;59(3):109–12.

56. Gunusen I, Karaman S, Nemli S, et al. Anesthetic management for cesarean delivery in a pregnant woman with polymyositis: a case report and review of literature. Cases J 2009;2:9107.

57. Nozaki Y, Ikoma S, Funauchi M, et al. Respiratory muscle weakness with dermatomyositis during pregnancy: successful treatment with intravenous immunoglobulin therapy. J Rheumatol 2008; 35(11):2289.

58. Luisiri P, Lance NJ, Curran JJ. Wegener's granulomatosis in pregnancy. Arthritis Rheum 1997;40(7): 1354–60.

59. Koukoura O, Mantas N, Linardakis H, et al. Successful term pregnancy in a patient with Wegener's granulomatosis: case report and literature review. Fertil Steril 2008;89(2):457, e1–5.

60. Auzary C, Huong DT, Wechsler B, et al. Pregnancy in patients with Wegener's granulomatosis: report of five cases in three women. Ann Rheum Dis 2000;59(10):800–4.

61. Jwarah E, Ashworth F. Wegener's granulomatosis in pregnancy. J Obstet Gynaecol 2006;26(4):368–70.

62. Parnham AP, Thatcher GN. Pregnancy and active Wegener granulomatosis. Aust N Z J Obstet Gynaecol 1996;36(3):361–3.

63. Lima F, Buchanan N, Froes L, et al. Pregnancy in granulomatous vasculitis. Ann Rheum Dis 1995; 54(7):604–6.

64. Kumar A, Mohan A, Gupta R, et al. Relapse of Wegener's granulomatosis in the first trimester of pregnancy: a case report. Br J Rheumatol 1998;37(3): 331–3.

65. Milford CA, Bellini M. Wegener's granulomatosis arising in pregnancy. J Laryngol Otol 1986; 100(4):475–6.

66. Corradi D, Maestri R, Facchetti F. Postpartum Churg-Strauss syndrome with severe cardiac involvement: description of a case and review of the literature. Clin Rheumatol 2009;28(6):739–43.

67. Bansal PJ, Tobin MC. Neonatal microscopic polyangiitis secondary to transfer of maternal myeloperoxidase-antineutrophil cytoplasmic antibody resulting in neonatal pulmonary hemorrhage and renal involvement. Ann Allergy Asthma Immunol 2004;93(4):398–401.

68. Milne KL, Stanley KP, Temple RC, et al. Microscopic polyangiitis: first report of a case with onset during pregnancy. Nephrol Dial Transplant 200◄ 19(1):234–7.

69. Gallaher JP, Douglass LH. Sarcoidosis and preg nancy. Obstet Gynecol 1953;2(6):590–2.

70. O'Leary JA. Ten-year study of sarcoidosis an pregnancy. Am J Obstet Gynecol 1962;84:462–6

71. Fried KH. Sarcoidosis and pregnancy. Acta Me Scand Suppl 1964;425:218–21.

72. Cipriani A, Casara D, Di VG, et al. Sarcoidosis an pregnancy. Sarcoidosis 1991;8(2):183–5.

73. Chapelon-Abric C, Ginsburg C, Biousse V, et a Sarcoïdose et grossesse. Etude rétrospectiv de 11 cas. Rev Med Interne 1998;19(5):305–1 [in French].

74. Abarquez C, Pandya K, Sharma OP. Sarcoidos and pregnancy. Clinical observation. Sarcoidos 1990;7(1):63–6.

75. Nordland M, Ylvisaker RS, Larson P, et al. Preg nancy complicated by idiopathic thrombocytc penic purpura and sarcoid disease of the spleen splenectomy subsequent normal delivery. Min Med 1946;29:166.

76. Mayock RL, Sullivan RD, Greening RR, et a Sarcoidosis and pregnancy. JAMA 1957;164(2 158–63.

77. Agha FP, Vade A, Amendola MA, et al. Effects c pregnancy on sarcoidosis. Surg Gynecol Obste 1982;155(6):817–22.

78. Miloskovic V. [Sarcoidosis in pregnancy–diag nostic, prognostic and therapeutic problems Med Pregl 2005;58(Suppl 1):51–4 [in Serbian].

79. Haynes de RR. Sarcoidosis and pregnancy. Obste Gynecol 1987;70(3 Pt 1):369–72.

80. King TE Jr. Restrictive lung disease in pregnanc Clin Chest Med 1992;13(4):607–22.

81. Cottin V. Update on bioagent therapy in sarcoic osis. F1000 Med Rep 2010;2:13.

82. Moller DR. Rare manifestations of sarcoidosis. Eu Respir Mon 2005;32:233–50.

83. Vahid B, Mushlin N, Weibel S. Sarcoidosis in preg nancy and postpartum period. Curr Respir Me Rev 2007;3:79–83.

84. Urban T, Lazor R, Lacronique J, et al. Pulmonar lymphangioleiomyomatosis. A study of 69 patient: Medicine (Baltimore) 1999;78(5):321–37.

85. Frognier R, Cottin V, Cordier JF. Women and inte stitial lung diseases. Eur Respir Mon 2003;2! 167–89.

86. Avila NA, Kelly JA, Chu SC, et al. Lymphangioleic myomatosis: abdominopelvic CT and US finding: Radiology 2000;216(1):147–53.

87. Johnson SR, Cordier JF, Lazor R, et al. Europea Respiratory Society guidelines for the diagnos and management of lymphangioleiomyomatosis Eur Respir J 2010;35(1):14–26.

88. Wahedna I, Cooper S, Williams J, et al. Relation c pulmonary lymphangio-leiomyomatosis to use c

the oral contraceptive pill and fertility in the UK: a national case control study. Thorax 1994;49(9): 910–4.

89. Johnson SR, Tattersfield AE. Clinical experience of lymphangioleiomyomatosis in the UK. Thorax 2000; 55(12):1052–7.

90. Johnson S. Lymphangioleiomyomatosis: clinical features, management and basic mechanisms. Thorax 1999;54(3):254–64.

91. Fujimoto M, Ohara N, Sasaki H, et al. Pregnancy complicated with pulmonary lymphangioleiomyomatosis: case report. Clin Exp Obstet Gynecol 2005;32(3):199–200.

92. Brunelli A, Catalini G, Fianchini A. Pregnancy exacerbating unsuspected mediastinal lymphangioleiomyomatosis and chylothorax. Int J Gynaecol Obstet 1996;52(3):289–90.

93. Cohen MM, Freyer AM, Johnson SR. Pregnancy experiences among women with lymphangioleiomyomatosis. Respir Med 2009;103(5):766–72.

94. Hassan W, Darwish A. Idiopathic pulmonary fibrosis and pregnancy: a case controlled study. [abstract]. Eur Respir J 2009;36:100s.

95. Sholapurkar SL, Vasishta K, Dhall GI, et al. Idiopathic pulmonary fibrosis (IPF) necessitating therapeutic midtrimester abortion: a case report. Asia Oceania J Obstet Gynaecol 1991;17(4):303–6.

96. Sharma CP, Aggarwal AN, Vashisht K, et al. Successful outcome of pregnancy in idiopathic pulmonary fibrosis. J Assoc Physicians India 2002;50:1446–8.

97. Ghidini A, Mariani E, Patregnani C, et al. Bronchiolitis obliterans organizing pneumonia in pregnancy. Obstet Gynecol 1999;94(5 Pt 2):843.

98. Adoun M, Ferrand E, Hira M, et al. Un cas atypique de pneumopathie organisée cryptogénique au cours d'une grossesse. Rev Mal Respir 2002;19(5 Pt 1): 638–40 [in French].

99. Ie S, Alper B, Szerlip HM. Respiratory bronchiolitis: an unusual cause of pulmonary infiltrates in a pregnant woman. Am J Med Sci 2000;320(3):219–21.

100. Tosoni C, Faden D, Cattaneo R, et al. Idiopathic eosinophilic pneumonia and pregnancy: report of a case. Int Arch Allergy Immunol 1995;106(2): 173–4.

101. Tohya T, Matsui K, Itoh M, et al. [A case of pulmonary infiltration with eosinophilia syndrome in pregnancy]. Nippon Sanka Fujinka Gakkai Zasshi 1990; 42(4):389–92 [in Japanese].

102. Dothager DW, Kollef MH. Postpartum pulmonary infiltrates with peripheral eosinophilia. Chest 1991;99(2):463–4.

103. Losa Garcia JE, Mateos RF, de la CB, et al. Neumonia eosinofila aguda en gestante. Arch Bronconeumol 1997;33(6):306–8 [in Spanish].

104. Kotani Y, Shiota M, Umemoto M, et al. Emergency cesarean section as a result of acute eosinophilic pneumonia during pregnancy. Tohoku J Exp Med 2009;219(3):251–5.

105. Davies CW, Mackinlay CI, Wathen CG. Recurrent post-partum pulmonary eosinophilia. Thorax 1997; 52(12):1095–6.

106. Christensen B. Which antibiotics are appropriate for treating bacteriuria in pregnancy? J Antimicrob Chemother 2000;46(Suppl 1):29–34.

107. Foucher P, Biour M, Blayac JP, et al. Drugs that may injure the respiratory system. Eur Respir J 1997;10(2):265–79.

108. Cottin V, Bonniaud P. Drug-induced infiltrative lung disease. Eur Respir Mon 2009;46:287–318.

109. Boggess KA, Benedetti TJ, Raghu G. Nitrofurantoin-induced pulmonary toxicity during pregnancy: a report of a case and review of the literature. Obstet Gynecol Surv 1996;51(6):367–70.

110. Poe RH, Condemi JJ, Weinstein SS, et al. Adult respiratory distress syndrome related to ampicillin sensitivity. Chest 1980;77(3):449–50.

111. Ramirez O, Martin B, Sancho B. Bronquiolitis obliterante con neumonia organizada inducida por carbamazepina. Med Clin (Barc) 2007;128(5):198–9 [in Spanish].

112. Banka R, Ward MJ. Bronchiolitis obliterans and organising pneumonia caused by carbamazepine and mimicking community acquired pneumonia. Postgrad Med J 2002;78(924):621–2.

113. Ben JM, Kammoun S, Kanoun F, et al. Manifestations respiratoires de la carbamazepine. A propos d'un cas. Rev Pneumol Clin 1997;53(6): 351–4 [in French].

114. Narita H, Ozawa T, Nishiyama T, et al. An atypical case of fulminant interstitial pneumonitis induced by carbamazepine. Curr Drug Saf 2009;4(1):30–3.

115. Matuschak GM, Owens GR, Rogers RM, et al. Progressive intrapartum respiratory insufficiency due to pulmonary alveolar proteinosis. Amelioration by therapeutic whole-lung bronchopulmonary lavage. Chest 1984;86(3):496–9.

116. Canto MJ, Vives MA, Carmona F, et al. Successful pregnancy after spontaneous remission of familial pulmonary alveolar proteinosis. Eur J Obstet Gynecol Reprod Biol 1995;63(2):191–3.

117. Heilbronn DB, Ridgway DN. Hand-Schueller-Christian disease and pregnancy. Report of a case. Am J Obstet Gynecol 1960;79:805–9.

118. Morrish JA, Newhall JF. Chronic histiocytosis X associated with pregnancy. Obstet Gynecol 1965; 26(4):504–7.

119. Mitra AG, Turpin SV, Cefalo RC. Pregnancy in a patient with eosinophilic granulomatosis of the lung: a case report. Obstet Gynecol 1994;83(5 Pt 2):811–3.

120. Tapia JE, Wagner HP, Altermatt HJ. [Pregnancy and childbirth in a mother with active histiocytosis]. Schweiz Med Wochenschr 1985;115(30):1060–4 [in German].

121. DiMaggio LA, Lippes HA, Lee RV. Histiocytosis X and pregnancy. Obstet Gynecol 1995;85(5 Pt 2):806–9.

122. Sharma R, Maplethorpe R, Wilson G. Effect of pregnancy on lung function in adult pulmonary Langerhans cell histiocytosis. J Matern Fetal Neonatal Med 2006;19(1):67–8.

123. Broscheit J, Eichelbroenner O, Greim C, et al. Anesthetic management of a patient with histiocytosis X and pulmonary complications during Caesarean section. Eur J Anaesthesiol 2004;21(11):919–21.

124. Bruce DM, Heys SD, Eremin O. Lymphangitis carcinomatosa: a literature review. J R Coll Surg Edinb 1996;41(1):7–13.

125. Venkatram S, Muppuri S, Niazi M, et al. A 24-year-old pregnant patient with diffuse alveolar hemorrhage. Chest 2010;138(1):220–3.

126. Gando S, Villarejo F, Maskin B, et al. A 37-year-old woman with multiple pulmonary nodular opacities and hemoptysis. Chest 2006;130(4):1241–3.

127. Seckl MJ, Sebire NJ, Berkowitz RS. Gestational trophoblastic disease. Lancet 2010;376(9742): 717–29.

128. Chittenden B, Ahamed E, Maheshwari A. Choriocarcinoma in a postmenopausal woman. Obstet Gynecol 2009;114(2 Pt 2):462–5.

129. Tidy JA, Rustin GJ, Newlands ES, et al. Presentation and management of choriocarcinoma after nonmolar pregnancy. Br J Obstet Gynaecol 1995;102(9):715–9.

130. Kumar J, Llancheran A, Ratnam SS. Pulmonary metastases in gestational trophoblastic disease: a review of 97 cases. Br J Obstet Gynaecol 1988; 95(1):70–4.

131. Mazur MT, Lurain JR, Brewer JI. Fatal gestational choriocarcinoma. Clinicopathologic study of patients treated at a trophoblastic disease center. Cancer 1982;50(9):1833–46.

132. de La CA, Benoit S, Bouregba M, et al. The treatment of severe pulmonary edema induced by beta adrenergic agonist tocolytic therapy with continuous positive airway pressure delivered by face mask. Anesth Analg 2002;94(6):1593–4, table

133. Pisani RJ, Rosenow EC 3rd. Pulmonary edema associated with tocolytic therapy. Ann Intern Med 1989;110(9):714–8.

134. Vaast P, Dubreucq-Fossaert S, Houfflin-Debarge V, et al. Acute pulmonary oedema during nicardipine therapy for premature labour; Report of five cases. Eur J Obstet Gynecol Reprod Biol 2004; 113(1):98–9.

135. Janower S, Carbonne B, Lejeune V, et al. Oedème pulmonaire aigu lors d'une menace d'accouchement prématuré: rôle de la tocolyse par la nicarpidine. J Gynecol Obstet Biol Reprod (Paris) 2005; 34(8):807–12 [in French].

136. Akerman G, Mignon A, Tsatsaris V, et al. L'oedème aigue du poumon chez des patientes en menace d'accouchement prématuré traitées par inhibiteur calcique: place de facteurs prédisposants ou pharmacologiques spécifiques? J Gynecol Obstet Biol Reprod (Paris) 2007;36(4):389–92 [in French].

137. Ogunyemi D. Risk factors for acute pulmonary edema in preterm delivery. Eur J Obstet Gynecol Reprod Biol 2007;133(2):143–7.

138. Gordon C. Pregnancy and autoimmune diseases. Best Pract Res Clin Rheumatol 2004;18(3):359–79.

139. Elefant E, Cournot MP, Assari F, et al. Immunosuppresseurs utilisés dans les maladies systémiques que faire en cas de grossesse? Presse Med 2008;37(11):1620–6 [in French].

140. Available at: www.Reprotox.org.distributed in Micromedix, Inc.'s TOMES Reprorisk module. Accessed November 8, 2010.

Peripartum Pulmonary Embolism

Margaret A. Miller, MD[a],*, Michel Chalhoub, MD[b],
Ghada Bourjeily, MD[c]

KEYWORDS

- Venous thromboembolism • Pulmonary embolism
- Pregnancy • Ventilation perfusion scan
- Multidetector computed tomography-pulmonary angiogram
- Heparin

Venous thromboembolism (VTE) is a relatively common complication of pregnancy. Maternal mortality is also increased as VTE is one of the leading causes of maternal deaths.[1–5] To prepare the mother for the blood losses associated with delivery, a state of hypercoagulability develops during pregnancy. This hypercoagulability, combined with other pregnancy-associated physiologic changes, may lead to the development of VTE, especially in the presence of additional risk factors. Given the higher risk of VTE and the significant mortality in pregnancy, a timely and accurate diagnosis of pulmonary embolism (PE) along with early institution of appropriate therapy are crucial in the management of these patients.

This review summarizes the physiologic factors predisposing to VTE, pregnancy-specific risk factors, limitations of available diagnostic tests as well as nuances in management.

EPIDEMIOLOGY

In the United States, the incidence of VTE is 0.6 to 2 per 1000 pregnancies.[6–11] Maternal mortality from VTE is 1.1 per 100,000 deliveries, making VTE one of the most common causes of maternal death during pregnancy in developed countries.[12] The case fatality rate of PE in pregnancy based on a recent query of the Nationwide Inpatient Sample from the Health care Cost and Use Project of the Agency for Health care Research and Quality was 2.4%.[9] In the postpartum period, VTE occurs at a rate of 3 to 7 events per 10,000 pregnancies.[6,7,13–15] Some studies have found higher antenatal incidence of VTE,[7,16] whereas other studies found higher incidence of VTE in the postnatal period,[8,11,13,15] and some studies found equal incidence of VTE in the postnatal and antenatal periods.[9,10] Given that the postpartum period (6 weeks) is significantly shorter than the antepartum period (around 40 weeks), the risk of VTE is several-fold higher in the postpartum period when corrected for time.[17] During pregnancy, VTE events occur at similar frequency during all 3 trimesters.[18] The increased risk of VTE decreases postpartum, and reaches the nonpregnant level after the sixth week postpartum.

Racial factors may play a role in the incidence of VTE. Asian and Hispanic pregnant women have significantly lower risk of VTE compared with white pregnant women (1.07 and 1.25 per 1000 deliveries compared with 1.75 per 1000 deliveries respectively), whereas African American pregnant women have the highest risk (2.64 per 1000 deliveries).[9]

Deep venous thrombosis (DVT) is the most common form of VTE in pregnancy[19] and it is found

The authors have nothing to disclose.
a Division of Obstetric and Consultative Medicine, Women and Infants' Hospital of Rhode Island, The Warren Alpert Medical School of Brown University, 100 Dudley Street, Suite 1100, Providence, RI 02905, USA
b Department of Medicine, Pulmonary and Critical Care Medicine, Staten Island University Hospital, 475 Seaview Avenue, Staten Island, NY 10305, USA
c Pulmonary and Critical Care Medicine, Department of Medicine, Women and Infants' Hospital of Rhode Island, The Warren Alpert Medical School of Brown University, 100 Dudley Street, Suite 1100, Providence, RI 02905, USA
* Corresponding author.
E-mail address: Mamiller@wihri.org

Clin Chest Med 32 (2011) 147–164
doi:10.1016/j.ccm.2010.11.005
0272-5231/11/$ – see front matter © 2011 Published by Elsevier Inc.

chestmed.theclinics.com

on the left side in 70% to 90% of cases.[7,18,20] The reason for the left side predilection is believed to be caused by compression of the left iliac vein by the right iliac artery and by the enlarged uterus. Isolated pelvic DVT occurs much more frequently in pregnancy[21] possibly suggesting a different anatomic source of lower extremity thrombosis in pregnancy compared with the nonpregnant population.[17] Women who undergo assisted reproductive techniques are at increased risk of developing upper extremity venous thrombosis.[22]

PATHOPHYSIOLOGY

During pregnancy, all Virchow triad elements are present. These include venous stasis, venous trauma, and hypercoagulability. Venous stasis is enhanced by venodilation that is caused by 2 mechanisms. The first is believed to be hormonal, possibly mediated by nitric oxide; the second mechanism is mechanical compression of pelvic veins by the gravid uterus and compression of the left iliac vein by the right iliac artery. Prenatal or postnatal immobilization contributes to venous stasis and further increases the risk of VTE.

Venous trauma mostly occurs during delivery, typically involves pelvic veins, and occurs during both vaginal and cesarean deliveries. The pulsatile compression of the left common iliac vein is believed to lead to vascular endothelial damage and predispose to thrombus formation. However, tissue factor, a coagulation initiator, is expressed in trophoblasts, amniotic fluid, and the uterine epithelium. It is possible that soluble circulating tissue factor levels increase close to delivery, with further release of tissue factor into the circulation when the placenta separates from the uterine wall.[23]

Alteration in coagulation factors during pregnancy has been reported in multiple studies.[6,24-27] These changes generate a prothrombotic state and are believed to prepare the pregnant woman for the stress of delivery. During gestation there is a significant increase in the levels of factors V, IX, X, VIII, as well as fibrinogen levels.[28,29] In addition, there is a decrease in protein S, and an increase in activated protein C resistance, plasminogen-activator inhibitor 1 (PAI-1) and PAI-2, and thrombin-activatable fibrinolysis inhibitor (TAFI).[30-32] These alterations enhance thrombosis and decrease clot lysis by the fibrinolytic system.

RISK FACTORS

Numerous risk factors for VTE in pregnancy have been evaluated.[9,14] Some have been identified as risk factors for antepartum VTE, and others have been associated with postpartum VTE. A history of thrombophilia (odds ratio [OR] 51.8, 95% confidence interval [CI] 38.7–69.2) and history of thrombosis (OR 24.8, 95% CI 17.1–36.0) have been associated with a significantly increased risk for VTE during pregnancy.[9] Body mass index (BMI, calculated as weight in kilograms divided by the square of height in meters) at the first prenatal visit greater than 25 kg/m² was associated with slight risk of VTE during pregnancy (OR 1.8, 95% CI 1.3–2.4) but when accompanied with antepartum immobilization, the risk of VTE increased significantly (OR 62.3, 95% CI 11.5–337.6).[14] The exact mechanisms by which obesity increases the risk of VTE in pregnancy are not clear. Possible explanations could be related to increased levels of PAI-1, fibrinogen, and serum viscosity.[33-36] In addition, insulin resistance along with hypertriglyceridemia are associated with increased levels of PAI- and alteration in the hemostatic system.[37] An increased risk for pregnancy-associated VTE has also been observed in patients with a history of heart disease (OR 7.1, 95% CI 6.2–8.3),[9] hypertension (OR 1.8, 95% CI 1.4–2.3),[9] and smoking (OR 2.1, 95% CI 1.3–3.4).[14] The chances of developing VTE increase with the number of cigarettes smoked per day. The risk of postpartum VTE is significantly higher in patients with a smoking history of 10 to 30 cigarettes per day at the start of the pregnancy (regardless of whether they continued to smoke during the pregnancy or not) (adjusted OR 2.1, 95% CI 2.1–3.4) compared with those who smoked 1 to 4 cigarettes per day (adjusted OR 1.1, 95% CI 0.5–2.4).[14] Age, parity, and cesarean deliveries have been associated with an increased risk for VTE in some studies but not in others. The adjusted OR of postpartum VTE is 3.1 for preeclampsia, and it increases to 5.8 if preeclampsia is accompanied by intrauterine growth retardation. The mechanisms by which preeclampsia increases the risk of VTE could be related to overstimulation of hepatic coagulation factors by hypoalbuminemia, intravascular hypovolemia, antithrombin loss, and hyperhomocysteinemia.[38] Other possible mechanism for this association could be that individuals with underlying thrombophilia develop thrombosis of placental vessels leading to preeclampsia.[39]

Assisted reproductive techniques (ART) have been associated with an increased risk for VTE.[1] This risk was higher in twin gestations after ART (adjusted OR 6.6, 95% CI 2.1–21.0) compared with single gestations after ART (adjusted OR 4.3, 95% CI 2.0–9.4) and with multiple gestations in spontaneous pregnancies (adjusted OR 2.6, 95% CI 1.1–6.2).[14] The exact mechanism behind the higher incidence of upper extremity DVT in women who have undergone ART is not well understood. A possible explanation suggests that the thoracic duct drains the estradiol-rich ascitic fluid into the subclavian veins, leading to a local reduction in thrombomodulin concentration, which affects the local antithrombotic activity of the endothelium.[22]

DIAGNOSIS

An accurate diagnosis of PE is important, as a false-negative diagnosis may be associated with unacceptably high mortality and a false-positive diagnosis would not only complicate labor and delivery plans but also lead to unnecessary prophylaxis in subsequent pregnancies and challenges with future contraception. Understanding the limitations of every step in the diagnostic tree helps the clinician optimize the management of pregnant women suspected of PE.

Clinical Presentation

In the nonpregnant population, clinical prediction models have been developed and validated, and are often used in combination with D-dimers and imaging to diagnose PE.[40,41] However, these tools have not been validated in the pregnant population and determinants of pretest probability for PE in pregnancy have not been clearly established. Both risk factors and clinical presentation of thrombosis are different in pregnancy. For example, pregnancy itself is a hypercoagulable state and an independent risk factor for thrombosis. DVT in pregnancy presents in the left leg in 85% of cases and many of the typical symptoms of PE (dyspnea, tachycardia, leg swelling) are common in normal pregnancy. None of the available clinical decision rules includes consideration of these differences.

Although some studies have shown that the clinical judgment of an expert provider may be as accurate as clinical prediction models in the general population,[42] no such study exists in pregnancy. Until clinical decision tools are developed for pregnant women, clinicians may need to rely more heavily on diagnostic imaging in making the diagnosis of PE.

Nonimaging Diagnostic Tools

Radiographic imaging remains the primary testing modality for diagnosing PE, but several adjunct tests have been used as well. In the nonpregnant population, the electrocardiographic changes historically considered to be suggestive of PE (S1Q1T3) occur only infrequently in acute PE[43] and the electrocardiogram is not considered to have a strong predictive value for PE. Tachycardia on electrocardiography or examination is often believed to be a more useful

indicator of PE and is included in both the Wells' criteria[40] and the Geneva criteria.[44] In pregnancy, however, the baseline heart rate may increase by 20% to 30%, therefore mild tachycardia is often seen in normal pregnancy and may not be a useful indicator of PE. Arterial blood gas values also change in pregnancy. The average Pao_2 is 105 mm Hg and based on a small retrospective analysis, the A-a gradient is normal in more than half of pregnant women with PE.[45] D-dimers carry a negative predictive value of 94% or better in the nonpregnant patient with a low clinical suspicion for PE.[46–48] Newer generations of D-dimers are more sensitive and may safely exclude the diagnosis of PE even when combined with moderate clinical pretest probability.[49] D-dimers are likely to perform differently in the pregnant population for many reasons. (1) D-dimer levels in asymptomatic pregnancies have consistently shown a significant increase as the pregnancy progresses.[50,51] (2) The incidence of PE in pregnant patients suspected of having the diagnosis is actually lower than the incidence of PE in nonpregnant patients being evaluated for the same diagnosis.[52] (3) Measurements of D-dimer levels must always be combined with validated tests to assign low or moderate clinical pretest probability to safely exclude PE. Although there have not been any diagnostic cohort studies evaluating D-dimers in the diagnosis of PE in pregnancy, a recent diagnostic cohort study confirmed an expected decrease in specificity of the test with each trimester in patients being evaluated for PE.[53] The investigators of this study have concluded that further studies need to be done before this test can be safely used to exclude a diagnosis of DVT in pregnancy.[53]

Imaging in Pregnancy

Both patients and providers are often anxious about the potential harmful effects of radiation on the fetus. The effects of radiation on the unborn child and the amount of radiation that follows diagnostic imaging studies are discussed in detail elsewhere in this issue. Counseling the patient about the risk of radiation must be balanced with an assessment of the risk of withholding the test. Virtually all diagnostic tests that use ionizing radiation for the diagnosis of PE expose the fetus to a radiation dose that is far less than the acceptable limit of radiation in pregnancy. The diagnosis and treatment of PE in pregnancy should not be delayed because of concerns about radiation exposure.

Despite the low dose of radiation associated with these diagnostic tests, practices to reduce exposure and limit unnecessary testing should obviously be considered. For example, abdominal shielding provides some protection to the fetus.[54]

In addition, automatic tube current modulation, faster table speed and higher pitch may improve dose efficiency in computed tomography (CT) scans. Radiation dose may be minimized with ventilation perfusion (VQ) scans by starting with a half-dose perfusion scan followed by a ventilation scan only if perfusion is abnormal. Other measures that would reduce fetal radiation exposure include hydration and advising the mother to void frequently to avoid pooling of the radioactive material in the bladder.

Chest radiography
Chest radiographs involve minimal radiation, may offer an alternative diagnosis,[55] rarely show signs suggestive of PE, and may potentially help the clinician decide on the type of further diagnostic studies.[56]

VQ scan
Data on the accuracy of VQ in pregnancy are not available and outcome studies are limited. The PIOPED study clearly established that the predictive value of the VQ scan in the general population is highly dependent on the pretest probability.[57] For example, the positive predictive value of a high probability VQ is much higher with a high, compared with a low, clinical suspicion (96% vs 56%, respectively). Several factors make it difficult to apply these results to a population of pregnant women. First, validated clinical prediction rules of PE are lacking in pregnancy. In addition, the prevalence of PE in pregnant women with suspicious symptoms is lower than the general population.[52] As a result, the positive predictive value of the lung scan is likely lower. The lower prevalence of PE in the pregnant population would also lead to a higher negative predictive value of normal/near normal scans.

Although a significant disadvantage of the use of VQ scan in the general population is the high rate of intermediate scans (39%),[57] the rate of intermediate scans in the pregnant population is close to 20% in 1 study,[52] and possibly lower in studies that use chest radiography before having a VQ scan or a multidetector computed tomography-pulmonary angiogram (MDCT-PA).[56] In addition, the rate of normal scans in pregnancy is significantly higher than in the general population (70% vs 14%, respectively).[52] This likely reflects the young age and low incidence of chronic lung disease in this population but may also be a reflection of the poor predictive power of the clinical presentation. The nondiagnostic scan rate in pregnancy varies between 7%[56] and 21%[52] leading to a need for additional testing and potential for further radiation exposure.

Fetal radiation exposure with a perfusion or a ventilation and perfusion scan is likely higher than with a MDCT-PA depending on the method used for absorbed radiation measurements,[54,58,59] however both studies are associated with radiation doses that are far less than the acceptable limit of 5 to 10 rad. On the other hand, maternal breast radiation exposure with a VQ scan is estimated to be 30 to 150 times lower than with a MDCT-PA, making VQ an attractive test for a young woman.[60]

MDCT-PA
Both outcome and accuracy data for the use of MDCT-PA are available for the general population, but no such data exist for the use of MDCT-PA in pregnancy. A clear advantage of MDCT-PA over a VQ scan is that MDCT-PA offers an alternative diagnosis. In 1 study of pregnant patients undergoing a reduced dose protocol MDCT in the diagnosis of PE, 19% had an alternative diagnosis by MDCT-PA.[55] In retrospective analyses of cost-effectiveness, MDCT-PA was found to be the most cost effective test in the evaluation of PE, whether it was used as the first-line test or whenever it was included at any point in the diagnostic approach.[61,62] The accuracy of technically adequate MDCT-PA in pregnancy is likely similar to that in the general population. However, the diagnostic approach in pregnancy uses nonvalidated clinical pretest probability, and D-dimer tests are likely to perform differently as well. Therefore, outcomes of MDCT in pregnancy should be tested further.

Technical limitations
Although the rate of technically limited studies in the nonpregnant population ranges between 2% and 9%,[63–65] technical limitations likely occur more frequently in pregnancy. Although no physiologic studies have been done to explain the higher likelihood of technical limitations, it is believed that normal physiologic changes in pregnancy may affect the quality of CT images. A significant increase in heart rate may affect the time between injection and appearance of contrast in the main pulmonary artery. Therefore, imaging protocols using a fixed time delay between the timing of the bolus injection and the initiation of scanning as used in the nonpregnant population may miss contrast opacification in the pulmonary vascular tree. Peak vascular enhancement is inversely proportional to cardiac output[66]; cardiac output is increased by 45% to 50% in pregnancy and is higher in multiple gestations. Increased weight and an enhanced Valsalva maneuver may also contribute to difficulties with vascular enhancement. Recent studies have shown that the rate of technical

imitations is 20.5% to 35.7%,[67–70] with a higher number of segments that are not properly evaluated.[70] However, other studies have shown no difference in quantitative measures of vascular enhancement between a pregnant and a nonpregnant group using a low-dose protocol.[55] These findings suggest that protocol modifications need to be performed in institutions imaging a large number of pregnant patients, not only to reduce the radiation dose but also to improve image quality and reduce the number of technically limited studies. In a recent survey-based study, 53% of the members of the Thoracic Radiology Society perform MDCT-PA as an initial test in pregnant patients but only 40% modify the imaging protocol.[71] Protocol modifications that could help with vascular enhancement include improving iodine delivery rates by changing the rate of injection from the standard 4 mL/s to 6 mL/s,[66] increasing contrast dose even in newer generation scanners that require a shorter scanning time, or using contrast medium with a higher iodine concentration.

Contrast media

Other concerns are related to iodinated contrast material. Contrast media are believed to cross the placenta because they are small molecules that redistribute in the extracellular space. Fetal gut opacification has been observed following intravenous administration of iodinated contrast to the pregnant woman. Iodine levels have also been detected in the amniotic fluid suggesting placental transfer and elimination by the fetal kidneys with a potential transfer back to the mother as some studies have shown a reduction in iodine levels with time. Despite documented placental transfer, no teratogenic effects have been reported. Concerns with iodine transfer across the placenta result from the potential effects of high doses of iodine on fetal thyroid. Although earlier small studies had suggested possible effects, more recent data showed normal thyroid function in 343 neonates exposed to iodinated contrast at various stages of gestation.[72] Controversy in the literature relates to the physical characteristics of the contrast material used, maternal thyroid and renal function, maternal iodine reserve, time of exposure to iodine during gestation, and duration of time between exposure and thyroid testing in the neonate.

Radiation exposure

Fetal radiation exposure following MDCT-PA was shown to be lower than exposure with a VQ scan at any gestational age.[59] Other studies using different methods to measure radiation absorption show slightly higher radiation with MDCT, which remains well below the acceptable limit of radiation.[54,58,59]

A significant concern in using MDCT-PA in this young patient population is breast radiation. Extrapolation of data from atomic bomb survivors suggests that exposure of the breasts before age 20 years and after age 35 years to a radiation dose of 1 Sv or higher was associated with an estimated excess relative risk of breast cancer of 14.6 and 2.0, respectively.[73,74] Extrapolating these estimates to North American women may be impractical because the rate of breast cancer in Japan is much lower than in the western world. In a 2005 report, the National Academy of Sciences Biologic Effects of Ionizing Radiation (BEIR) VII reported on an absolute risk model derived from A-bomb survivors as well as 3 US cohorts exposed to ionizing radiation.[75] Using this model, a recent estimate of the relative risk of breast cancer following CT coronary angiography was 1 in 143 at age 20 years and a lifetime relative risk of 0.7% after exposure to an average of 0.05 to 0.08 rad.[76] MDCT-PA done without breast shields exposes the breast to an average of 2 to 5 rad.[77,78] Bismuth shields have been shown to reduce the amount of radiation exposure from an average of 0.022 rad to 0.01 Gy,[77] although breast shielding is not used routinely in adult women in the United States. The authors' (MAM, GB) institution uses breast shields routinely on all women undergoing CT of the chest, abdomen, or pelvis.

Compression ultrasonography

Compression ultrasonography (CUS) has a low yield in the evaluation of PE as an initial test in patients without leg symptoms.[79] In the nonpregnant population, proximal thrombus is found on CUS in 23% to 52% of patients with confirmed PE,[79–82] with most manifesting signs and symptoms of DVT. For several reasons, CUS as an initial test may perform even more poorly in the diagnosis of PE in pregnant women. Sensitivity of CUS is likely lower in pregnancy because isolated pelvic vein thrombi are more common in pregnancy[21] and CUS have a low yield in detecting these thrombi. The frequency of lower extremity thrombi in pregnant patients with PE is unknown. The clinical significance of positive compression ultrasounds in asymptomatic patients is unclear.

In pregnant patients with signs and/or symptoms of DVT in addition to suspected PE, it is reasonable to use CUS to exclude DVT as the initial test of choice. However, prompt evaluation of pregnant women with symptoms of PE, but not DVT with radiologic tests should not be avoided because of concerns about radiation exposure.

Magnetic resonance imaging

Magnetic resonance (MR) is in its early stages in the diagnosis of PE. The use of gadolinium-enhanced MR angiography has been evaluated in the PIOPED III trial,[83] but, unfortunately, pregnant women were excluded from this trial. MR angiography was technically inadequate in 25% of patients because of poor quality. The rate of technically inadequate studies varied by clinical center from 11% to 51%. Among the technically adequate studies, the sensitivity of MR angiography was 78% and the specificity was 99%. Combined MR angiography and MR venography had a higher sensitivity (92%) and similar specificity (96%).

The use of MR is limited in pregnancy when gadolinium is necessary for the imaging protocol. Studies regarding the safety of this agent in human pregnancy are very limited.[84] Gadolinium crosses the placenta but its effects on the fetus are not well studied. Non–gadolinium-enhanced techniques such as time-of-flight angiography and MR direct thrombus imaging do not involve gadolinium or ionizing radiation but these techniques have not been appropriately studied yet and can not be recommended for routine use in or outside pregnancy.

Non–gadolinium-enhanced MR venography also plays an important role in the diagnosis of pelvic clots in patients with negative ultrasounds and a high index of suspicion for thrombi. MR detects clots in the inferior vena cava and in the abdomen and does not involve ionizing radiation.

Other imaging studies

Pulmonary angiogram was considered the gold standard test in the diagnosis of PE for many years but has clearly been replaced by MDCT-PA in recent years. Pulmonary angiograms are now rarely used in most institutions. The disadvantage of this test in pregnancy is the relatively high level of fetal radiation exposure (0.0005 Gy by brachial route) compared with MDCT-PA (0.000003–0.000131 Gy)[59] and its invasive nature.

Conventional venograms have been considered the gold standard in the evaluation of lower extremity veins[85] for many years. Their use in the general population is now quite limited because of the wide availability of less invasive testing. Conventional venograms are also an option in pregnancy but less invasive techniques such as MR venography may offer an alternative that is associated with no radiation exposure to the fetus.

CT venography is easy to perform with 3- to 4-minute delayed images during a MDCT-PA study with the dual advantage of evaluating the pulmonary tree and the leg veins. In the PIOPED II trial,[6] CT venography improved the sensitivity of MDCT-PA from 83% to 90%. Other studies have shown a sensitivity of 93% to 100%, a specificity of 97% to 100%,[86–88] a negative predictive value of 100% and a positive predictive value of 71%.[89] A major disadvantage is the added fetal radiation exposure, estimated to be close to 0.05 Gy.[90,91] Having not been studied in the pregnant population, the routine use of CT venography in these patients is rarely justified.

Impedance plethysmography has been used in the past as a first-line noninvasive test. Sensitivity of this test in the detection of proximal venous thrombi is lower than leg ultrasounds and approaches 65%.[92,93] Serial impedance plethysmography has been evaluated in a cohort study of 152 pregnant patients and was shown to safely exclude DVT.[94] However, this diagnostic tool is no longer in use.

PROGNOSIS

Prognostic rules predicting short-term mortality have been developed in the general population but have not been validated in pregnancy. The Geneva prognostic criteria[95] include heart rate greater than 110 beats per minute at presentation and both this prognostic tool and the PE severity index (PESI)[96] include systolic blood pressure less than 100 mm Hg as part of the adverse prognostic criteria. Given the increase in heart in pregnancy by 20% to 30% by the third trimester and the reduction in systemic vascular resistance resulting in a physiologic reduction in blood pressure, these criteria may not be as predictive of mortality in this population. A review of consecutive autopsies in Brazil has identified 512 deaths related to pulmonary thromboembolism and a review of potential predictors has identified pelvic vein thrombosis as a mortality predictor.[9] It is not clear whether this holds true in pregnancy given that the rate of isolated pelvic vein thrombosis is significantly higher than in the nonpregnant population.[21]

Two-dimensional Echocardiography

Echocardiography is an insensitive tool in the diagnosis of PE.[46] However, echocardiography helps assess right ventricular function and can provide prognostic clues relating to in-hospital mortality from massive PE,[98,99] but more so in hemodynamically unstable patients.[100] In patients with PE, echocardiography helps evaluate right atrial and ventricular dilation, paradoxic septal motion, pulmonary hypertension, and tricuspid regurgitation

Nonetheless, it is important to know that the hyperdynamic state of a normal pregnancy may affect the reading of echocardiography. For instance, both the systolic and the diastolic dimensions and systolic function are slightly increased in pregnancy. There is also a moderate increase in the size of the right chambers and the left atrium, progressive dilation of pulmonary, tricuspid and mitral valve annuli, and some degree of pulmonary, tricuspid and mitral regurgitation.[101] Hence, interpretation of two-dimensional echocardiograms should preferably be performed by a cardiologist experienced in reading those for pregnant women.

APPROACH TO DIAGNOSIS OF PE IN PREGNANCY

A diagnostic approach to suspected PE in pregnancy is suggested in **Figs. 1–3**. In patients who present with symptoms of PE and DVT, compression ultrasound is the best initial test. If there are no signs or symptoms of DVT, immediate VQ scan or MDCT-PA should be done, considering the advantages and disadvantages of each test. If imaging is not immediately available, full-dose anticoagulation therapy should be started.

An initial indeterminate VQ scan result should prompt evaluation with MDCT-PA. If an intraluminal filling defect in at least a segmental or greater vessel appears in the same distribution as the matched perfusion defect on the VQ scan, then the result is considered positive and the patient should be treated for PE.

The management of subsegmental emboli is quite challenging both during and outside of pregnancy. There are insufficient data regarding outcomes of patients with subsegmental emboli in whom anticoagulation has been withheld. Recommendations in the literature[102,103] are based on limited outcome data and expert opinion rather than randomized studies. Given that normal VQ scans can safely exclude PE,[57] the finding of normal perfusion on a perfusion scan in patients with an isolated subsegmental intraluminal filling defect on MDCT is likely reassuring. However, if a perfusion defect is noted in the same vascular distribution, PE can be diagnosed. Although this approach has not been demonstrated to be safe during pregnancy or outside pregnancy, the investigators suggest performing a perfusion scan in patients with an isolated subsegmental embolus on MDCT before deciding to commit the patient to unnecessary anticoagulation or unsafely withholding it.

MANAGEMENT
Acute PE

Heparins
Acute treatment of PE can be done with low-molecular-weight heparin (LMWH) or unfractionated heparin (UFH). LMWH is first-line therapy for the treatment of acute PE in the general population and in pregnancy. Both LMWH and UFH potentiate antithrombin's anti-activated coagulation factor activity (including anti-Xa and anti-IIa activity), limit further thrombus formation, and permit time for fibrinolysis of the established thrombus.

Advantages of LMWH compared with UFH in the general population are summarized in **Table 1** and include (1) longer half-life and better bioavailability[104]; (2) comparable efficacy and safety[105,106]; and (3) a lower risk of heparin-induced thrombocytopenia,[107] a rare but serious complication resulting from the development of platelet activating anti-PF4/heparin complex antibodies potentially leading to arterial and venous thrombosis.[108] A randomized study evaluating the use of LMWH compared with UFH and untreated controls in pregnant women has shown no difference in bone density in the LMWH group compared with the untreated group but showed significantly lower measurements of bone density in the group treated with UFH compared with untreated patients and patients treated with LMWH.[109] Rare osteoporotic fractures were also reported in a systematic review (0.04%).[19] The

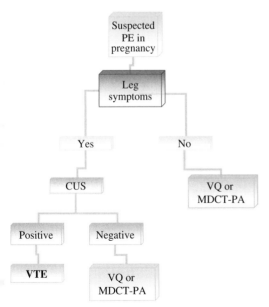

Fig. 1. Suggested algorithm for suspected PE and leg symptoms suggestive of DVT. (*Adapted from* Bourjeily G, Paidas M, Khalil H, et al. Pulmonary embolism in pregnancy. Lancet 2010;375:500–12; with permission.)

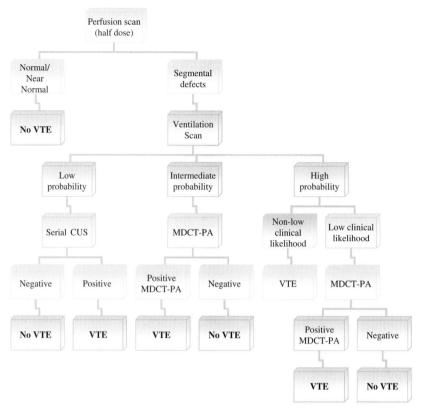

Fig. 2. Suggested algorithm for VQ scan. (*Adapted from* Bourjeily G, Paidas M, Khalil H, et al. Pulmonary embolism in pregnancy. Lancet 2010;375:500–12; with permission.)

risk of bleeding with LMWH is not increased in pregnancy compared with the general population. In a systematic review,[19] the risk of antepartum bleeding was 0.43%, risk of postpartum bleeding was 0.94% and 0.61% for wound hematoma. The risk of skin allergies was 1.8%,[19] similar to the risk in the nonpregnant population.

No adequately powered studies have been done to determine differences in efficacy and safety of LMWH compared with UFH in pregnancy. One study and a small series suggest equivalence.[110] LMWHs do not cross the placenta and a systematic review showed that 94.7% of 2215 pregnancies treated with LMWH had successful outcomes, defined as live birth.[19]

Of particular concern in pregnant women is the potential for limited options for regional anesthesia. Because of reports of epidural hematomas and hemiplegia in nonobstetric patients on anticoagulants undergoing epidural anesthesia, the American Society of Regional Anesthesia (ASRA) recommends that regional anesthesia should be avoided in patients who have received LMWH within the previous 12 to 24 hours.[111]

Heparins (both UFH and LMWH) do not cross the placenta so there is no risk of fetal teratogenicity or fetal bleeding. For this reason, it is necessary to use heparins to treat and prevent thrombosis throughout pregnancy.

Dosing and monitoring of LMWH in pregnancy must account for changes in pharmacokinetics. Studies of LMWH suggest that drug clearance is dependent on gestational age,[112,113] with increasing doses of LMWH being required to maintain a therapeutic level as pregnancy progresses.[113,114] Other small series suggest that prolonged use may result in an accumulation of dose effect.[115] Treatment should be initiated with standard dosing as in the nonpregnant population, but monitoring of drug effect is advised.[116] Weekly anti-Xa levels performed 3 to 6 hours after dosing with a target level of 0.5 to 1.1 are likely warranted until therapeutic, with subsequent monthly monitoring in patients on full anticoagulation after the first month.

Intravenous UFH should be considered in the treatment of acute PE in pregnancy in patients with renal failure, or when urgent reversal of anticoagulation may be required (eg, high bleeding risk or imminent surgery or delivery). A weight-based bolus should be calculated using the patient's current weight. Monitoring with partial thromboplastin time (PTT) may be inadequate in

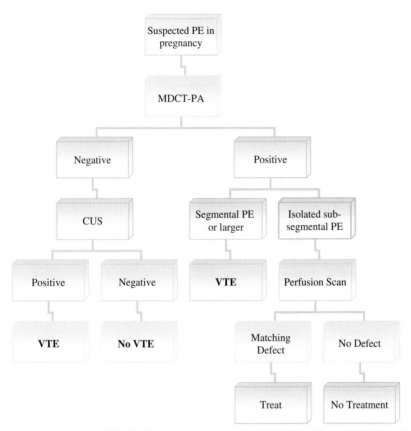

Fig. 3. Diagnostic algorithm for MDCT-PA. (*Adapted from* Bourjeily G, Paidas M, Khalil H, et al. Pulmonary embolism in pregnancy. Lancet 2010;375:500–12, with permission.)

the pregnant woman for several reasons. Activated partial thromboplastin time (aPTT) likely performs differently in pregnancy as a result of increased heparin-binding proteins, factor VIII levels, and fibrinogen. Reduced heparin bioavailability, increased dose-response variability, and dissociation of heparin levels and PTT among pregnant patients[117] suggest that heparin anti-Xa monitoring may be preferable.[118] Because of the difficulty in obtaining this test in a timely manner, PTT is still the primary monitoring tool in most institutions.

Thrombolysis

Thrombolytic therapy has been used in pregnancy with a risk of bleeding that is similar to the risk observed outside of pregnancy. Thirty-two cases of thrombolysis in pregnancy have been reported (10 with PE) followed by additional case reports (3 with PE), with major nonfatal bleeding reported in 2 of 32 cases.[119] There may be a risk of obstetric and neonatal complications such as pregnancy loss, abruption, and preterm labor. However, it is hard to ascertain whether these complications are a result of the underlying disease, the therapy, or neither. With such limited data, the use of thrombolytics in pregnancy should be reserved for women with PE who are hemodynamically unstable or with refractory hypoxemia. Data on nonpregnant

Table 1
Use of LMWH versus UFH in pregnancy

	LMWH Versus UFH
Bioavailability	Better with LMWH
Efficacy	Comparable
Safety	Comparable
Likelihood of regional anesthesia	Likely lower with LMWH
Risk of HIT	Lower with LMWH
Heparin-induced osteopenia	Lower with LMWH
Monitoring	Anti-Xa level with LMWH, target level 0.5–1.1 Heparin anti-Xa level with UFH preferred, target 0.35–0.67

Abbreviation: HIT, heparin-induced thrombocytopenia.

patients had not shown a mortality benefit in patients with large PE with right ventricular dysfunction, but without hemodynamic compromise or hypoxemia treated with thrombolytics[120]; therefore the use of these agents under these circumstances should be discouraged.

Subacute PE

Heparins should also be used as subacute and chronic anticoagulation therapy in pregnant women. Coumarin crosses the placenta and is an established teratogen. Fetal exposure to coumarin between weeks 5 and 12 causes a distinctive embryopathy when the small facial bones are forming in 5% to 10% of infants.[121] Exposure later in gestation has also been associated with an increased risk of fetal hemorrhage and a 2% to 3% risk of central nervous system malformations. Unlike patients with valvular heart disease, LMWH is at least as effective as coumarins in preventing recurrent thromboembolic disease. For this reason, LMWH is the drug of choice for the treatment of thrombosis throughout pregnancy and the use of coumarins for this indication cannot be justified. Although warfarin crosses into the breast milk, the infant's exposure is minimal and there is no change in the infant's coagulation profile.

Duration of Therapy

There are no adequately designed studies available to guide the duration of therapy and this issue remains controversial. Although data on patients with cancer with VTE suggest that dose reduction after 1 month of therapy with full-dose anticoagulation may be safe,[122] the safety of this approach in pregnancy has not been established. Although malignancy is likely associated with a higher risk of recurrence than pregnancy, pharmacokinetic properties of LMWH in pregnancy make this approach harder to apply without further studies establishing its safety. It is unclear whether pregnancy should be considered a temporary risk factor and pregnancy-associated VTE treated for 3 months. There is a general agreement that patients should be treated at least for 6 weeks postpartum. Recent guidelines from the American College of Chest Physicians recommends the use of anticoagulation for 6 months and at least in the postpartum period.[123] Although some patients may be candidates for long-term anticoagulation (antiphospholipid antibody syndrome, recurrent VTE), most require a total of 3 to 6 months of therapy.

Labor and Delivery

Management of patients with acute PE can be challenging around the time of labor and delivery.

Delivery in a patient on full-dose anticoagulation may be associated with significant bleeding risk. Decisions regarding discontinuation of anticoagulation for delivery must consider the type of anticoagulation, the timing of the PE, the risk of VTE recurrence, and nonanalgesic indications of regional anesthesia (**Table 2**). UFH has a shorter half-life and is more easily reversed with protamine than LMWH. This approach is advantageous in terms of reducing the risk of bleeding as well as the improved chances of regional anesthesia. Some experts recommend switching patients on full-dose LMWH to a therapeutic dose of UFH at 36 weeks in anticipation of delivery, whereas others continue LMWH and discontinue only around delivery. In patients with acute PE near term (>37 weeks), placement of an inferior vena cava filter should be considered as any duration off anticoagulation may carry excessive risk.[124] For all patients on full-dose anticoagulation in pregnancy, a planned induction of labor provides an opportunity to discontinue anticoagulation before delivery. With a remote clot, patients should be instructed to stop anticoagulation 12 to 24 hours before the start of the induction. However, even if induction of labor is planned, the onset of labor can be unpredictable and the duration variable.

Reinitiation of anticoagulation should be individualized with the patient's risk of recurrent VTE weighed against the risk of bleeding. In patients with high risk of recurrent VTE, intravenous heparin or LMWH should be started as soon as hemostasis is achieved with subsequent overlap with warfarin. Average-risk patients may be restarted on anticoagulation within 24 hours.

Prevention

Large-scale studies on prophylaxis of VTE in pregnancy are limited so recommendations regarding prophylaxis of VTE in pregnancy are based primarily on case series, consensus statements, and studies done in the nonpregnant population. Without clear data regarding level of risk of VTE in any given clinical scenario in pregnancy, it is difficult to consider the risk versus benefit of prophylactic anticoagulation. Estimates of major bleeding risk with prophylactic anticoagulation in pregnancy are around 0.4% to 1.5%.[19] Therefore the rate of VTE needs to approach the bleeding rate before prophylactic anticoagulation is warranted. In many clinical scenarios where VTE risk is believed to be low (<1.5%), avoidance of immobilization and compression stockings is likely all that is needed. In patients with previous VTE, data regarding recurrence in pregnancy is inconsistent

Table 2
Suggested management of anticoagulation for labor and delivery

Clinical Scenario	Plan for Labor and Delivery
Patient on prophylactic dose of LMWH for remote clot	Switch to UFH 10,000 units twice a day at 36 weeks' gestation or continue LMWH until induction. Disadvantages of the latter include reversal difficulties if labor occurs before planned induction date Discontinue UFH 12 h before procedure
Patient on therapeutic dose of LMWH VTE >1 month before EDD	Switch to UFH at 36 weeks' gestation Discontinue UFH 12–24 h before scheduled procedure Restart IV UFH or subcutaneous LMWH 12–24 h after delivery
Patient with VTE 2–4 wk before EDD	Initiate treatment with intravenous UFH. Once therapeutic, switch to subcutaneous heparin (total daily IV dose divided into twice daily dosing) Discontinue subcutaneous UFH heparin 24 h before procedure and initiate intravenous heparin Discontinue UFH 6 h before anticipated delivery. Restart IV heparin 6 h after delivery if possible Consider IVC filter given the unpredictable nature of labor
Patient with VTE <2 weeks before delivery	Place IVC filter (preferably retrievable) Initiate IV UFH using standard weight-based dosing Discontinue UFH 6 hours before anticipated procedure Restart IV heparin 6 hours after delivery if possible
In all cases	Anesthesia consult regarding anesthetic and analgesic options Monitor platelets closely when changing to UFH Consider cesarean delivery only if obstetric or indications other than anticoagulation Consider planned induction for all patients on therapeutic anticoagulation Discontinue heparin at the first sign of labor Weigh risk of recurrence with discontinuation of anticoagulation against the risk of obstetric hemorrhage and epidural/spinal hematoma Check coagulation profile on admission

Abbreviations: EDD, estimated due date; IV, intravenous; IVC, inferior vena cava.

Available randomized trials on risk of recurrence following thromboprophylaxis compared with no therapy or placebo are limited by their very small numbers[125,126] and most recommendations are based on a known risk of recurrence of 1.4% to 11.4%[127,128] and the following data. In a prospective study, women with a single prior VTE associated with a temporary risk factor (including pregnancy and oral contraceptives) and no thrombophilia have been shown to have a recurrence risk of 0%.[127] In the same study, women with a single prior unprovoked VTE with a thrombophilia had a risk of recurrent thrombosis in pregnancy of 5.9%. However, a retrospective study of 155 pregnancies found that the rate of recurrent VTE in pregnancy was similar in women with prior VTE associated with pregnancy or oral contraceptives and those with unprovoked VTE.[129]

National and International Guidelines on prevention of thrombosis in pregnancy differ widely and are summarized in **Table 3**. A reasonable approach to prevention is to consider thrombosis prophylaxis

Table 3
Summary of guidelines for prevention of thrombosis in pregnancy

	Source of Recommendation/ Level of Evidence	Antepartum	Postpartum
Single VTE Transient risk (nonhormonal) No thrombophilia	ACCP (Grade 1C) RCOG C ACOG	Surveillance	Anticoagulant prophylaxis
Single VTE Transient risk (hormonal) No thrombophilia	ACCP (Grade 2C) ACOG C RCOG	Surveillance or anticoagulant prophylaxis Anticoagulant prophylaxis	Anticoagulant prophylaxis Anticoagulant prophylaxis
Single VTE Idiopathic No thrombophilia	ACCP (Grade 1C) ACOG RCOG C	Anticoagulant prophylaxis or surveillance	Anticoagulant prophylaxis
Single VTE Thrombophilia	ACCP (Grade 1C) ACOG RCOG B	Anticoagulant prophylaxis or surveillance Anticoagulant prophylaxis	Anticoagulant prophylaxis Anticoagulant prophylaxis
Single VTE Higher risk thrombophilia	ACCP (Grade 2C) RCOG C ACOG	Anticoagulant prophylaxis	Anticoagulant prophylaxis
Multiple VTE	ACCP (Grade 2C) RCOG C ACOG	Anticoagulant prophylaxis	Anticoagulant prophylaxis

Abbreviations: ACCP, American College of Chest Physicians[123]; ACOG, American College of Obstetrics and Gynecology[134]; RCOG, Royal College of Physicians.[135]

in all women with a history of previous DVT in the context of other risk factors. Those with single VTE provoked by factors other than pregnancy or exogenous estrogen and with no thrombophilia may not benefit from thromboprophylaxis. Thrombophilia alone with no prior history of VTE may represent varying degrees of risk but methodological limitations clearly affect the accuracy of these estimates. A recent systematic review of 9 studies[130] has shown that the highest risks for VTE were associated with homozygosity for factor V Leiden (OR 34.40, 95% CI 9.86–120.05) and homozygosity of the prothrombin G20210A variant (OR 26.36, 95% CI 1.24–559.20). The most common inherited thrombophilias were associated with lower risks (heterozygosity for factor V Leiden, OR 8.32, 95% CI 5.44–12.70; and heterozygosity for the prothrombin G20210A variant, OR 6.80, 95% CI 2.46–18.77). Patients with compound heterozygosity for factor V Leiden and prothrombin gene mutation are also at very high risk of recurrence. On the other hand, factor V Leiden was found to have 0% antepartum risk in some cohorts[131] but higher in others.[132,133] Patients

Table 4
Typical dosing of anticoagulation in pregnancy

	Prophylactic	Therapeutic
UFH	5000 units SQ twice a day, first trimester 7500 units SQ twice a day, second trimester 10,000 units SQ twice a day, third trimester	Total daily requirement of IV heparin divided into twice daily dosing
LMWH	Standard daily dosing <20 weeks' gestation Double the dose after 20 weeks	Standard therapeutic dosing, titrate to anti-Xa level

Abbreviations: IV, intravenous; SQ, subcutaneously.

with BMI greater than 25 kg/m^2 and immobilization for more than 1 week may have a particularly high risk (adjusted OR 62.3, 95% CI 11.5–337.6).[14]

Typical dosing for anticoagulation in pregnancy is summarized in **Table 4**.

SUMMARY

The poor predictive value of the clinical presentation of PE in the pregnant women can make the diagnosis particularly challenging. With no validated clinical decision rules and lack of established usefulness of D-dimer in pregnancy, a working knowledge of the normal physiologic changes of pregnancy is critical in interpreting symptoms of PE in the parturient. Apprehension about radiologic procedures in pregnancy may lead to unnecessary delay in diagnosis and clinicians should be aware that the risk of missed diagnosis is significantly higher than the risk of radiation from diagnostic radiologic procedures. A paucity of data makes it difficult to define the test of choice for diagnosis of PE in pregnancy. Several options have been discussed in this review. Considerations in treating a pregnant woman with anticoagulation include pharmacokinetic changes, potential teratogenicity, and bleeding risk during labor and delivery.

Further research is needed to be able to confidently make recommendations regarding the management of venous thromboembolism in pregnancy. Nevertheless, PE remains a leading cause of maternal mortality and an understanding of the presentation of PE in pregnancy and the risk/benefit of diagnostic tests and treatment is required for prompt diagnosis and prevention of this condition.

REFERENCES

1. al-Meshari A, Chattopadhyay SK, Younes B, et al. Trends in maternal mortality in Saudi Arabia. Int J Gynaecol Obstet 1996;52:25–32.
2. Kobayashi T, Nakabayashi M, Ishikawa M, et al. Pulmonary thromboembolism in obstetrics and gynecology increased by 6.5-fold over the past decade in Japan. Circ J 2008;72:753–6.
3. Legnain M, Singh R, Busarira MO. Maternal mortality in Benghazi: a clinicoepidemiological study. East Mediterr Health J 2000;6:283–92.
4. Panting-Kemp A, Geller SE, Nguyen T, et al. Maternal deaths in an urban perinatal network, 1992–1998. Am J Obstet Gynecol 2000;183:1207–12.
5. Sullivan EA, Ford JB, Chambers G, et al. Maternal mortality in Australia 1973–1996. Aust N Z J Obstet Gynaecol 2004;44:452–7.
6. Andersen BS, Steffensen FH, Sorensen HT, et al. The cumulative incidence of venous thromboembolism during pregnancy and puerperium–an 11 year Danish population-based study of 63,300 pregnancies. Acta Obstet Gynecol Scand 1998;77:170–3.
7. Gherman RB, Goodwin TM, Leung B, et al. Incidence, clinical characteristics, and timing of objectively diagnosed venous thromboembolism during pregnancy. Obstet Gynecol 1999;94:730–4.
8. Heit JA, Kobbervig CE, James AH, et al. Trends in the incidence of venous thromboembolism during pregnancy or postpartum: a 30-year population-based study. Ann Intern Med 2005;143:697–706.
9. James AH, Jamison MG, Brancazio LR, et al. Venous thromboembolism during pregnancy and the postpartum period: incidence, risk factors, and mortality. Am J Obstet Gynecol 2006;194:1311–5.
10. Lindqvist P, Dahlback B, Marsal K. Thrombotic risk during pregnancy: a population study. Obstet Gynecol 1999;94:595–9.
11. Simpson EL, Lawrenson RA, Nightingale AL, et al. Venous thromboembolism in pregnancy and the puerperium: incidence and additional risk factors from a London perinatal database. BJOG 2001;108:56–60.
12. European perinatal health report by the Euro-Peristat project: [better statistics for better health for pregnant women and their babies]: data from 2004. 2008. Available at: http://www.europeristat.com/index.shtml. Accessed July 22, 2010.
13. Danilenko-Dixon DR, Heit JA, Silverstein MD, et al. Risk factors for deep vein thrombosis and pulmonary embolism during pregnancy or post partum: a population-based, case-control study. Am J Obstet Gynecol 2001;184:104–10.
14. Jacobsen AF, Skjeldestad FE, Sandset PM. Ante- and postnatal risk factors of venous thrombosis: a hospital-based case-control study. J Thromb Haemost 2008;6:905–12.
15. Treffers PE, Huidekoper BL, Weenink GH, et al. Epidemiological observations of thrombo-embolic disease during pregnancy and in the puerperium, in 56,022 women. Int J Gynaecol Obstet 1983;21:327–31.
16. McColl MD, Ramsay JE, Tait RC, et al. Risk factors for pregnancy associated venous thromboembolism. Thromb Haemost 1997;78:1183–8.
17. Bourjeily G, Paidas M, Khalil H, et al. Pulmonary embolism in pregnancy. Lancet 2010;375:500–12.
18. Ray JG, Chan WS. Deep vein thrombosis during pregnancy and the puerperium: a meta-analysis of the period of risk and the leg of presentation. Obstet Gynecol Surv 1999;54:265–71.
19. Greer IA, Nelson-Piercy C. Low-molecular-weight heparins for thromboprophylaxis and treatment of

venous thromboembolism in pregnancy: a systematic review of safety and efficacy. Blood 2005;106:401–7.

20. Greer IA. Thrombosis in pregnancy: maternal and fetal issues. Lancet 1999;353:1258–65.

21. James AH, Tapson VF, Goldhaber SZ. Thrombosis during pregnancy and the postpartum period. Am J Obstet Gynecol 2005;193:216–9.

22. Bauersachs RM, Manolopoulos K, Hoppe I, et al. More on: the 'ART' behind the clot: solving the mystery. J Thromb Haemost 2007;5:438–9.

23. Boer K, den Hollander IA, Meijers JC, et al. Tissue factor-dependent blood coagulation is enhanced following delivery irrespective of the mode of delivery. J Thromb Haemost 2007;5:2415–20.

24. Cumming AM, Tait RC, Fildes S, et al. Development of resistance to activated protein C during pregnancy. Br J Haematol 1995;90:725–7.

25. Greer IA. The challenge of thrombophilia in maternal-fetal medicine. N Engl J Med 2000;342:424–5.

26. Hellgren M, Blomback M. Studies on blood coagulation and fibrinolysis in pregnancy, during delivery and in the puerperium. I. Normal condition. Gynecol Obstet Invest 1981;12:141–54.

27. Stirling Y, Woolf L, North WR, et al. Haemostasis in normal pregnancy. Thromb Haemost 1984;52:176–82.

28. Clark P, Brennand J, Conkie JA, et al. Activated protein C sensitivity, protein C, protein S and coagulation in normal pregnancy. Thromb Haemost 1998;79:1166–70.

29. Rosenkranz A, Hiden M, Leschnik B, et al. Calibrated automated thrombin generation in normal uncomplicated pregnancy. Thromb Haemost 2008;99:331–7.

30. Comp PC, Thurnau GR, Welsh J, et al. Functional and immunologic protein S levels are decreased during pregnancy. Blood 1986;68:881–5.

31. Kruithof EK, Tran-Thang C, Gudinchet A, et al. Fibrinolysis in pregnancy: a study of plasminogen activator inhibitors. Blood 1987;69:460–6.

32. Ku DH, Arkel YS, Paidas MP, et al. Circulating levels of inflammatory cytokines (IL-1 beta and TNF-alpha), resistance to activated protein C, thrombin and fibrin generation in uncomplicated pregnancies. Thromb Haemost 2003;90:1074–9.

33. Eliasson M, Evrin PE, Lundblad D. Fibrinogen and fibrinolytic variables in relation to anthropometry, lipids and blood pressure. The Northern Sweden MONICA Study. J Clin Epidemiol 1994;47:513–24.

34. Ernst E, Resch KL. Fibrinogen as a cardiovascular risk factor: a meta-analysis and review of the literature. Ann Intern Med 1993;118:956–63.

35. Landin K, Stigendal L, Eriksson E, et al. Abdominal obesity is associated with an impaired fibrinolytic activity and elevated plasminogen activator inhibitor-1. Metabolism 1990;39:1044–8.

36. Yarnell JW, Sweetnam PM, Rumley A, et al. Lifestyle and hemostatic risk factors for ischemic heart disease: the Caerphilly Study. Arterioscler Thromb Vasc Biol 2000;20:271–9.

37. Lee KW, Lip GY. Effects of lifestyle on hemostasis, fibrinolysis, and platelet reactivity: a systematic review. Arch Intern Med 2003;163:2368–92.

38. Sanchez SE, Zhang C, Rene Malinow M, et al. Plasma folate, vitamin B(12), and homocyst(e)ine concentrations in preeclamptic and normotensive Peruvian women. Am J Epidemiol 2001;153:474–80.

39. van Walraven C, Mamdani M, Cohn A, et al. Risk of subsequent thromboembolism for patients with pre-eclampsia. BMJ 2003;326:791–2.

40. Wells PS, Anderson DR, Rodger M, et al. Derivation of a simple clinical model to categorize patients probability of pulmonary embolism: increasing the models utility with the SimpliRED D-dimer. Thromb Haemost 2000;83:416–20.

41. Wells PS, Anderson DR, Rodger M, et al. Excluding pulmonary embolism at the bedside without diagnostic imaging: management of patients with suspected pulmonary embolism presenting to the emergency department by using a simple clinical model and d-dimer. Ann Intern Med 2001;135:98–107.

42. Carrier M, Wells PS, Rodger MA. Excluding pulmonary embolism at the bedside with low pre-test probability and D-dimer: safety and clinical utility of 4 methods to assign pre-test probability. Thromb Res 2006;117:469–74.

43. Panos RJ, Barish RA, Whye DW Jr, et al. The electrocardiographic manifestations of pulmonary embolism. J Emerg Med 1988;6:301–7.

44. Le Gal G, Righini M, Roy PM, et al. Prediction of pulmonary embolism in the emergency department: the revised Geneva score. Ann Intern Med 2006;144:165–71.

45. Powrie RO, Larson L, Rosene-Montella K, et al. Alveolar-arterial oxygen gradient in acute pulmonary embolism in pregnancy. Am J Obstet Gynecol 1998;178:394–6.

46. Roy PM, Colombet I, Durieux P, et al. Systematic review and meta-analysis of strategies for the diagnosis of suspected pulmonary embolism. BMJ 2005;331:259.

47. van Belle A, Buller HR, Huisman MV, et al. Effectiveness of managing suspected pulmonary embolism using an algorithm combining clinical probability, D-dimer testing, and computed tomography. JAMA 2006;295:172–9.

48. Kline JA, Runyon MS, Webb WB, et al. Prospective study of the diagnostic accuracy of the simplify D-dimer assay for pulmonary embolism in emergency department patients. Chest 2006;129:1417–23.

49. Perrier A, Roy PM, Sanchez O, et al. Multidetector-row computed tomography in suspected pulmonary embolism. N Engl J Med 2005;352:1760–8.

50. Morse M. Establishing a normal range for D-dimer levels through pregnancy to aid in the diagnosis of pulmonary embolism and deep vein thrombosis. J Thromb Haemost 2004;2:1202–4.

51. Eichinger S. D-dimer testing in pregnancy. Pathophysiol Haemost Thromb 2003;33:327–9.

52. Chan WS, Ray JG, Murray S, et al. Suspected pulmonary embolism in pregnancy: clinical presentation, results of lung scanning, and subsequent maternal and pediatric outcomes. Arch Intern Med 2002;162:1170–5.

53. Chan WS, Chunilal S, Lee A, et al. A red blood cell agglutination D-dimer test to exclude deep venous thrombosis in pregnancy. Ann Intern Med 2007; 147:165–70.

54. Doshi SK, Negus IS, Oduko JM. Fetal radiation dose from CT pulmonary angiography in late pregnancy: a phantom study. Br J Radiol 2008;81:653–8.

55. Litmanovich D, Boiselle PM, Bankier AA, et al. Dose reduction in computed tomographic angiography of pregnant patients with suspected acute pulmonary embolism. J Comput Assist Tomogr 2009;33:961–6.

56. Scarsbrook AF, Bradley KM, Gleeson FV. Perfusion scintigraphy: diagnostic utility in pregnant women with suspected pulmonary embolic disease. Eur Radiol 2007;17:2554–60.

57. Value of the ventilation/perfusion scan in acute pulmonary embolism. Results of the prospective investigation of pulmonary embolism diagnosis (PIOPED). The PIOPED Investigators. JAMA 1990;263:2753–9.

58. Hurwitz LM, Yoshizumi T, Reiman RE, et al. Radiation dose to the fetus from body MDCT during early gestation. AJR Am J Roentgenol 2006;186:871–6.

59. Winer-Muram HT, Boone JM, Brown HL, et al. Pulmonary embolism in pregnant patients: fetal radiation dose with helical CT. Radiology 2002; 224:487–92.

60. Groves AM, Yates SJ, Win T, et al. CT pulmonary angiography versus ventilation-perfusion scintigraphy in pregnancy: implications from a UK survey of doctors' knowledge of radiation exposure. Radiology 2006;240:765–70.

61. van Erkel AR, van Rossum AB, Bloem JL, et al. Spiral CT angiography for suspected pulmonary embolism: a cost-effectiveness analysis. Radiology 1996;201:29–36.

62. Doyle NM, Ramirez MM, Mastrobattista JM, et al. Diagnosis of pulmonary embolism: a cost-effectiveness analysis. Am J Obstet Gynecol 2004;191:1019–23.

63. Moores LK, Jackson WL Jr, Shorr AF, et al. Meta-analysis: outcomes in patients with suspected pulmonary embolism managed with computed tomographic pulmonary angiography. Ann Intern Med 2004;141:866–74.

64. Quiroz R, Kucher N, Zou KH, et al. Clinical validity of a negative computed tomography scan in patients with suspected pulmonary embolism: a systematic review. JAMA 2005;293:2012–7.

65. Stein PD, Fowler SE, Goodman LR, et al. Multidetector computed tomography for acute pulmonary embolism. N Engl J Med 2006;354:2317–27.

66. Schaefer-Prokop C, Prokop M. CTPA for the diagnosis of acute pulmonary embolism during pregnancy. Eur Radiol 2008;18:2705–8.

67. Andreou AK, Curtin JJ, Wilde S, et al. Does pregnancy affect vascular enhancement in patients undergoing CT pulmonary angiography? Eur Radiol 2008;18:2716–22.

68. Khalil H, Bourjeily G, Lazarus E, et al. Multidetector CT pulmonary angiograms in pregnant patients: the "limited, no central PE" - how limited? Chicago: Radiological Society of North America; 2007.

69. Ridge CA, McDermott S, Freyne BJ, et al. Pulmonary embolism in pregnancy: comparison of pulmonary CT angiography and lung scintigraphy. AJR Am J Roentgenol 2009;193:1223–7.

70. U-King-Im J, Freeman SJ, Boylan T, et al. Quality of CT pulmonary angiography for suspected pulmonary embolus in pregnancy. Eur Radiol 2008;18: 2709–15.

71. Schuster ME, Fishman JE, Copeland JF, et al. Pulmonary embolism in pregnant patients: a survey of practices and policies for CT pulmonary angiography. AJR Am J Roentgenol 2003;181:1495–8.

72. Bourjeily G, Chalhoub M, Phornphutkul C, et al. Neonatal thyroid function: effect of a single exposure to iodinated contrast medium in utero. Radiology 2010;256(3):744–50.

73. Land CE, Tokunaga M, Tokuoka S, et al. Early-onset breast cancer in A-bomb survivors. Lancet 1993; 342:237.

74. Tokunaga M, Land CE, Tokuoka S, et al. Incidence of female breast cancer among atomic bomb survivors, 1950–1985. Radiat Res 1994;138:209–23.

75. National Research Council (US) Committee to Assess Health Risks from Exposure to Low Level of Ionizing Radiation. Health risks from exposure to low levels of ionizing radiation: BEIR VII Phase 2. Washington, DC: National Academies Press; 2006. Available at: http://www.nap.edu/catalog/11340.html. Accessed July 1, 2010.

76. Einstein AJ, Henzlova MJ, Rajagopalan S. Estimating risk of cancer associated with radiation exposure from 64-slice computed tomography coronary angiography. JAMA 2007;298:317–23.

77. Hopper KD, King SH, Lobell ME, et al. The breast: in-plane x-ray protection during diagnostic thoracic CT–shielding with bismuth radioprotective garments. Radiology 1997;205:853–8.

78. Parker MS, Hui FK, Camacho MA, et al. Female breast radiation exposure during CT pulmonary

angiography. AJR Am J Roentgenol 2005;185: 1228–33.

79. Turkstra F, Kuijer PM, van Beek EJ, et al. Diagnostic utility of ultrasonography of leg veins in patients suspected of having pulmonary embolism. Ann Intern Med 1997;126:775–81.

80. Torres JA, Aracil E, Puras E, et al. Role of venous duplex imaging of lower extremity for pulmonary embolism diagnosis. Angiologia 1999;51:71–6.

81. Mac Gillavry MR, Sanson BJ, Buller HR, et al. Compression ultrasonography of the leg veins in patients with clinically suspected pulmonary embolism: is a more extensive assessment of compressibility useful? Thromb Haemost 2000;84:973–6.

82. Barrellier MT, Lezin B, Landy S, et al. [Prevalence of duplex ultrasonography detectable venous thrombosis in patients with suspected or acute pulmonary embolism]. J Mal Vasc 2001;26:23–30 [in French].

83. Stein PD, Chenevert TL, Fowler SE, et al. Gadolinium-enhanced magnetic resonance angiography for pulmonary embolism: a multicenter prospective study (PIOPED III). Ann Intern Med 2010;152:434–43.

84. Marcos HB, Semelka RC, Worawattanakul S. Normal placenta: gadolinium-enhanced dynamic MR imaging. Radiology 1997;205:493–6.

85. Hull R, Hirsh J, Sackett DL, et al. Clinical validity of a negative venogram in patients with clinically suspected venous thrombosis. Circulation 1981;64: 622–5.

86. Garg K, Kemp JL, Wojcik D, et al. Thromboembolic disease: comparison of combined CT pulmonary angiography and venography with bilateral leg sonography in 70 patients. AJR Am J Roentgenol 2000;175:997–1001.

87. Loud PA, Katz DS, Bruce DA, et al. Deep venous thrombosis with suspected pulmonary embolism: detection with combined CT venography and pulmonary angiography. Radiology 2001;219:498–502.

88. Coche EE, Hamoir XL, Hammer FD, et al. Using dual-detector helical CT angiography to detect deep venous thrombosis in patients with suspicion of pulmonary embolism: diagnostic value and additional findings. AJR Am J Roentgenol 2001; 176:1035–9.

89. Garg K, Kemp JL, Russ PD, et al. Thromboembolic disease: variability of interobserver agreement in the interpretation of CT venography with CT pulmonary angiography. AJR Am J Roentgenol 2001;176: 1043–7.

90. Rademaker J, Griesshaber V, Hidajat N, et al. Combined CT pulmonary angiography and venography for diagnosis of pulmonary embolism and deep vein thrombosis: radiation dose. J Thorac Imaging 2001;16:297–9.

91. Scarsbrook AF, Evans AL, Owen AR, et al. Diagnosis of suspected venous thromboembolic disease in pregnancy. Clin Radiol 2006;61:1–12.

92. Ginsberg JS, Wells PS, Hirsh J, et al. Reevaluation of the sensitivity of impedance plethysmography for the detection of proximal deep vein thrombosis. Arch Intern Med 1994;154:1930–3.

93. Heijboer H, Buller HR, Lensing AW, et al. A comparison of real-time compression ultrasonography with impedance plethysmography for the diagnosis of deep-vein thrombosis in symptomatic outpatients. N Engl J Med 1993;329:1365–9.

94. Hull RD, Raskob GE, Carter CJ. Serial impedance plethysmography in pregnant patients with clinically suspected deep-vein thrombosis. Clinical validity of negative findings. Ann Intern Med 1990; 112:663–7.

95. Wicki J, Perrier A, Perneger TV, et al. Predicting adverse outcome in patients with acute pulmonary embolism: a risk score. Thromb Haemost 2000;84: 548–52.

96. Aujesky D, Obrosky DS, Stone RA, et al. Derivation and validation of a prognostic model for pulmonary embolism. Am J Respir Crit Care Med 2005;172: 1041–6.

97. Yoo HH, De Paiva SA, Silveira LV, et al. Logistic regression analysis of potential prognostic factors for pulmonary thromboembolism. Chest 2003;123: 813–21.

98. Sukhija R, Aronow WS, Lee J, et al. Association of right ventricular dysfunction with in-hospital mortality in patients with acute pulmonary embolism and reduction in mortality in patients with right ventricular dysfunction by pulmonary embolectomy. Am J Cardiol 2005;95:695–6.

99. Binder L, Pieske B, Olschewski M, et al. N-terminal pro-brain natriuretic peptide or troponin testing followed by echocardiography for risk stratification of acute pulmonary embolism. Circulation 2005;112: 1573–9.

100. ten Wolde M, Sohne M, Quak E, et al. Prognostic value of echocardiographically assessed right ventricular dysfunction in patients with pulmonary embolism. Arch Intern Med 2004;164:1685–9.

101. Elkayam U, Gleicher N. Cardiac evaluation during pregnancy. In: Elkayam U, Gleicher N, editors. Cardiac problems in pregnancy: diagnosis and management of maternal and fetal disease. 3rd edition. New York (NY): Wiley-Liss; 1998. p. 33–7.

102. Goodman LR. Small pulmonary emboli: what do we know? Radiology 2005;234:654–8.

103. Remy-Jardin M, Pistolesi M, Goodman LR, et al. Management of suspected acute pulmonary embolism in the era of CT angiography: a statement from the Fleischner Society. Radiology 2007;245: 315–29.

104. Couturaud F, Julian JA, Kearon C. Low molecular weight heparin administered once versus twice daily in patients with venous thromboembolism: a meta-analysis. Thromb Haemost 2001;86:980–4.

105. Gould MK, Dembitzer AD, Doyle RL, et al. Low-molecular-weight heparins compared with unfractionated heparin for treatment of acute deep venous thrombosis. A meta-analysis of randomized, controlled trials. Ann Intern Med 1999;130:800–9.

106. Dolovich LR, Ginsberg JS, Douketis JD, et al. A meta-analysis comparing low-molecular-weight heparins with unfractionated heparin in the treatment of venous thromboembolism: examining some unanswered questions regarding location of treatment, product type, and dosing frequency. Arch Intern Med 2000;160:181–8.

107. Martel N, Lee J, Wells PS. Risk for heparin-induced thrombocytopenia with unfractionated and low-molecular-weight heparin thromboprophylaxis: a meta-analysis. Blood 2005;106:2710–5.

108. Warkentin TE, Greinacher A. Heparin-induced thrombocytopenia: recognition, treatment, and prevention: the Seventh ACCP Conference on Antithrombotic and Thrombolytic Therapy. Chest 2004;126:311S–37S.

109. Pettila V, Leinonen P, Markkola A, et al. Postpartum bone mineral density in women treated for thromboprophylaxis with unfractionated heparin or LMW heparin. Thromb Haemost 2002;87:182–6.

110. Malcolm JC, Keely EJ, Karovitch AJ, et al. Use of low molecular weight heparin in acute venous thromboembolic events in pregnancy. J Obstet Gynaecol Can 2002;24:568–71.

111. Horlocker TT, Wedel DJ, Rowlingson JC, et al. Regional anesthesia in the patient receiving antithrombotic or thrombolytic therapy: American Society of Regional Anesthesia and Pain Medicine Evidence-Based Guidelines (Third Edition). Reg Anesth Pain Med 2010;35:64–101.

112. Casele HL, Laifer SA, Woelkers DA, et al. Changes in the pharmacokinetics of the low-molecular-weight heparin enoxaparin sodium during pregnancy. Am J Obstet Gynecol 1999;181:1113–7.

113. Hunt BJ, Doughty HA, Majumdar G, et al. Thromboprophylaxis with low molecular weight heparin (Fragmin) in high risk pregnancies. Thromb Haemost 1997;77:39–43.

114. Abou-Nassar K, Kovacs MJ, Kahn SR, et al. The effect of dalteparin on coagulation activation during pregnancy in women with thrombophilia. A randomized trial. Thromb Haemost 2007;98:163–71.

115. Brieger D, Dawes J. Long-term persistence of biological activity following administration of Enoxaparin sodium (clexane) is due to sequestration of antithrombin-binding low molecular weight fragments–comparison with unfractionated heparin. Thromb Haemost 1996;75:740–6.

116. Hirsh J, Bauer KA, Donati MB, et al. Parenteral anticoagulants: American College of Chest Physicians Evidence-Based Clinical Practice Guidelines (8th Edition). Chest 2008;133:141S–59S.

117. Chunilal SD, Young E, Johnston MA, et al. The APTT response of pregnant plasma to unfractionated heparin. Thromb Haemost 2002;87:92–7.

118. Levine MN, Hirsh J, Gent M, et al. A randomized trial comparing activated thromboplastin time with heparin assay in patients with acute venous thromboembolism requiring large daily doses of heparin. Arch Intern Med 1994;154:49–56.

119. Leonhardt G, Gaul C, Nietsch HH, et al. Thrombolytic therapy in pregnancy. J Thromb Thrombolysis 2006;21:271–6.

120. Konstantinides S, Geibel A, Heusel G, et al. Heparin plus alteplase compared with heparin alone in patients with submassive pulmonary embolism. N Engl J Med 2002;347:1143–50.

121. Hall JG, Pauli RM, Wilson KM. Maternal and fetal sequelae of anticoagulation during pregnancy. Am J Med 1980;68:122–40.

122. Prandoni P, Lensing AW, Piccioli A, et al. Recurrent venous thromboembolism and bleeding complications during anticoagulant treatment in patients with cancer and venous thrombosis. Blood 2002;100:3484–8.

123. Bates SM, Greer IA, Pabinger I, et al. Venous thromboembolism, thrombophilia, antithrombotic therapy, and pregnancy: American College of Chest Physicians Evidence-Based Clinical Practice Guidelines (8th Edition). Chest 2008;133:844S–86S.

124. Jamjute P, Reed N, Hinwood D. Use of inferior vena cava filters in thromboembolic disease during labor: case report with a literature review. J Matern Fetal Neonatal Med 2006;19:741–4.

125. Gates S, Brocklehurst P, Ayers S, et al. Thromboprophylaxis and pregnancy: two randomized controlled pilot trials that used low-molecular-weight heparin. Am J Obstet Gynecol 2004;191:1296–303.

126. Howell R, Fidler J, Letsky E, et al. The risks of antenatal subcutaneous heparin prophylaxis: a controlled trial. Br J Obstet Gynaecol 1983;90:1124–8.

127. Brill-Edwards P, Ginsberg JS, Gent M, et al. Safety of withholding heparin in pregnant women with a history of venous thromboembolism. Recurrence of clot in this pregnancy study group. N Engl J Med 2000;343:1439–44.

128. Pabinger I, Grafenhofer H, Kaider A, et al. Risk of pregnancy-associated recurrent venous thromboembolism in women with a history of venous thrombosis. J Thromb Haemost 2005;3:949–54.

129. De Stefano V, Martinelli I, Rossi E, et al. The risk of recurrent venous thromboembolism in pregnancy and puerperium without antithrombotic prophylaxis. Br J Haematol 2006;135:386–91.

130. Robertson L, Wu O, Langhorne P, et al. Thrombophilia in pregnancy: a systematic review. Br J Haematol 2006;132:171–96.

131. Dizon-Townson D, Miller C, Sibai B, et al. The relationship of the factor V Leiden mutation and pregnancy outcomes for mother and fetus. Obstet Gynecol 2005;106:517–24.

132. Martinelli I, Legnani C, Bucciarelli P, et al. Risk of pregnancy-related venous thrombosis in carriers of severe inherited thrombophilia. Thromb Haemost 2001;86:800–3.

133. Middeldorp S, Libourel EJ, Hamulyak K, et al. The risk of pregnancy-related venous thromboembolism in women who are homozygous for factor V Leiden. Br J Haematol 2001;113:553–5.

134. American College of Obstetricians and Gynecologists Practice Bulletin. Inherited thrombophilias in pregnancy. New York. Number 113, 2010.

135. Royal College of Obstetricians and Gynaecologists. Reducing the risk of thrombosis and embolism during pregnancy and the puerperium. London. Greep Top Guideline No. 37, 2009.

Pregnancy and Pulmonary Hypertension

C. Randall Lane, MD[a], Terence K. Trow, MD[b],*

KEYWORDS

- Pulmonary hypertension • Pregnancy • Management
- Conception counseling

Pulmonary arterial hypertension (PAH) is a rare disorder that can affect women of child-bearing age. When it is complicated by pregnancy, it is associated with increased mortality, and as such is considered a contraindication to becoming pregnant. This conclusion is drawn from several observational studies that have demonstrated mortality as high as 60% in women with pulmonary hypertension (PH) who undergo pregnancy.[1] Although the use of newer vasodilator therapy in the last decade has resulted in improved outcomes in patients with PAH, overall this disorder still carries a substantial risk of maternal death, and avoidance of pregnancy and consideration of termination should it occur are the current recommendations.

PHYSIOLOGY

The physiologic changes of pregnancy are poorly tolerated by women with PAH. During pregnancy, cardiac output increases by 50% from baseline. This is accomplished by several mechanisms. Blood volume increases in the early stages, leading to an increase in stroke volume. This is further enhanced by a reduction in afterload secondary to decreased peripheral vascular resistance.[2] Later in pregnancy, cardiac output is augmented by an increase in heart rate. Under normal conditions, there is a decrease in pulmonary vascular resistance (PVR) to accommodate these changes. However, patients with preexisting PAH are unable to make this adjustment. The right ventricle, which now faces increased afterload from higher PVR, cannot accommodate the increase in cardiac output and becomes overloaded. This can result in progressive right ventricular failure and sudden death from arrhythmia. During delivery, the pain of parturition is associated with stimulation of the sympathetic nervous system and dramatic increases in heart rate, blood pressure, and myocardial oxygen consumption, and can be associated with vagal responses that can lead to hypotension and sudden death.[3] Valsalva maneuvers also exaggerate the increase in blood pressure and myocardial oxygen consumption. In addition, with every uterine contraction, approximately 500 mL of blood is diverted from the uterine to the maternal circulation, with a resultant increase in cardiac output and blood pressure. After delivery, there is significant autotransfusion from the uterine circulation and an additional increase in venous return from the relief of vena caval obstruction by the gravid uterus with concomitant fluid shifts into the intravascular space, which can add to a state of right ventricular volume overload. In addition, pregnancy is associated with a hypercoagulable state, resulting from increased fibrin levels, reduced fibrinolytic activity, increased procoagulant activity with higher resistance to activated protein C, lower protein S, and increases in clotting factor activity.[4] Thromboembolic disease is very poorly tolerated in these patients, who already have compromised right

[a] Section of Pulmonary and Critical Care Medicine, Yale University School of Medicine, 333 Cedar Street, PO Box 208057, New Haven, CT 06520-8057, USA
[b] Yale Pulmonary Hypertension Center, Section of Pulmonary and Critical Care Medicine, Yale University School of Medicine, 333 Cedar Street, PO Box 28057, LLCI 105D, New Haven, CT 06520-8057, USA
* Corresponding author.
E-mail address: terence.trow@yale.edu

Clin Chest Med 32 (2011) 165–174
doi:10.1016/j.ccm.2010.10.006
0272-5231/11/$ – see front matter © 2011 Elsevier Inc. All rights reserved.

ventricular function. These physiologic maladaptations help to explain the high mortality that has been associated with PH during pregnancy.

CLASSIFICATION OF PH

According to the latest World Health Organization criteria, PAH is defined by a mean pulmonary artery (PA) pressure greater than 25 mm Hg at rest, a normal PA occlusion pressure ($\leq$15 mm Hg), and increased PVR.[5] Current categorization of PAH includes patients with idiopathic or heritable PH, PH associated with congenital heart disease, as well as PH in the setting of connective tissue disease, human immunodeficiency virus (HIV), portal hypertension, anorexigen use, or pulmonary venoocclusive disease (**Box 1**).[6] Other categories of PH, such as PH caused by lung disease, acquired left-sided heart disease, or chronic thromboembolic disease can also occur in pregnant women but there is considerably less literature describing these entities in pregnancy. There are several possible reasons for this. PH is often a marker of the severity of other types of lung disease or acquired cardiac disease, which often occurs with advanced age or heavy disease burden, both of which are less likely to have developed in women of child-bearing age. An exception is rheumatic valvular disease, which has been reported and is seen relatively frequently in pregnancy in the developing world. This review focuses on PAH in pregnancy, although the literature regarding other categories of PH in pregnancy is also discussed when available.

DIAGNOSIS AND SCREENING

The availability and improved technique of transthoracic echocardiography (TTE) has led to its widespread use as a screening tool for PH. Good correlation has been demonstrated between PA pressures measured by right heart catheterization (RHC) and the right ventricular systolic pressure measured by TTE, but many factors, such as advanced lung disease, premature ventricular contractions, and inaccurate estimates of right atrial pressure in the modified Bernoulli equation, can lead to discrepancies and misdiagnosis.[7] The use of TTE to diagnose PH during pregnancy has been evaluated in 2 case series. Penning and colleagues[8] found that TTE overestimated pulmonary artery pressures in a retrospective review of 27 pregnant patients who were evaluated for cardiac disease with both a TTE and an RHC. Of the 25 patients found to have PH by TTE, 8 patients (33%) had normal PA pressures when measured by RHC. More recently, Wylie

---

Box 1
Updated clinical classification of pulmonary hypertension (Dana Point)

Class 1: Pulmonary Arterial Hypertension

Idiopathic

Heritable

Associated with:

> Congenital heart disease
>
> Drug use
>
> HIV
>
> Connective tissue disease
>
> Portal hypertension
>
> Schistosomiasis
>
> Chronic hemolytic anemia

Persistent pulmonary hypertension of the newborn

Pulmonary venoocclusive disease and pulmonary capillary hemangiomatosis

Class 2: Pulmonary Hypertension Caused by Left Heart Disease

Systolic dysfunction

Diastolic dysfunction

Valvular disease

Class 3: Pulmonary Hypertension Caused by Lung Disease and/or Hypoxia

Chronic obstructive pulmonary disease (COPD)

Interstitial lung disease

Sleep-disordered breathing

Alveolar hypoventilation

High-altitude exposure

Class 4: Chronic Thromboembolic Pulmonary Hypertension (CTEPH)

Chronic pulmonary embolism

Class 5: Pulmonary Hypertension with Unclear Multifactorial Mechanisms

Metabolic disorders: Gaucher disease, thyroid disease, glycogen storage disease

> Hematologic disorders: myeloproliferative disorders, splenectomy
>
> Systemic disorders: sarcoidosis, pulmonary Langerhans cell histiocytosis, vasculitis
>
> Others: fibrosing mediastinitis, chronic renal failure on dialysis, tumoral obstruction

Adapted from Simonneu G, Robbins IM, Beghetti M, et al. Updated clinical classification of pulmonary hypertension. JACC 2009; 54(Suppl 1):S45; with permission.

and colleagues[9] found good statistical correlation between TTE and RHC (r = 0.70, P<.0001), however, similar to the study by Penning and colleagues, the diagnosis of PH made by TTE was not confirmed in one-third of the patients. Conversely, in 5 of 18 patients, RHC measurements revealed more severe PH than was determined by TTE, thus demonstrating the risk of both over- and underestimating PA pressures with TTE during pregnancy, despite an overall good correlation. Possible explanations for the discrepancy include inaccuracies in estimating the right atrial pressure from the size of the inferior vena cava (IVC) in pregnancy because of difficulty visualizing the IVC, or to a falsely increased tricuspid jet in the setting of lower blood viscosity caused by physiologic anemia of pregnancy or higher blood flow.[9] Other findings on echocardiography that should be interpreted with caution are the physiologic increase in chamber size in pregnancy. Even when PH is confirmed on RHC, it is important to underscore that PH does not mean PAH is present, and as such, a careful assessment of PA occlusion pressure and PVR must occur on every RHC. Given the gravity of the diagnosis of PAH during pregnancy, and the ramifications with respect to continuation of the pregnancy, the diagnosis of PAH must be confirmed by RHC before recommendations are made.

PREGNANCY OUTCOMES AND MORTALITY

PH complicates a relatively small number of pregnancies. The true incidence of PH in pregnancy has not been reported, but studies have attempted to estimate the effect of PH on maternal outcomes. Between 2002 and 2004, there were an estimated 14 million hospitalizations related to pregnancy, based on extrapolations from the Nationwide Inpatient Sample database.[10] Of these, 407 (0.003%) were to the result of a diagnosis of idiopathic pulmonary arterial hypertension (IPAH). In this study, PAH was also associated with a significantly longer hospital stay, but there were not enough events to draw conclusions about maternal death rates.

The reported mortality of PH has ranged from nearly 60% in early reports, to as low as 25% more recently. These discrepancies likely reflect data collection methods and study design, as well as advances made in the care of patients with PH in recent years. McCaffery and Dunn[1] compiled 23 pregnancies in 16 patients with primary PH in 1963, including previously reported cases, and some from their own institution. Nine of the 16 women died during the course of those pregnancies, thus suggesting a mortality that exceeded 50%. This was the agreed consensus for many years. Weiss and colleagues[11] reviewed 125 published cases of PH reported during pregnancy and separated them into 3 groups: primary PH, congenital heart disease associated PH with Eisenmenger syndrome, and secondary PH. Notably, secondary PH included mostly patients who would be described as PAH under the current World Health Organization (WHO) classification system (HIV-related, connective tissue disease (CTD)-related, or anorexigen associated), in addition to patients with chronic thromboembolic PH. Patients with PH secondary to lung disease or acquired left heart disease were not included. This was the first study to investigate mortality for different causes of PH. In their report, Eisenmenger syndrome and primary PH (now referred to as IPAH) had similar mortality in pregnant women (36% and 30%, respectively); however, their entity of secondary PH had a mortality of 56%. Of these patients, nearly all those with systemic disease or anorexigen-related PH died. During the period of this study, the use of vasodilators had not become a standard part of the management of PH.

The most recent report[12] assessing mortality was collected and analyzed similarly to the study by Weiss and colleagues[11] with the goal of determining if any progress had been made in management of PH in pregnancies using newer therapies. It similarly divided patients into IPAH, congenital heart disease (CHD)-associated PAH, and PAH of other causes (including CTD, HIV, anorexigens, and so forth). Like the Weiss study, it found a trend toward lower rates of mortality in patients with IPAH and CHD-PAH, compared with patients with other causes of PAH, although this trend was not statistically significant. In each group, however, mortality was lower than in the study by Weiss and colleagues, with rates of 17%, 28%, and 33%, respectively. In this analysis, patients with IPAH demonstrated the largest reduction in mortality, perhaps a reflection of the use of PAH-specific therapy, which is used more frequently for IPAH than for other causes of PH. A significant limitation of these studies is the determination of mortality by compiling cases from the literature, increasing the likelihood of reporting bias. Particularly with regard to the use of newer therapies, successful outcomes may be more likely to be reported, thus skewing the results to make it seem that mortality has improved. Both of these review studies are also limited by lower numbers of patients with IPAH and secondary PAH than patients with Eisenmenger syndrome. However, given the relative rarity of PAH, and the small number of cases during pregnancy, prospective studies are difficult. To enroll enough patients to have significant power would require a long-term multicenter study.

To avoid the pitfall of reporting bias, some groups have published consecutive case series from single institutions, reviewing data from all patients presenting with PH during pregnancy from a defined period. The first such report was a series of 8 patients presenting in a 10-year period.[13] Despite being performed before the era of vasodilator therapy, only 1 death was reported. More recently, a French group reported a series of 15 pregnancies complicated by PH.[14] Five deaths were reported, consistent with the previously described rates in the range of 30%. Mortality occurred most often late in pregnancy or postpartum. Zwicke and Buggy[15] reported 37 consecutive cases of PH during pregnancy (33 cases of PAH, 4 of mitral stenosis). In their series, all 37 mothers survived, and 36 live infants were delivered, with 1 therapeutic termination. This study used a new management strategy with regular assessment of right ventricular (RV) function, which is described in more detail later in the article. These case series are from large centers with significant expertise in the management of PH, and likely represent the most idealized management of such patients. The small number of patients also limits the conclusions that can be drawn about mortality in the population at large. Data regarding the mortality of pregnant women with PH secondary to lung or left-sided acquired heart disease is currently lacking. A small series looked at 168 cases of maternal cardiac disease.[16] Of those, 20 patients (11.9%) had PH and their outcomes were compared with age-matched controls who had cardiac disease without PH. Most patients (12/20) had noncongenital valvular disease, and the remainder had Eisenmenger physiology from CHD. There was only 1 maternal death, which occurred in a patient with Eisenmenger syndrome. Mode of delivery (vaginal vs operative) did not differ between the 2 groups, nor did maternal mortality. There was 1 perinatal death in each group, and there was a significantly higher incidence of low birthweight in babies born to mothers with PH. This study is limited by its small size, making it difficult to draw definitive conclusions. Our review of the literature did not reveal any studies comparing outcomes of women with lung disease in the presence or absence of secondary PH.

PH DEVELOPING DURING PREGNANCY

The onset of PH during pregnancy can be a first manifestation of previously undiagnosed or asymptomatic PH, which becomes unmasked under the stress of pregnancy. PH can also develop acutely during the course of pregnancy. The presence of severe dyspnea, syncope, or chest pain during pregnancy should prompt immediate investigation. The diagnosis of acute pulmonary embolism should always be suspected in such patients. If excluded, a TTE should be done to look for cardiac disease, including PH. If present on TTE, the diagnosis of PH should be confirmed by RHC because of the previously outlined limitations of TTE, and the ramifications on the pregnancy. The workup for causes of PH should proceed as it would in a nonpregnant patient, beginning with a detailed history and physical examination followed by appropriate laboratory and imaging studies based on those findings.[17] However, certain causes that are particular to pregnancy must be considered.

Worldwide, mitral stenosis is the most common cardiac valvular disease seen in pregnant women.[18] The presence of PH increases the risk of pregnancy in patients with mitral stenosis. In the nonpregnant state, mitral stenosis may be well tolerated or even asymptomatic in young, otherwise healthy women. However, the normal increase in heart rate during pregnancy allows for less left ventricular filling time. In the setting of the increased blood volume seen in pregnancy and significant mitral stenosis, pulmonary venous hypertension (PVH) can develop from back pressure. The presence of pulmonary edema and left atrial enlargement helps to distinguish mitral stenosis from other causes of sudden onset PH in pregnancy. Rate control is essential to allow for adequate left ventricular filling and preload. Diuresis prevents left atrial overdistension, which in turn can result in atrial fibrillation and PVH. However, this must be done cautiously to preserve preload, bearing in mind that pregnant women may have a higher glomerular filtration rate and generally respond to lower doses of diuretics. Ten milligrams of furosemide is a reasonable starting dose, with up-titration as needed based on the response. In mild cases of mitral stenosis (New York Heart Association [NYHA] class I or II), diuresis and beta blockade result in good outcomes.[19] If medical therapy fails, or in patients who are more symptomatic at baseline (NYHA III or IV), percutaneous balloon valvulotomy is the procedure of choice. It has been shown to be as effective as mitral valve commissurotomy in pregnancy[20] and a long-term follow-up study showed good fetal outcomes as well as durable symptomatic improvement for the mother.[21]

Tumor emboli syndrome is a rare cause of PH, associated with several different types of malignancies, but more commonly with germ cell tumors. Choriocarcinoma is a malignancy of trophoblastic tissue that can occur after a spontaneous abortion, or less frequently after a normal pregnancy. It can present with amenorrhea and a positive pregnancy test, which can lead the patient and physician to initially suspect pregnancy. Acute PH from choriocarcinoma is rare, but has been reported.[22,23] Because choriocarcinoma is very responsive to chemotherapy, the resulting tumor emboli syndrome and its attendant PH can be essentially cured with chemotherapy treatment. This entity should suspected in acute development of PH in women of child-bearing age.[24]

Amniotic fluid embolism (AFE) can present with sudden cardiopulmonary decompensation, usually occurring during labor and delivery, or in the immediate postpartum period.[25] AFE results in sudden vasoconstriction of the pulmonary vasculature leading to increased PVR with right heart failure, in addition to coagulopathy and disseminated intravascular coagulation. The mechanism behind the increased PVR is not simply the presence of fluid emboli in the pulmonary circulation, but the attendant release of biochemical mediators, including endothelin-1.[26–28] Management is generally supportive, consisting of resuscitation with mechanical ventilation, vasopressor use, and ionotropic support, along with replacement of blood products. It stands to reason that if the mechanism of increased PVR is similar to that of PAH, then AFE-associated PH would potentially respond to PAH-specific therapy. Both inhaled nitric oxide and aerosolized prostacyclin have been reported to successfully reverse the hemodynamic compromise and impaired oxygenation of AFE.[27,29]

CONCEPTION COUNSELING

Despite possible improvements in pregnancy outcomes in woman with PH, the risk of death is still high enough to warrant a recommendation to avoid pregnancy. Contraception is indicated in women of child-bearing age with PH, but the modality must be chosen carefully. Combined hormonal contraceptives (oral, implanted, or transdermal) increase the risk of thrombosis, and are therefore contraindicated in woman with PH in whom this could represent a life-threatening complication. In patients with IPAH on therapeutic warfarin therapy as part of their treatment regimen,[30] combined hormonal contraceptives may be acceptable. Progestin-only methods are generally safe and well tolerated. Progestin-eluting implantable intrauterine devices are an option, however, their insertion requires a procedure, which carries a risk of a vagal reaction that could be poorly tolerated in the presence of PH.[31] Operative sterilization to avoid pregnancy is an option, and has been done successfully,[32] however, the mortality of such a procedure could be as high as 6%.[33] Should pregnancy occur, early termination may be advisable, especially if clinical deterioration is seen early in the course of the pregnancy. In the French series previously cited,[14] 1 patient underwent therapeutic termination at 21 weeks after decompensating early in the second trimester, improving significantly with this intervention. The risk of death from therapeutic abortion in women with PH has not been determined, but may be higher if performed late in gestation. Individual decisions should be based on the gestational age at diagnosis, fetal viability, and the anticipated physiologic stressors such as a peak in plasma volume around 22 to 24 weeks and a peak in cardiac output around 32 weeks. The use of spinal or epidural anesthesia, rather than general anesthesia with intubation, may help to reduce risk, but rigorous evidence from the literature is lacking. Given the mortality described in pregnancy with PH, and the likely lower rate of mortality during an early termination procedure, if therapeutic abortion is agreeable to the patient, it should be offered.

MANAGEMENT OF PH DURING PREGNANCY

For many different reasons, neither contraception nor termination of pregnancy is an option for some patients. Although it is unclear to what extent current strategies used to manage PH in pregnancy have had an effect on mortality, successful outcomes have been described with a variety of medical and surgical approaches. When a woman with known PH becomes pregnant, or if PH is newly discovered during pregnancy, the patient should be referred to a center that has expertise in managing PH. Collaborations between the obstetricians, PH specialists, intensivists, and anesthesiologists are most important. Patients should be seen frequently during pregnancy, and hospitalization should be done early in the event of severe symptoms. Urgent delivery may become necessary in the event of evolving right heart failure and may allow better outcomes by intervening before the right ventricle has lost all compensatory ability.[15] Physiologically it would seem reasonable to limit cardiac demands by reducing activity, and avoiding hypoxemia with supplemental oxygen, although being aware of the increased risk of venous thromboembolism (VTE) with antepartum immobilization.

Delivery and Anesthesia

The optimal mode of delivery for patients with PH is not established by the available literature. Earlier reports suggested a higher mortality when cesarean section was used.[11] This was believed to be a result of increased fluid shifts from abdominal surgery, as well as increased PVR and increased RV afterload imparted by positive pressure ventilation in the setting of endotracheal intubation, which can precipitate acute right heart failure. Since that study, many case reports have described successful cesarean deliveries in patients with PAH, using regional anesthesia, as well as proactive use of pulmonary vasodilators such as nitric oxide via the endotracheal tube or nasal canula.[34,35] The central alpha agonist dexmedtomidine has the advantage of providing pain relief with less effect on hemodynamics than other agents, and its successful use in managing cesarean delivery in PH patients has been reported.[36] In the most recent long-term systematic review by Bedard and colleagues,[12] the rate of cesarean delivery was higher, perhaps reflecting trends in the field. This study yielded lower mortality, however there are numerous other possible explanations for the improved mortality including more frequent use of PAH-specific therapy as well as closer monitoring leading to delivery before maternal decompensation. Although cesarean delivery may avoid labor and the autotransfusion associated with contractions, this mode of delivery is associated with more venous thromboembolic complications and more fluid shifts, and should be reserved for patients with obstetric indications for an operative delivery. In addition, most maternal deaths occur postpartum, and are likely influenced more by fluid status and hemodynamics rather than the mode of delivery. If vaginal delivery is chosen, effective analgesia is of utmost importance to prevent the sudden increases in cardiac output or dangerous vasovagal response that can occur with pain during parturition. This is best achieved with epidural anesthesia, although there is still a risk of hypotension. Maternal death occurs most commonly in the postpartum period, and it is unclear how the choice of individual anesthetic drug effects the outcome.[37,38]

In the abstract by Zwicke and Buggy[15] a protocol approach was taken to management of the prepartum period and delivery. Beginning at 28 weeks, regular assessment of RV function was done with echocardiography, prompting early delivery if RV dysfunction was detected. Of 37 patients, 5 underwent cesarean section, 1 had a therapeutic abortion, and the remainder delivered vaginally with spinal and epidural anesthesia. Each mother survived, as did all 36 infants delivered. If the condition of the mother warrants urgent delivery, induction of vaginal delivery may be an option. However, oxytocin carries a theoretic risk of increasing PVR, a phenomenon demonstrated in animal models.[39,40] Nonetheless, oxytocin has been used safely to induce labor in women with PH.[13] During delivery, systemic hypotension may result from the many therapies needed to manage patients with PH, including oxytocin, pulmonary vasodilator drugs, ionotropes such as dobutamine, and analgesic agents. The use of vasopressin, which preferentially causes an increase in systemic vascular resistance without increasing PVR is an option to support systemic blood pressure without worsening RV function.[41]

Monitoring

Although the diagnosis of PAH in pregnancy, as in all patients, should be established with an RHC, the role of invasive monitoring techniques during the period of delivery in patients with PH is controversial, and there are insufficient data to either recommend or discourage pulmonary arterial catheter (PAC) use. Several case studies of successful cesarean deliveries report the use of vasodilator and ionotropic support guided by PACs. Some investigators who advocate for their use utilize vasodilators and ionotropes, using measurements of PA pressure and cardiac output to titrate.[42] However, in the 2 large case series that exist in the literature,[11,12] the use of PACs did not influence maternal or fetal outcomes. PACs carry a risk of thrombosis and infection, and in patients who are already in a decompensated state, these risks need to be weighed carefully against the potential benefit of the information obtained.

Medical Therapy

This discussion focuses on the management of PAH during pregnancy. The management of PH secondary to chronic lung disease is not well described in the literature. This is perhaps because this is a diagnosis of a population that is either older and beyond reproductive age (eg, COPD or idiopathic pulmonary fibrosis) or very ill with disease burden that makes pregnancy unlikely. Because the use of vasodilator drugs in nonpregnant patients with PH from chronic lung disease has been studied with discouraging results,[43,44] they are not likely to benefit pregnant patients with this condition.

RV failure is the most common cause of death in pregnant patients with PH. Increases in PVR lead to difficulty for the RV in handling the increased venous return that occurs in pregnancy. The cornerstone of management is to lower the PVR and maintain ideal intravascular volumes best tolerated by a challenged RV. Volume management with diuretics must be done cautiously to avoid depriving the RV of adequate preload leading to a decrease in cardiac output, but aggressively enough to avoid hepatic congestion and bowel wall edema from advancing right heart failure.

The introduction of vasodilators in the 1990s had a dramatic effect on hemodynamics, short-term survival, and quality of life for patients with PAH, particularly in the case of IPAH.[45–47] As mentioned before, some of the reduced mortality seen in more recent studies of PH in pregnancy may be the result of vasodilator therapy, although no clear evidence exists in the literature that PAH-specific therapies are responsible for reduced mortality. The only large analysis to include patients treated with newer vasodilators showed the lowest mortality of any study overall.[12] Several agents are available for use. The management of PH in pregnant patients with prostanoids has been described in numerous case studies.[42,48–50] Prostacyclin analogues can be given by the inhaled or intravenous route. Available parenteral agents include epoprostenol (Flolan) and treprostinil (Remodulin). Ilosprost (Ventavis) is given by the inhaled route. There are reports of successful use of each in pregnant women, but there are insufficient data to recommend one over the other. The use of the inhaled route results in concentration of the prostacyclin analogue in the pulmonary circulation, and has a theoretic advantage of avoiding some of the systemic side effects, particularly inhibition of platelet aggregation, which can lead to significant bleeding during the delivery and postpartum period. Inhaled nitric oxide is also an option that has been used frequently in the case of acute cardiopulmonary decompensation during pregnancy or in the postpartum period.[51–53]

Oral vasodilators have become a more manageable alternative to intravenous and inhaled therapy, and have demonstrated improved outcomes in PAH. The agents available in the United States are the phosphodiesterase-5 inhibitors sildenafil (Revatio) and tadalafil (Adcirca), the endothelin-1 receptor antagonists bosentan (Tracleer) and ambrisentan (Letaris), and calcium channel blockers. High-dose calcium channel blockers have been used to treat PAH, and are relatively safe in pregnancy provided hypotension is avoided, but are effective only in a limited number of patients with PAH who are proven responders to a vasodilator challenge at the time of RHC.

Prostacyclin use may be associated with systemic arteriolar dilatation and shunting of blood away from the uterine circulation or may lead to paradoxic placental arteriolar constriction in animal models.[54] Although no reports of adverse fetal outcomes are available, this lack in the limited number of cases reported in the literature does not guarantee drug safety in pregnancy. However, in conditions with high maternal mortality such as PAH, risks and benefits assessment should take into consideration the effect of the disease in question against the small possibility of adverse fetal effects related to exposure to the drug. Iloprost has shown neonatal anomalies in some animal species but not in others and has limited safety reports in human pregnancies. The endothelin-1 antagonist bosentan has been shown to have deleterious effects on the fetus in animal studies including facial and blood vessel abnormalities. However, there are case reports of bosentan use during pregnancy, even in the early developmental phase, in patients who were not aware of their pregnancy, which describe successful maternal and fetal outcomes.[55] It should only be used if PH cannot be managed with other agents. Animal data for sildenafil do not show adverse fetal effects in most species studied. Sildenafil has been used successfully to manage PH in pregnancy, but experience is limited and the literature consists only of case reports[51,56] The largest trial of sildenafil in pregnancy investigated its use in preeclampsia, and did not show any adverse fetal outcomes, however the sample size was small (35 patients).[57]

Antithrombotic Treatment

In addition to managing the hemodynamics of PH in pregnant patients, the problem of hypercoagulability and thromboprophylaxis must also be addressed. The use of anticoagulation in PH in nonpregnant patients has been shown to be beneficial in several small nonrandomized studies.[58–61] Its use during pregnancy with PH has not been studied prospectively, and there are no trials comparing different agents in this setting. A single-center series of 7 patients with Eisenmenger syndrome was remarkable for bleeding complications in 3 of 5 patients receiving heparin prophylaxis.[62] Hemoptysis and bleeding diatheses more commonly complicate Eisenmenger syndrome than other forms of pulmonary vascular disease[33] making individualization of prophylaxis appropriate. In the large case review by Bedard and colleagues,[12] 2 out of 8 maternal deaths in Eisenmenger syndrome were secondary to thromboembolism in patients who did not receive prophylaxis. In this study, there were no VTE events among patients with a diagnosis of IPAH, perhaps because this population had a higher rate of thromboprophylaxis.

The choice of agents for use includes warfarin, unfractionated heparin (UFH), and low-molecular-weight heparin (LMWH). Comparative studies have not been done, and the choice of agent is left to the discretion of the physician. Warfarin should be avoided during the early development of the fetus as it is associated with embryonic toxicity, usually between the sixth and twelfth week of pregnancy.[4,63] Later in pregnancy, there is a small risk of central nervous system abnormalities. The risk of fetal hemorrhage is present throughout pregnancy. Regular blood test monitoring is inconvenient. Given that heparins are associated with similar or better efficacy in thromboprophylaxis, a lower rate of complications and no teratogenicity, the use of warfarin for this indication cannot be justified. UFH and LMWH are larger molecules that do not cross the placenta. LMWH is associated with a lower risk of heparin-induced thrombocytopenia[64] and less osteopenia.[65,66] As the time of delivery approaches, use of UFH is preferred because it is more readily reversible in the event of hemorrhage. Although the limited use of fondiparinux (Arixtra), a factor Xa inhibitor, has not been associated with adverse fetal effects,[67] there are limited data to support or recommend against its use in pregnancy. It may be useful as a prophylactic agent in patients with heparin-induced thrombocytopenia. Thomboprophylaxis is discussed in more detail in the article on pulmonary embolism in pregnancy by Miller and colleagues elsewhere in this issue.

SUMMARY AND RECOMMENDATIONS

The diagnosis of PH by TTE is not uncommon in pregnancy. Because of the high output state of pregnancy, PH on a TTE should never be misconstrued as diagnostic of PAH. In approximately one-third of cases, the TTE finding represents a false-positive. Those with true arteriopathy and PAH are at increased risk for mortality as a result of the physiologic stresses of pregnancy, labor, and delivery. Recently published data that take newer therapies into account suggest that the mortality of PH in pregnancy may have decreased to as low as 25% from earlier studies that suggested rates as high as 60%, but all data may be subject to reporting bias. Despite this advancement, the risk of maternal death is still unacceptably high, and patients with PH should be advised to avoid pregnancy. Progestin-only methods of contraception are safe to use in such

patients. Although therapeutic abortion carries a risk of death for the mother, this risk remains lower than that of continuing the pregnancy to term. If a patient opts to become pregnant and carry the child to term, there are options available to optimize the chance of a successful maternal and fetal outcome. These include traditional therapies such as oxygen, rest, and early hospitalization of symptomatic patients, as well as the proactive use of parenteral, inhaled, or oral PAH-specific therapies. Although there are very limited safety data on any of these treatment options, the risk of untreated disease on maternal mortality outweighs the risk of potential teratogenicity. The most effective drugs with the lowest likelihood of teratogenicity should obviously be chosen. Decisions regarding thromboprophylaxis must individualized to the patient and their disease. Vaginal delivery with early regional anesthesia seems to have theoretic advantages over cesarean delivery. The latter is mostly reserved for obstetric indications or the emergent need for an intervention because of fetal compromise. Collaboration between high-risk obstetricians, anesthesiologists, and PH specialists is necessary to help coordinate the treatment of PH during pregnancy and optimize the timing and mode of delivery to ensure the best fetal and maternal outcomes.

REFERENCES

1. Mccaffrey R, Dunn L. Primary pulmonary hypertension in pregnancy. Obstet Gynecol Surv 1964;19:567.
2. Madden B. Pulmonary hypertension and pregnancy. Int J Obstet Anesth 2009;18:156.
3. Warnes C. Pregnancy and pulmonary hypertension. Int J Cardiol 2004;97(Suppl 1):11.
4. Marik P, Plante L. Venous thromboembolic disease and pregnancy. N Engl J Med 2008;359:2025.
5. Badesch D, Raskob G, Elliott C, et al. Pulmonary arterial hypertension: baseline characteristics from the REVEAL Registry. Chest 2010;137:376.
6. Simonneau G, Robbins I, Beghetti M, et al. Updated clinical classification of pulmonary hypertension. J Am Coll Cardiol 2009;54:S43.
7. Arcasoy S, Christie J, Ferrari V, et al. Echocardiographic assessment of pulmonary hypertension in patients with advanced lung disease. Am J Respir Crit Care Med 2003;167:735.
8. Penning S, Robinson K, Major C, et al. A comparison of echocardiography and pulmonary artery catheterization for evaluation of pulmonary artery pressures in pregnant patients with suspected pulmonary hypertension. Am J Obstet Gynecol 2001;184:1568.
9. Wylie B, Epps K, Gaddipati S, et al. Correlation of transthoracic echocardiography and right heart catheterization in pregnancy. J Perinat Med 2007;35:497.

10. Chakravarty E, Khanna D, Chung L. Pregnancy outcomes in systemic sclerosis, primary pulmonary hypertension, and sickle cell disease. Obstet Gynecol 2008;111:927.

11. Weiss B, Zemp L, Seifert B, et al. Outcome of pulmonary vascular disease in pregnancy: a systematic overview from 1978 through 1996. J Am Coll Cardiol 1998;31:1650.

12. Bédard E, Dimopoulos K, Gatzoulis M. Has there been any progress made on pregnancy outcomes among women with pulmonary arterial hypertension? Eur Heart J 2009;30:256.

13. Smedstad K, Cramb R, Morison D. Pulmonary hypertension and pregnancy: a series of eight cases. Can J Anaesth 1994;41:502.

14. Bonnin M, Mercier F, Sitbon O, et al. Severe pulmonary hypertension during pregnancy: mode of delivery and anesthetic management of 15 consecutive cases. Anesthesiology 2005;102:1133.

15. Zwicke DL, Buggy BP. Pregnancy and pulmonary arterial hypertension: successful management of 37 consecutive patients [abstract]. Chest 2008; 134:64002S.

16. Tahir H. Pulmonary hypertension, cardiac disease and pregnancy. Int J Gynaecol Obstet 1995;51:109.

17. Trow T, McArdle J. Diagnosis of pulmonary arterial hypertension. Clin Chest Med 2007;28:59.

18. Siva A, Shah A. Moderate mitral stenosis in pregnancy: the haemodynamic impact of diuresis. Heart 2005;91:e3.

19. Bonow R, Carabello B, Chatterjee K, et al. 2008 focused update incorporated into the ACC/AHA 2006 guidelines for the management of patients with valvular heart disease: a report of the American College of Cardiology/American Heart Association Task Force on Practice Guidelines (Writing Committee to revise the 1998 guidelines for the management of patients with valvular heart disease). Endorsed by the Society of Cardiovascular Anesthesiologists, Society for Cardiovascular Angiography and Interventions, and Society of Thoracic Surgeons. J Am Coll Cardiol 2008;52:e1.

20. de Souza J, Martinez EJ, Ambrose J, et al. Percutaneous balloon mitral valvuloplasty in comparison with open mitral valve commissurotomy for mitral stenosis during pregnancy. J Am Coll Cardiol 2001;37:900.

21. Sivadasanpillai H, Srinivasan A, Sivasubramoniam S, et al. Long-term outcome of patients undergoing balloon mitral valvotomy in pregnancy. Am J Cardiol 2005;95:1504.

22. Kelly M, Rustin G, Ivory C, et al. Respiratory failure due to choriocarcinoma: a study of 103 dyspneic patients. Gynecol Oncol 1990;38:149.

23. Seckl M, Rustin G, Newlands E, et al. Pulmonary embolism, pulmonary hypertension, and choriocarcinoma. Lancet 1991;338:1313.

24. Gangadharan V, Chitrathara K, Sivaramakrishnan R, et al. Pulmonary hypertension—a rare presentation of choriocarcinoma. Acta Oncol 1993;32:461.

25. Conde-Agudelo A, Romero R. Amniotic fluid embolism: an evidence-based review. Am J Obstet Gynecol 2009;201:445, e1.

26. Khong T. Expression of endothelin-1 in amniotic fluid embolism and possible pathophysiological mechanism. Br J Obstet Gynaecol 1998;105:802.

27. McDonnell N, Chan B, Frengley R. Rapid reversal of critical haemodynamic compromise with nitric oxide in a parturient with amniotic fluid embolism. Int J Obstet Anesth 2007;16:269.

28. O'Shea A, Eappen S. Amniotic fluid embolism. Int Anesthesiol Clin 2007;45:17.

29. Van Heerden P, Webb S, Hee G, et al. Inhaled aerosolized prostacyclin as a selective pulmonary vasodilator for the treatment of severe hypoxaemia. Anaesth Intensive Care 1996;24:87.

30. Galiè N, Seeger W, Naeije R, et al. Comparative analysis of clinical trials and evidence-based treatment algorithm in pulmonary arterial hypertension. J Am Coll Cardiol 2004;43:81S.

31. Thorne S, Nelson-Piercy C, MacGregor A, et al. Pregnancy and contraception in heart disease and pulmonary arterial hypertension. J Fam Plann Reprod Health Care 2006;32:75.

32. Temelcos C, Kuhn R, Stribley C. Sterilization of women with Eisenmenger syndrome: report of 4 cases. Aust N Z J Obstet Gynaecol 1997;37:121.

33. Weiss B, Hess O. Pulmonary vascular disease and pregnancy: current controversies, management strategies, and perspectives. Eur Heart J 2000;21:104.

34. Robinson J, Banerjee R, Landzberg M, et al. Inhaled nitric oxide therapy in pregnancy complicated by pulmonary hypertension. Am J Obstet Gynecol 1999;180:1045.

35. Weiss B, Maggiorini M, Jenni R, et al. Pregnant patient with primary pulmonary hypertension: inhaled pulmonary vasodilators and epidural anesthesia for cesarean delivery. Anesthesiology 2000; 92:1191.

36. Toyama H, Wagatsuma T, Ejima Y, et al. Cesarean section and primary pulmonary hypertension: the role of intravenous dexmedetomidine. Int J Obstet Anesth 2009;18:262.

37. Abboud T, Raya J, Noueihed R, et al. Intrathecal morphine for relief of labor pain in a parturient with severe pulmonary hypertension. Anesthesiology 1983;59:477.

38. Martin J, Tautz T, Antognini J. Safety of regional anesthesia in Eisenmenger's syndrome. Reg Anesth Pain Med 2002;27:509.

39. Johnstone M. The cardiovascular effects of oxytocic drugs. Br J Anaesth 1972;44:826.

40. Roberts N, Keast P, Brodeky V, et al. The effects of oxytocin on the pulmonary and systemic circulation

in pregnant ewes. Anaesth Intensive Care 1992;20: 199.

41. Price L, Forrest P, Sodhi V, et al. Use of vasopressin after Caesarean section in idiopathic pulmonary arterial hypertension. Br J Anaesth 2007;99:552.

42. Stewart R, Tuazon D, Olson G, et al. Pregnancy and primary pulmonary hypertension: successful outcome with epoprostenol therapy. Chest 2001;119:973.

43. Rietema H, Holverda S, Bogaard H, et al. Sildenafil treatment in COPD does not affect stroke volume or exercise capacity. Eur Respir J 2008;31:759.

44. Stolz D, Rasch H, Linka A, et al. A randomised, controlled trial of bosentan in severe COPD. Eur Respir J 2008;32:619.

45. Badesch D, Tapson V, McGoon M, et al. Continuous intravenous epoprostenol for pulmonary hypertension due to the scleroderma spectrum of disease. A randomized, controlled trial. Ann Intern Med 2000;132:425.

46. Barst R, Rubin L, McGoon M, et al. Survival in primary pulmonary hypertension with long-term continuous intravenous prostacyclin. Ann Intern Med 1994;121:409.

47. Rubin L, Mendoza J, Hood M, et al. Treatment of primary pulmonary hypertension with continuous intravenous prostacyclin (epoprostenol). Results of a randomized trial. Ann Intern Med 1990;112:485.

48. Bendayan D, Hod M, Oron G, et al. Pregnancy outcome in patients with pulmonary arterial hypertension receiving prostacyclin therapy. Obstet Gynecol 2005;106:1206.

49. Bildirici I, Shumway J. Intravenous and inhaled epoprostenol for primary pulmonary hypertension during pregnancy and delivery. Obstet Gynecol 2004;103:1102.

50. Easterling T, Ralph D, Schmucker B. Pulmonary hypertension in pregnancy: treatment with pulmonary vasodilators. Obstet Gynecol 1999;93:494.

51. Lacassie H, Germain A, Valdés G, et al. Management of Eisenmenger syndrome in pregnancy with sildenafil and L-arginine. Obstet Gynecol 2004; 103:1118.

52. Lam G, Stafford R, Thorp J, et al. Inhaled nitric oxide for primary pulmonary hypertension in pregnancy. Obstet Gynecol 2001;98:895.

53. Lust K, Boots R, Dooris M, et al. Management of labor in Eisenmenger syndrome with inhaled nitric oxide. Am J Obstet Gynecol 1999;181:419.

54. Parisi V, Walsh S. Fetal vascular responses to prostacyclin. Am J Obstet Gynecol 1989;160:871.

55. Molelekwa V, Akhter P, McKenna P, et al. Eisenmenger's syndrome in a 27 week pregnancy—management with bosentan and sildenafil. Ir Med J 2005;98:87.

56. Goland S, Tsai F, Habib M, et al. Favorable outcome of pregnancy with an elective use of epoprostenol and sildenafil in women with severe pulmonary hypertension. Cardiology 2010;115:205.

57. Samangaya R, Mires G, Shennan A, et al. A randomised, double-blinded, placebo-controlled study of the phosphodiesterase type 5 inhibitor sildenafil for the treatment of preeclampsia. Hypertens Pregnancy 2009;28:369.

58. Barst R, Gibbs J, Ghofrani H, et al. Updated evidence-based treatment algorithm in pulmonary arterial hypertension. J Am Coll Cardiol 2009;54: S78.

59. Frank H, Mlczoch J, Huber K, et al. The effect of anticoagulant therapy in primary and anorectic drug-induced pulmonary hypertension. Chest 1997;112:714.

60. Fuster V, Steele P, Edwards W, et al. Primary pulmonary hypertension: natural history and the importance of thrombosis. Circulation 1984;70:580.

61. Rich S, Kaufmann E, Levy P. The effect of high doses of calcium-channel blockers on survival in primary pulmonary hypertension. N Engl J Med 1992;327:76.

62. Pitts J, Crosby W, Basta L. Eisenmenger's syndrome in pregnancy: does heparin prophylaxis improve the maternal mortality rate? Am Heart J 1977;93:321.

63. Oakley C. Anticoagulation and pregnancy. Eur Heart J 1995;16:1317.

64. Greer I, Nelson-Piercy C. Low-molecular-weight heparins for thromboprophylaxis and treatment of venous thromboembolism in pregnancy: a systematic review of safety and efficacy. Blood 2005;106:401.

65. Carlin A, Farquharson R, Quenby S, et al. Prospective observational study of bone mineral density during pregnancy: low molecular weight heparin versus control. Hum Reprod 2004;19:1211.

66. Pettilä V, Leinonen P, Markkola A, et al. Postpartum bone mineral density in women treated for thromboprophylaxis with unfractionated heparin or LMW heparin. Thromb Haemost 2002;87:182.

67. Mazzolai L, Hohlfeld P, Spertini F, et al. Fondaparinux is a safe alternative in case of heparin intolerance during pregnancy. Blood 2006;108:1569.

Sleep-disordered Breathing in Pregnancy

Ghada Bourjeily, MD[a],*, Gina Ankner, RN, MSN[b],
Vahid Mohsenin, MD[c]

KEYWORDS

- Sleep-disorderd breathing • Pregnancy
- Treatment • Outcome

Many women report alterations in their sleep during pregnancy. Changes in sleep pattern and duration are common, as are sleep complaints associated with the physical changes of pregnancy. Physiologic changes of pregnancy not only are associated with sleep fragmentation but may also either protect against or predispose to the development of sleep-disordered breathing (SDB). This diagnosis is important in the pregnant population because a few studies now suggest a significant association between habitual snoring and adverse pregnancy outcomes[1–3] such as gestational hypertensive disorders and gestational diabetes, with some suggesting adverse fetal or neonatal outcomes.[3] The purpose of this article is to discuss the pathophysiology of SDB in pregnancy, review the available literature evaluating associations with adverse outcomes, and discuss the subtleties in the management of these patients.

FACTORS PREDISPOSING TO SDB IN PREGNANCY

During pregnancy, airway mucosa undergoes changes that lead to edema and friability.[4] These changes are believed to be related to increased plasma volume and capillary engorgement, as well as the higher levels of estrogens. These changes may be accentuated by a mild respiratory tract infection, fluid overload, preeclampsia, and other factors. In some patients, changes in the nasal mucosa lead to the development of gestational rhinitis, which consists of symptomatic nasal congestion that invariably improves almost immediately after delivery. Given that nocturnal nasal congestion is a risk factor for SDB,[5,6] it is possible that gestational rhinitis could predispose to the development of this disease.

Airway patency is an important predictor of SDB. Mucosal edema occurs in both normal pregnant women and women with preeclampsia. Preeclampsia, a multisystem disorder characterized by systemic endothelial dysfunction, hypertension, and proteinuria, is also associated with marked fluid retention that affects the upper airway resulting in pharyngolaryngeal edema. Pharyngeal dimensions assessed using the Mallampati scoring system are reduced in pregnancy.[7] Measures of upper airway size using acoustic reflectance show a significant reduction in upper airway size at various sites including the oropharyngeal junction in pregnant women compared with nonpregnant controls.[8] This reduction in airway size is even more explicit in patients with preeclampsia.[9] Airway narrowing that

[a] Pulmonary and Critical Care Medicine, Department of Medicine, Women and Infants Hospital of Rhode Island, The Warren Alpert Medical School of Brown University, 100 Dudley Street, Suite 1100, Providence, RI 02905, USA
[b] Department of Medicine, Women and Infants Hospital of Rhode Island, 100 Dudley Street, Suite 1100, Providence, RI 02905, USA
[c] Yale Center for Sleep Medicine, Division of Pulmonary, Critical Care and Sleep Medicine, Yale University School of Medicine, 333 Cedar Street, New Haven, CT 06520, USA
* Corresponding author.
E-mail address: GBourjeily@wihri.org

Clin Chest Med 32 (2011) 175–189
doi:10.1016/j.ccm.2010.11.003
0272-5231/11/$ – see front matter © 2011 Elsevier Inc. All rights reserved.

occurs in normal pregnancy seems to resolve after delivery.[8]

In addition, late in pregnancy, the gravid uterus causes diaphragmatic elevation, which causes functional residual capacity (FRC) to be reduced approximately 20% by term. This reduction in FRC may result in less caudal traction of the trachea and pharynx, potentially leading to increased airway collapsibility[10] but this effect has not been studied specifically in pregnancy. Further contributing to this collapsibility is the increased ventilatory drive associated with increased levels of progesterone in pregnancy that may cause a vacuum effect on the edematous upper airway.[11,12] Both minute ventilation and arterial oxygen tension increase in normal gravidas. However, the literature suggests a mild increase in the alveolar-arterial gradient in late pregnancy[13] and potential oxygen desaturations while lying in the supine position because of early airway closing during tidal breathing[14] or positional changes in cardiac output.

FACTORS PROTECTING AGAINST SDB IN PREGNANCY

Factors that may protect against the development of SDB in pregnancy include increased minute ventilation,[15] as well as a preference for the lateral sleeping position in late gestation[16] and decreases in rapid eye movement (REM) sleep.[17]

Progesterone stimulates the ventilatory drive and increases electromyographic activity of the upper airway dilator muscle.[18] Progesterone's stimulating properties enhance the responsiveness of the upper airway dilator muscles to chemical stimuli during sleep.[19,20] This progesterone effect theoretically protects against the development of SDB, with less obstructive events observed in high progesterone periods of the menstrual cycle.[21] However, this effect may be offset by augmented respiratory drive and increased negative intraluminal pressure promoting narrowing and collapse of airways as mentioned earlier.

The effect of estrogen on apneic/hypopneic episodes is not entirely clear because estrogen replacement therapy reduced the apneic/hypopneic index (AHI) in patients with mild to moderate SDB[22]; however evidence of sleep fragmentation or significant change in the AHI was not observed in drug-induced menopause in healthy premenopausal women.[23]

In summary, pregnancy may either protect against or predispose to the development of SDB[24]; studies evaluating predictors of SDB in pregnancy are very limited. Although some factors such as body mass index (BMI, calculated as weight in kilograms divided by the square of height

in meters) have been associated with symptoms of SDB in pregnancy in multiple studies[1,25] and SDB in others,[26] these studies were not designed to longitudinally evaluate whether SDB develops during pregnancy or predates pregnancy in these women. Prepregnancy BMI, weight gain during pregnancy, and BMI at delivery have all been associated with loud snoring.[1] In addition, age and neck circumference measured around delivery have been associated with snoring, gasping, and witnessed apneas.[1]

EPIDEMIOLOGY

The prevalence of SDB in pregnancy has not yet been studied but a few studies report the incidence of symptoms of SDB in this population. As a general rule, women tend to under-report snoring. Many studies suggest that snoring occurs in 14% to 45% of pregnant women[1,2,27] as opposed to 4% of premenopausal, nonpregnant women. Pregnant women are more likely to have a bed partner, and therefore could possibly be more likely to report awareness of their snoring. In a large epidemiologic study of symptoms of SDB during pregnancy, women with a bed partner tended to report snoring in pregnancy more frequently than those without a bed partner ($P = .05$).[1] The overall incidence of snoring in this cohort was 35%. Pregnant women with a higher BMI are more likely to snore than women with a lower BMI.[1,26] Small case-controlled studies show a higher prevalence of obstructive sleep apnea (OSA) by polysomnography in obese pregnant patients than in nonobese pregnant controls.[26] Furthermore, symptoms of daytime hypersomnolence increase in pregnancy[25,28,29] with reported abnormally high Epworth sleepiness scale (ESS) scores in close to 25% of pregnant patients.[28] Although there are many reasons that could potentially lead to sleep disruption in pregnancy resulting in daytime hypersomnolence, a study based on a cross-sectional survey showed that ESS scores correlated with both snoring and gasping ($P = .0008$ and $P = .001$, respectively) but not with nocturnal micturition or gastroesophageal reflux disease.[28]

MATERNAL OUTCOMES
Gestational Hypertensive Disorders

Associations between SDB symptoms and gestational hypertensive disorders have been shown in multiple studies[1–3,27,30] after correction for other risk factors (**Table 1**). In addition, polysomnographically diagnosed SDB was found significantly more frequently in women with gestational hypertensive disorders.[31] Another study showed a significantly higher rate of preeclampsia in women with OSA compared with normal weight pregnant controls but not compared with pregnant obese controls.[32] However, pregnant obese controls did not have the diagnosis of OSA excluded in that study and this limitation was acknowledged by the investigators.

Preeclampsia is a significant cause of maternal and fetal morbidity and mortality. The underlying mechanism for the association of SDB with gestational hypertensive disorders has not been elucidated. Hypoxemia is a possible factor as data from high-altitude residents suggest higher rates of preeclampsia and fetal growth restriction compared with low-altitude residents, which is believed to be related to chronic hypoxia.[33,34] There are limited data on the effect of intermittent hypoxia on pregnancy outcomes; however, intermittent hypoxia may lead to endothelial dysfunction. Recent studies have shown that endothelial dysfunction is present in patients with OSA in all severity categories.[35,36] On the other hand, angiogenic-antiangiogenic disequilibrium and endothelial dysfunction are implicated as underlying mechanisms of preeclampsia. A recent study showed a significant association between preeclampsia, OSA, and endothelial dysfunction in pregnant women.[37] Pregnant snorers were also found to have higher levels of oxidative stress markers such as malondialdehyde compared with nonsnoring pregnant controls.[38] These data suggest a potential link between preeclampsia and OSA; intermittent hypoxia may lead to placental hypoxemia that triggers a cascade of events leading to preeclampsia.

Air flow limitations during sleep without outright apneas are another possible mechanism in the development of gestational hypertensive disorders. Frequent, prolonged air flow limitations that are not associated with significant desaturations were identified in patients with preeclampsia compared with normal pregnant and nonpregnant women.[39] Air flow limitations were also present in a noncontrolled study of patients with risk factors for preeclampsia.[40] In addition, a case-control study evaluating women with gestational hypertensive disorders by polysomnography showed a crude odds ratio of 5.6 for OSA in these women compared with pregnant nonhypertensive controls.[31] However, OSA was defined in this study as having an AHI >15 events per hour without a requirement for desaturation.[31] Given the lack of consensus criteria for air flow limitations, the definition has varied significantly between studies, with inter-reader agreement being a potential issue. Treatment of patients with risk factors for preeclampsia and air flow limitations (but no SDB) with continuous positive airway pressure (CPAP) starting in early pregnancy has shown beneficial effects on blood pressure control[40,41] and improved fetal outcomes when compared with controls.[41] These findings indirectly suggest that even in the absence of hypoxia and reoxygenation, air flow limitation may have a role in causing hemodynamic changes in patients without outright apneas or hypopneas.

An alternative explanation is that preeclampsia predisposes to the development of SDB. Patients with preeclampsia have lower oncotic pressures than normal pregnant women and have a larger neck circumference and a smaller upper airway size[8]; these factors are known predictors of SDB. Additional studies are needed to evaluate this theory further.

Given that preeclampsia is now being considered a precursor of cardiovascular disease, and that SDB is associated with cardiovascular disease in the nonpregnant population, it is possible that the constellation of symptoms of SDB and the development of preeclampsia may have significant implications on future cardiovascular health. Pregnancy has been implicated as a stressor for many chronic diseases[42] and some investigators have suggested that pregnancy may accelerate the development of SDB.[3] Although no comparative longitudinal studies exist to support these statements, future research on the natural history of SDB around childbearing years would help answer some of these questions.

Gestational Diabetes

Multiple studies have shown an association between SDB, diabetes mellitus, and abnormal glucose metabolism outside of pregnancy. For example, snoring has been associated with a higher risk of increased glycosylated hemoglobin in premenopausal women.[43] In the Sleep AHEAD trial, a subgroup of the Look AHEAD trial, investigating the long-term health effect of an intensive lifestyle intervention in more than 5000 overweight and obese adults with type 2 diabetes, OSA was diagnosed in 86% (262/305) of obese or overweight subjects with type 2 diabetes.[44] However, there may be a potential for a selection bias in this sample because the subgroup of patients in the Sleep AHEAD trial had a small but significant difference in the frequency of snoring compared with the larger Look AHEAD sample, suggesting that participants with sleep complaints were more likely to enroll in the Sleep AHEAD trial. OSA has been linked to decreased insulin sensitivity[45] and multiple studies using the homeostasis model assessment of insulin resistance[46] have correlated the severity of SDB with the

Table 1
Literature review: symptoms of SDB and gestational hypertensive disorders

	Publication Year	Design	Number of Patients	Variable Tested	Significant Association With GHD	OR, CI	Multivariable Regression Analysis	Comments
Franklin et al[3]	2000	Cross-sectional, retrospective	502	Symptoms	Yes, nonproteinuric HTN	2.03, $P<.05$	Weight, age, smoking habits	Not corrected for many risk factors for GHD
Calaora-Tournadre et al[2]	2006	Cross-sectional	438	Symptoms	Yes, (combined snoring and vigilance trouble)	2.6		Excluded multiple gestations
Perez-Chada et al[30]	2007	Cross-sectional	456	Symptoms	Yes	1.82, 1.16–2.84	BMI, weight gain, neck circumference, smoking, alcohol and age	Not corrected for many risk factors for GHD
Yin et al[57]	2008	Cross-sectional	178 pregnant and 50 nonpregnant controls	Symptoms and oxygen desaturation	No			Women with adverse pregnancy or fetal outcomes selected
Ursavas et al[27]	2008	Cross-sectional	469 pregnant and 208 nonpregnant controls	Symptoms	Yes, nonproteinuric HTN			Study excluded women at high risk for adverse outcomes and GHD
Ayrim et al[97]	2009	Cross-sectional	200 pregnant and 200 nonpregnant age-matched controls	Symptoms	No			Study does not clarify whether subject selection was random

Study	Year	Design	N	SDB	Association	OR, CI	Adjusted factors	Comments
Champagne et al[31]	2009	Case-control	17 pregnant with GHD and 33 without HTN	OSA	Yes	7.5, 3.5–16.2	Age, gestational age, prepregnancy BMI, prior pregnancies, and previous live births	OSA defined as AHI ≥15 events/h without requirement for desaturation
Louis et al[32]	2010	Case-control	57 subjects (68 pregnancies)	OSA	Yes, compared with normal weight but not compared with obese controls			Obese controls not excluded for OSA
Olivarez et al[53]	2010	Prospective	100	OSA	No			Women recruited during antepartum hospitalization. Association with GHD was not the main outcome
Bourjeily et al[1]	2010	Cross-sectional	1000	Snoring	Yes	2.3, 1.4–4.0	DM, chronic HTN, renal disease, multiple gestation, prior preeclampsia, BMI at delivery, age, smoking	Study excluded women with fetal losses, potentially negatively affecting association

Abbreviations: AHI, apnea/hypopnea index; BMI, body mass index; CI, confidence interval; DM, diabetes mellitus; GHD, gestational hypertensive disorders; HTN, hypertension; OR, odds ratio; OSA, obstructive sleep apnea.

degree of insulin resistance.[47,48] A recent study[49] showed that patients with various degrees of SDB had a significant reduction in insulin sensitivity that was independent of age, sex, race, and body fat when compared with controls. There was also a reduction in pancreatic β-cell function in those with moderate and severe disease. Both insulin sensitivity and the glucose disposition index correlate with the average degree of oxyhemoglobin desaturation index.[49]

A recent systematic review and meta-analysis found that women with gestational diabetes were at significantly higher risk of developing subsequent type 2 diabetes than women with normoglycemic pregnancies (relative risk 7.43, 95% confidence interval [CI] 4.79–11.51).[50] Despite the increased risk of type 2 diabetes in patients with gestational diabetes, and the association of the former with SDB, there are limited studies evaluating the association of gestational diabetes with SDB. A recent large study evaluating symptoms of SDB and their association with pregnancy and neonatal outcomes has shown a significant association of symptoms of SDB with gestational diabetes that was independent of age, BMI at delivery, multifetal pregnancy, and smoking (adjusted odds ratio [OR] 2.1, 95% CI 1.3–3.4).[1] When snoring, gasping, and apnea symptoms were combined, the association was stronger (adjusted OR 4.0, 95% CI 1.4–11.1) suggesting that the association is greater with a higher likelihood of OSA.[1] Future studies are needed to further elucidate the association and explore the potential underlying mechanism.

Delivery Mode

Cesarean deliveries are operative deliveries that may be associated with a higher rate of complications compared with vaginal deliveries, and should be avoided when possible. Cesarean deliveries are usually performed electively for obstetric causes that may hinder a successful vaginal delivery or emergently for causes such as fetal compromise. Complications of cesarean deliveries include higher rates of medical complications such as venous thromboembolism, as well as obstetric complications and longer hospital stay.

Associations between sleep and delivery mode have been evaluated in a few studies. The effects of sleep duration on labor and delivery outcomes have been inconsistent in the literature.[51,52] Early studies did not show any significant effect of sleep duration on delivery outcomes.[51] More recent studies using actigraphy showed that women with sleep deprivation at term had significantly longer labor and more cesarean deliveries.[52] Emerging data focusing on SDB suggest an

association between habitual snoring,[1] OSA,[32] and unplanned cesarean deliveries even after adjusting for BMI, multifetal gestations, newborn weight, gestational hypertensive disorders, and gestational diabetes.[1] None of these studies have examined the potential mechanism underlying this association and further studies assessing polysomnographic parameters and anthropometric data are needed.

FETAL OUTCOMES
Preterm Birth

Preterm labor is one of the most common complications of pregnancy, potentially resulting in preterm delivery. Preterm birth is defined as birth occurring before 37 weeks' gestation and occurs in about 12% of deliveries in the United States. Prematurity is a significant cause of morbidity and mortality. Preterm birth may result from conditions such as preterm premature rupture of membranes, preterm labor, infection, or may be induced for fetal or maternal well-being. Preliminary data show that preterm delivery is more likely to occur in snorers compared with nonsnorers and in patients with OSA compared with an obese group without a diagnosis of OSA.[32] Other studies comparing a group of 20 women with OSA diagnosed using a single channel device to a group of 80 women who were excluded for OSA, all admitted to an inpatient ward for unrelated causes at or after 26 weeks' gestation, showed only a trend toward statistical significance for preterm labor.[53]

Growth Restriction

A few studies have evaluated the association between SDB symptoms and fetal outcomes[1–3,27,54–56] and are somewhat conflicting (**Table 2**). Although the study by Franklin and colleagues[3] showed an association of loud snoring with growth restriction, the study did not adjust for confounders such as hypertensive disorders or diabetes. Many other studies have not shown such an association.[1,2,54,57] Definitions of outcomes may contribute to the inconsistency and future studies with an emphasis on appropriate dating of pregnancies and serial fetal growth assessments should be performed to ensure accuracy of birth weight for gestational age and avoid overlooking fetal growth stunting.

Intermittent hypoxia may be the most plausible mechanism for potential adverse effects on the fetus. Human studies exploring this phenomenon are lacking but limited animal studies show a reduction in birth weight[58] in rat pups exposed to intermittent hypoxia in utero, which resolved fter 15 days of age. Although epidemiologic data om chronically hypoxic pregnant women living at igh altitudes strongly suggest a negative effect on trauterine growth, it is not entirely clear whether he effect of chronic intermittent hypoxia would ave the same effect.

Associations of symptoms of SDB with lower pgar scores measured at 1 minute and 5 minutes fter birth have also been inconsistent in the terature.[1,3]

etal Heart Rate Response

)ther potential effects of SDB on fetal well-being clude the direct effect of apneas on fetal heart rate esponse. Case reports suggest acute fetal decelera- ons during maternal apneic episodes[56,59,60] but hese reports were based on clinical observations of pneas and not on polysomnographic data. One ecent study looked at simultaneous polysomnogra- hy and fetal nonstress testing in a series of 4 preg- ant women with OSA and suggested late fetal ecelerations accompanying the apneic episodes.[55] lowever, the study did not show the temporal rela- onship between apneas, desaturations, and decel- rations, and did not adjust for associated medical roblems in the 3 pregnant women with OSA and fetal ecelerations (2 with gestational diabetes mellitus nd 1 with cardiovascular disease). Another study as synchronized fetal heart rate and uterine contrac- ons monitoring with nasal flow, heart rate, and xygen saturation measurements using a single hannel device.[53] This study did not show evidence f abnormal decelerations associated with obstruc- ve events or desaturations.

)IAGNOSIS OF SDB IN PREGNANCY
:linical Risk Assessment

everal clinical diagnostic tools have been devel- ped for the evaluation of SDB. For instance, the Ierlin Questionnaire is a 10-item survey that was leveloped for the primary care setting and consists f 3 categories related to the risk of having sleep pnea.[61] Other questionnaires have been devel- ped for the preoperative population.[62] Many of hese tools include weight in risk assessment. Preg- ancy is associated with weight gain that varies rom an increase in plasma volume and fat deposi- ion in the early stages of pregnancy to weight gain rom placental and fetal growth, and accumulation f amniotic fluid in the second part of gestation. Although weight is considered an important vari- ble in predicting SDB outside of pregnancy, it nay have a different predictive value in pregnancy. t is not clear whether it is a woman's weight gain luring pregnancy or her prepregnancy weight that ; more predictive of SDB, but prepregnancy weight

seemed to be more predictive of symptoms of SDB in 1 study.[1]

In a recent study aimed at investigating polysom- nography and fetal monitoring, pregnant women were screened with the Berlin Questionnaire before polysomnography. Only 11% of patients with suspicion of SDB were found to have that diagnosis at polysomnography.[55] Another more recent study specifically evaluated the Berlin Questionnaire in pregnancy, which also showed a poor predictive value.[53] Available data suggest that clinical evalua- tion tools may be less predictive in pregnancy than outside pregnancy. Tools taking into account pregnancy-specific factors need to be developed specifically for this population.

Polysomnography

Polysomnography remains the gold standard test in diagnosing SDB. Snoring and air flow limitation with or without a diagnosis of OSA are associated with adverse pregnancy outcomes[1–3,27,30,31,39–41] raising the question of whether milder forms of SDB could be important to diagnose in this popula- tion. Whether the same criteria for diagnosing sleep apnea should be used in pregnancy is not yet known.

Normal pregnancy
Some sleep and respiratory parameters have been studied in normal pregnancies. Total sleep time is increased in early pregnancy but sleep efficiency is reduced.[63] In late pregnancy, although nocturnal sleep time is reduced, total sleep time is increased, mainly because of daytime naps. REM sleep seems to be reduced in pregnancy.[17] Some studies have shown no oxygen desaturation during sleep in normal pregnant women,[64,65] whereas others suggest significant desaturations.[66,67]

Circulating levels of progesterone increase very early in gestation. Progesterone acts as a strong respiratory stimulant augmenting the ventilatory drive by stimulating the chemoreceptors located on the ventrolateral surface of the medulla.[68,69] In response to this stimulation, arterial carbon dioxide pressure ($Paco_2$) is reduced and respiratory alka- losis ensues with a mean arterial pH during preg- nancy of about 7.44. This respiratory alkalosis is likely to result in instability of the respiratory control system during sleep.[11] In the nonpregnant popula- tion, hypocapnia and respiratory alkalosis may lead to central apneas during non-REM sleep.[70] No conclusive evidence currently exists to establish whether respiratory alkalosis seen in pregnancy is also associated with central apneas.

Maternal response to apnea
Respiratory and cardiac physiologic changes may affect the maternal response to apnea. Expiratory

Table 2
Literature review: SDB and adverse fetal outcomes

	Year	Design	Number of Patients	Variable Tested	Significant Association With Adverse Fetal Outcomes	Comment
Loube et al[54]	1996	Prospective, nonrandomized screening	350	Symptoms	No	Outcomes included birth weight, Apgar
Franklin et al[3]	2000	Cross-sectional, retrospective	502	Symptoms	Yes, IUGR, Apgar	Study did not adjust for risk factors
Leung et al[25]	2005	Prospective	247	Symptoms	No	Outcomes included birth weight, Apgar, gestational age at delivery
Calaora-Tournadre et al[2]	2006	Cross-sectional	438	Symptoms	No	Excluded multiple births
Sahin et al[55]	2008	Prospective observational	35 (4 with OSA)	OSA	Yes Apgar scores	Outcomes evaluated included fetal decelerations, Apgar and birth weight. Note small number of patients and comorbidities in patients with OSA
Yin et al[57]	2008	Cross-sectional	178 pregnant and 50 nonpregnant controls	Snoring and oxygen desaturations	No	Women with adverse pregnancy or fetal outcomes selected

	Year	Design		Symptoms		
Ayrim et al[97]	2009	Cross-sectional	200 pregnant and 200 nonpregnant age-matched controls	Symptoms	No	Outcomes included birth weight, gestational age at birth, Apgar score
Olivarez et al[53]	2010	Prospective	100	Apneas	No	Outcomes included abnormal fetal decelerations
Louis et al[32]	2010	Retrospective	57	OSA	Yes	Outcomes significant for preterm birth. No evidence of growth restriction in OSA group
Bourjeily et al[1]	2010	Cross-sectional	1000	Snoring	Yes	Study excluded women with fetal losses, potentially negatively affecting association. Preterm birth but association no longer significant in multivariable regression. No difference in birthweight

Abbreviations: IUGR, intrauterine growth restriction; OSA, obstructive sleep apnea.

reserve volume and FRC decrease in pregnancy[15,71]; FRC is about 20% lower by term than before conception[15] and lower in the supine position.[72] In addition, oxygen consumption increases by close to 20% as a result of the demand of fetal conception products and maternal organs. The disproportionate increase in minute ventilation results in an increase in oxygen tension in the awake resting state. However, women near term lying in the supine position have been shown to have a significant decrease in their oxygen saturation while awake.[73] This decrease has been attributed to early closing volume. Cardiac output is increased by 45% in pregnancy[74] as a result of an increase in stroke volume early in pregnancy and an increase in heart rate later in pregnancy with a peak early in the third trimester. However, given the compression of the inferior vena cava by the gravid uterus in the supine position, venous return can be significantly hindered resulting in a 20% to 30% reduction in cardiac output.[75,76] This reduction is improved when the pregnant woman lies in the left lateral decubitus position. These changes are dynamic and progress with the pregnancy, possibly leading to different responses to obstructive events depending on gestational age and body position during sleep.

Response to obstructive events in pregnancy has not been well studied. Limited data from case-control studies have shown that the hemodynamic response to apneas in pregnancy is potentiated by hypertensive disorders of pregnancy. Fluctuations in blood pressure readings in response to apneic episodes are more pronounced in women with preeclampsia and OSA compared with women with OSA without hypertension.[77] Hypertensive fluctuations seem to improve in untreated women postpartum.[78]

Few studies have examined the immediate effect of apneas on oxygen desaturation and $Paco_2$ changes in pregnant women. Available data show a significantly more rapid rate of decline in oxygen saturation after sedation and neuromuscular blockade in a group of pregnant women compared with a nonpregnant group (3.6% ± 0.8%/min vs 7.5% ± 0.9%/min, respectively)[79,80] and a faster increase in $Paco_2$ (6.8 ± 1.8 mm Hg/min vs 2.8 ± 1.2 mm Hg/min, respectively).[80] However, sedation, paralysis, and induced apneas are not an optimal model for OSA because sedation and paralysis eliminate the effect of the central respiratory drive during obstructive events.

With the increase in heart rate in the second part of pregnancy, it is not clear whether the heart rate response to obstructive events is different in these patients.

TREATMENT

Just like the nonpregnant population, the diagnosis of OSA should be firmly established and its severity determined before making further decisions regarding management. Once the diagnosis is established, patients should be educated about risk factors, natural history, and consequences of OSA. Although outcome studies for pregnancy associated complications are mainly based on studies of symptoms of SDB rather than polysomnography-confirmed SDB, it is possible that these outcomes are at least as likely to occur in patients with an established diagnosis of SDB. Although there are currently no available randomized trials evaluating the effect of treatment of SDB on pregnancy outcomes, it remains reasonable to treat pregnant patients for the same indications as nonpregnant patients. Successful treatment of OSA has been shown to lead to clinical improvement including better quality of life, decreased daytime sleepiness, lower blood pressure,[81–85] and decreased vascular morbidity and mortality.[86–88] Treatment of OSA has also resulted in a reduction in health care use.[89,90]

Treatment Indications

The American Academy of Sleep Medicine recommends therapy for patients with a respiratory disturbance index (RDI) of 5 to 14 events per hour in addition to daytime hypersomnolence, loud snoring, witnessed apneas, or awakenings caused by gasping or choking; or for patients with an RDI of 15 or more events per hour without regard to the presence or absence of symptoms or comorbidities. There is no consensus regarding whether patients with an RDI between 5 and 14 events per hour performing mission-critical work or those with objectively measured daytime hypersomnolence or cardiovascular disease would require therapy. However, the Center for Medicare and Medicaid stipulates the need for treatment of patients with AHI between 5 and 14 with cognitive deficit and cardiovascular comorbidities.[91] With regard to pregnancy, several questions remain:

1. Given the association between SDB (with or without OSA) and gestational hypertensive disorders should pregnant patients with an RDI of 5 to 14 and a current or prior history of gestational hypertensive disorders be treated?
2. Should patients with risk factors for preeclampsia and snoring or flow limitation be treated with CPAP? A small, randomized, controlled study of pregnant patients with risk factors for preeclampsia and loud snoring (but no SDB) who were treated with CPAP in early pregnancy

showed improved blood pressure control compared with the untreated group.[41] Similarly, CPAP treatment was shown to improve blood pressure in all sleep stages in a group of women with severe preeclampsia compared with a nontreatment night in the same group.[92] These findings need to be confirmed in larger trials before treatment with CPAP can be recommended for this group of patients.

These questions are interesting considerations that warrant further research before they can be implemented.

Behavior Modification

Behavior modification is usually a necessary component in the management of OSA. Weight loss has been shown to improve OSA and type 2 diabetes mellitus in obese patients.[44,93] However, weight loss should not be started during pregnancy; and although bariatric surgery has been shown to reduce the severity of OSA, it is not a treatment option during pregnancy. Patients and clinicians should be aware that bariatric surgery performed before pregnancy may be associated with complications including anemia resulting from malabsorption of iron and cyanocobalamin, fat-soluble vitamin deficiency, as well as potential surgical complications with the progression of the pregnancy such as band migration and balloon defects.

In patients with positional OSA, changes in sleep position can be advised during pregnancy. The left lateral position improves cardiac output by about 20% to 30% in pregnancy and may not only contribute to a reduced disease severity but also has the potential to improve oxygenation. Although reasonable, this hypothesis has not been proved.

In addition to avoiding alcohol for the obvious reasons of worsening OSA, hypersomnolence, and central nervous system depression, alcohol should be avoided in pregnancy to decrease the risk of fetal complications. A systematic review of medications should be done in all patients to discontinue those with central nervous system effects. This strategy is notably more complicated in pregnancy because the potential teratogenicity of certain medications limits treatment options.

OSA-specific Therapy

Positive airway pressure is the first-line treatment of OSA. Positive airway pressure reduces the frequency of respiratory events during sleep, decreases daytime hypersomnolence and improves quality of life.[83,84] Positive airway pressure can be delivered using CPAP, bilevel positive airway pressure, or autotitrating positive airway pressure (APAP). With the anticipated weight gain of pregnancy, pressure requirements may increase by 1 to 2 cm.[94] Therefore, APAP may prove to be a more effective option; however, no studies have shown improved adherence or cost reduction. Many women with young children prefer the APAP option because it may eliminate the need for another night away from home. Alternatively, a repeat titration study may be performed around midgestation.

Although pregnant women have a greater tendency to aspirate, no reports have been published regarding the use of noninvasive positive airway pressure and increased risk for aspiration. Nocturnal CPAP treatment has been shown to improve blood pressure in all sleep stages in a group of women with severe preeclampsia compared with a nontreatment night in the same group.[92] A randomized controlled trial of 24 women with preeclampsia and 15 pregnant controls showed reduction in cardiac output in the group with preeclampsia but not in the control group.[95] When the group with preeclampsia was randomized to either CPAP or no CPAP, there was a significant improvement in cardiac output in the treatment group.[95] There was no significant effect of CPAP on cardiac output in pregnant women without preeclampsia in that study.[95]

Oral appliances such as mandibular advancement splints have been shown to reduce the frequency of respiratory events, arousals, and episodes of oxyhemoglobin desaturation compared with no treatment or sham interventions.[96] This mode of treatment should be considered in pregnancy if there are issues with adherence or potential problems with positive airway pressure treatment. A follow-up with portable respiratory monitoring is required to assess the efficacy of the oral appliance.

Elective surgical procedures are usually deferred until the postpartum period, therefore, upper airway surgery is rarely (if ever) justifiable in pregnancy. However, pregnant women with life-threatening apnea that cannot be controlled with other interventions and who would be candidates for a tracheotomy outside of pregnancy, should have the procedure done while pregnant.

SDB tends to improve in the postpartum period in untreated patients.[78] It is reasonable to repeat a sleep study 3 to 6 months after pregnancy to assess the need for continuation of therapy or to titrate CPAP if needed after the loss of the weight gained during pregnancy.

SCREENING FOR SDB

It is reasonable to screen pregnant patients with gestational hypertensive disorders for the presence of symptoms suggestive of SDB. However, given the lack of validated clinical tools and the poor positive predictive value of existing questionnaires in pregnancy,[53,55] screening may not yet prove to be cost-effective.

SUMMARY

Pregnant women may be predisposed to the development of SDB given the physiologic changes of pregnancy. Evidence suggests an association of symptoms of SDB in pregnancy and adverse outcomes. Validation of clinical tools is needed in pregnancy given that current tools do not have an adequate predictive power. Treatment of SDB with CPAP in pregnancy is efficacious, with positive hemodynamic effects in women with preeclampsia. Pressure requirements may increase slightly during the course of the pregnancy and repeat titration should be considered as the pregnancy progresses. Alternatively, autotitrating positive airway pressure may be used. The severity of SDB may improve after delivery.

REFERENCES

1. Bourjeily G, Raker CA, Chalhoub M, et al. Sleep disordered breathing symptoms in pregnancy and adverse pregnancy and fetal outcomes. Eur Respir J 2010;36(4):849–55.
2. Calaora-Tournadre D, Ragot S, Meurice JC, et al. [Obstructive sleep apnea syndrome during pregnancy: prevalence of main symptoms and relationship with pregnancy-induced hypertension and intra-uterine growth retardation]. Rev Med Interne 2006;27:291–5 [in French].
3. Franklin KA, Holmgren PA, Jonsson F, et al. Snoring, pregnancy-induced hypertension, and growth retardation of the fetus. Chest 2000;117:137–41.
4. Camann WR, Ostheimer GW. Physiological adaptations during pregnancy. Int Anesthesiol Clin 1990; 28:2–10.
5. Young T, Finn L, Kim H. Nasal obstruction as a risk factor for sleep-disordered breathing. The University of Wisconsin Sleep and Respiratory Research Group. J Allergy Clin Immunol 1997;99:S757–62.
6. Young T, Finn L, Palta M. Chronic nasal congestion at night is a risk factor for snoring in a population-based cohort study. Arch Intern Med 2001;161: 1514–9.
7. Pilkington S, Carli F, Dakin MJ, et al. Increase in Mallampati score during pregnancy. Br J Anaesth 1995; 74:638–42.
8. Izci B, Vennelle M, Liston WA, et al. Sleep-disordered breathing and upper airway size in pregnancy and post-partum. Eur Respir J 2006;27:321–7.
9. Izci B, Riha RL, Martin SE, et al. The upper airway in pregnancy and pre-eclampsia. Am J Respir Cr. Care Med 2003;167:137–40.
10. White DP. Pathogenesis of obstructive and central sleep apnea. Am J Respir Crit Care Med 2005 172:1363–70.
11. Edwards N, Middleton PG, Blyton DM, et al. Sleep disordered breathing and pregnancy. Thorax 2002 57:555–8.
12. Santiago JR, Nolledo MS, Kinzler W, et al. Sleep and sleep disorders in pregnancy. Ann Intern Med 2001 134:396–408.
13. Crapo RO. Normal cardiopulmonary physiology during pregnancy. Clin Obstet Gynecol 1996;39:3–16
14. Garrard GS, Littler WA, Redman CW. Closing volume during normal pregnancy. Thorax 1978;33 488–92.
15. Cugell DW, Frank NR, Gaensler EA, et al. Pulmonary function in pregnancy. I. Serial observations in normal women. Am Rev Tuberc 1953;67:568–97.
16. Mills GH, Chaffe AG. Sleeping positions adopted by pregnant women of more than 30 weeks gestation Anaesthesia 1994;49:249–50.
17. Driver HS, Shapiro CM. A longitudinal study of sleep stages in young women during pregnancy and post partum. Sleep 1992;15:449–53.
18. Popovic RM, White DP. Upper airway muscle activity in normal women: influence of hormonal status J Appl Physiol 1998;84:1055–62.
19. Parisi RA, Santiago TV, Edelman NH. Genioglossal and diaphragmatic EMG responses to hypoxia during sleep. Am Rev Respir Dis 1988;138:610–6.
20. Wheatley JR, White DP. The influence of sleep on pharyngeal reflexes. Sleep 1993;16:S87–9.
21. Stahl ML, Orr WC, Males JL. Progesterone levels and sleep-related breathing during menstrual cycles of normal women. Sleep 1985;8:227–30.
22. Manber R, Kuo TF, Cataldo N, et al. The effects of hormone replacement therapy on sleep-disordered breathing in postmenopausal women: a pilot study Sleep 2003;26:163–8.
23. D'Ambrosio C, Stachenfeld NS, Pisani M, et al. Sleep, breathing, and menopause: the effect of fluctuating estrogen and progesterone on sleep and breathing in women. Gend Med 2005;2:238–45.
24. Bourjeily G, Mohsenin V. Sleep physiology in pregnancy. In: Bourjeily G, Rosene-Montella K, editors Pulmonary problems in pregnancy. New York Humana Press; 2009. p. 37–55.
25. Leung PL, Hui DS, Leung TN, et al. Sleep disturbances in Chinese pregnant women. BJOG 2005 112:1568–71.
26. Maasilta P, Bachour A, Teramo K, et al. Sleep-related disordered breathing during pregnancy in obese women. Chest 2001;120:1448–54.
27. Ursavas A, Karadag M, Nalci N, et al. Self-reported snoring, maternal obesity and neck circumference

as risk factors for pregnancy-induced hypertension and preeclampsia. Respiration 2008;76:33–9.

28. Bourjeily G, Raker CA. Epworth sleepiness score in pregnancy. Toronto: American Thoracic Society International Conference; 2008.

29. Pien GW, Fife D, Pack AI, et al. Changes in symptoms of sleep-disordered breathing during pregnancy. Sleep 2005;28:1299–305.

30. Perez-Chada D, Videla AJ, O'Flaherty ME, et al. Snoring, witnessed sleep apnoeas and pregnancy-induced hypertension. Acta Obstet Gynecol Scand 2007;86:788–92.

31. Champagne K, Schwartzman K, Opatrny L, et al. Obstructive sleep apnoea and its association with gestational hypertension. Eur Respir J 2009;33:559–65.

32. Louis JM, Auckley D, Sokol RJ, et al. Maternal and neonatal morbidities associated with obstructive sleep apnea complicating pregnancy. Am J Obstet Gynecol 2010;202(3):261, e1–5.

33. Jensen GM, Moore LG. The effect of high altitude and other risk factors on birthweight: independent or interactive effects? Am J Public Health 1997;87:1003–7.

34. Miller S, Tudor C, Nyima, et al. Maternal and neonatal outcomes of hospital vaginal deliveries in Tibet. Int J Gynaecol Obstet 2007;98:217–21.

35. Jelic S, Padeletti M, Kawut SM, et al. Inflammation, oxidative stress, and repair capacity of the vascular endothelium in obstructive sleep apnea. Circulation 2008;117:2270–8.

36. Kohler M, Craig S, Nicoll D, et al. Endothelial function and arterial stiffness in minimally symptomatic obstructive sleep apnea. Am J Respir Crit Care Med 2008;178:984–8.

37. Yinon D, Lowenstein L, Suraya S, et al. Pre-eclampsia is associated with sleep-disordered breathing and endothelial dysfunction. Eur Respir J 2006;27:328–33.

38. Koken G, Sahin FK, Cosar E, et al. Oxidative stress markers in pregnant women who snore and fetal outcome: a case control study. Acta Obstet Gynecol Scand 2007;86:1317–21.

39. Connolly G, Razak AR, Hayanga A, et al. Inspiratory flow limitation during sleep in pre-eclampsia: comparison with normal pregnant and nonpregnant women. Eur Respir J 2001;18:672–6.

40. Guilleminault C, Palombini L, Poyares D, et al. Pre-eclampsia and nasal CPAP: Part 1. Early intervention with nasal CPAP in pregnant women with risk-factors for pre-eclampsia: preliminary findings. Sleep Med 2007;9:9–14.

41. Poyares D, Guilleminault C, Hachul H, et al. Pre-eclampsia and nasal CPAP: part 2. Hypertension during pregnancy, chronic snoring, and early nasal CPAP intervention. Sleep Med 2007;9:15–21.

42. Kaaja RJ, Greer IA. Manifestations of chronic disease during pregnancy. JAMA 2005;294:2751–7.

43. Joo S, Lee S, Choi HA, et al. Habitual snoring is associated with elevated hemoglobin A1c levels in non-obese middle-aged adults. J Sleep Res 2006;15:437–44.

44. Foster G, Borradaile K, MH S, et al. A randomized study on the effect of weight loss on obstructive sleep apnea among obese patients with type 2 diabetes: the Sleep AHEAD study. Arch Intern Med 2009;169:1619–26.

45. Theorell-Haglow J, Berne C, Janson C, et al. Obstructive sleep apnoea is associated with decreased insulin sensitivity in females. Eur Respir J 2008;31:1054–60.

46. Matthews DR, Hosker JP, Rudenski AS, et al. Homeostasis model assessment: insulin resistance and beta-cell function from fasting plasma glucose and insulin concentrations in man. Diabetologia 1985;28:412–9.

47. Otake K, Sasanabe R, Hasegawa R, et al. Glucose intolerance in Japanese patients with obstructive sleep apnea. Intern Med 2009;48:1863–8.

48. Peled N, Kassirer M, Shitrit D, et al. The association of OSA with insulin resistance, inflammation and metabolic syndrome. Respir Med 2007;101:1696–701.

49. Punjabi NM, Beamer BA. Alterations in glucose disposal in sleep-disordered breathing. Am J Respir Crit Care Med 2009;179:235–40.

50. Bellamy L, Casas JP, Hingorani AD, et al. Type 2 diabetes mellitus after gestational diabetes: a systematic review and meta-analysis. Lancet 2009;373:1773–9.

51. Evans ML, Dick MJ, Clark AS. Sleep during the week before labor: relationships to labor outcomes. Clin Nurs Res 1995;4:238–49.

52. Lee KA, Gay CL. Sleep in late pregnancy predicts length of labor and type of delivery. Am J Obstet Gynecol 2004;191:2041–6.

53. Olivarez SA, Maheshwari B, McCarthy M, et al. Prospective trial on obstructive sleep apnea in pregnancy and fetal heart rate monitoring. Am J Obstet Gynecol 2010;202(6):552, e1–7.

54. Loube DI, Poceta JS, Morales MC, et al. Self-reported snoring in pregnancy. Association with fetal outcome. Chest 1996;109:885–9.

55. Sahin FK, Koken G, Cosar E, et al. Obstructive sleep apnea in pregnancy and fetal outcome. Int J Gynaecol Obstet 2008;100:141–6.

56. Joel-Cohen SJ, Schoenfeld A. Fetal response to periodic sleep apnea: a new syndrome in obstetrics. Eur J Obstet Gynecol Reprod Biol 1978;8:77–81.

57. Yin TT, Williams N, Burton C, et al. Hypertension, fetal growth restriction and obstructive sleep apnoea in pregnancy. Eur J Obstet Gynecol Reprod Biol 2008;141:35–8.

58. Gozal D, Reeves SR, Row BW, et al. Respiratory effects of gestational intermittent hypoxia in the

developing rat. Am J Respir Crit Care Med 2003; 167:1540–7.

59. Charbonneau M, Falcone T, Cosio MG, et al. Obstructive sleep apnea during pregnancy. Therapy and implications for fetal health. Am Rev Respir Dis 1991;144:461–3.

60. Roush SF, Bell L. Obstructive sleep apnea in pregnancy. J Am Board Fam Pract 2004;17:292–4.

61. Netzer NC, Stoohs RA, Netzer CM, et al. Using the Berlin Questionnaire to identify patients at risk for the sleep apnea syndrome. Ann Intern Med 1999; 131:485–91.

62. Ramachandran SK, Kheterpal S, Consens F, et al. Derivation and validation of a simple perioperative sleep apnea prediction score. Anesth Analg 2010; 110:1007–15.

63. Lee KA, Zaffke ME, McEnany G. Parity and sleep patterns during and after pregnancy. Obstet Gynecol 2000;95:14–8.

64. Nikkola E, Ekblad U, Ekholm E, et al. Sleep in multiple pregnancy: breathing patterns, oxygenation, and periodic leg movements. Am J Obstet Gynecol 1996;174:1622–5.

65. Trakada G, Tsapanos V, Spiropoulos K. Normal pregnancy and oxygenation during sleep. Eur J Obstet Gynecol Reprod Biol 2003;109:128–32.

66. Bourne T, Ogilvy AJ, Vickers R, et al. Nocturnal hypoxaemia in late pregnancy. Br J Anaesth 1995;75: 678–82.

67. Feinsilver SH, Hertz G. Respiration during sleep in pregnancy. Clin Chest Med 1992;13:637–44.

68. Lyons HA. Centrally acting hormones and respiration. Pharmacol Ther B 1976;2:743–51.

69. White DP, Douglas NJ, Pickett CK, et al. Sexual influence on the control of breathing. J Appl Physiol 1983;54:874–9.

70. Javaheri S. A mechanism of central sleep apnea in patients with heart failure. N Engl J Med 1999;341: 949–54.

71. Alaily AB, Carrol KB. Pulmonary ventilation in pregnancy. Br J Obstet Gynaecol 1978;85:518–24.

72. Norregaard O, Schultz P, Ostergaard A, et al. Lung function and postural changes during pregnancy. Respir Med 1989;83:467–70.

73. Ang CK, Tan TH, Walters WA, et al. Postural influence on maternal capillary oxygen and carbon dioxide tension. Br Med J 1969;4:201–3.

74. Hunter S, Robson SC. Adaptation of the maternal heart in pregnancy. Br Heart J 1992;68:540–3.

75. Katz VL. Physiologic changes during normal pregnancy. Curr Opin Obstet Gynecol 1991;3: 750–8.

76. Pirhonen JP, Erkkola RU. Uterine and umbilical flow velocity waveforms in the supine hypotensive syndrome. Obstet Gynecol 1990;76:176–9.

77. Edwards N, Blyton DM, Kirjavainen TT, et al. Hemodynamic responses to obstructive respiratory events during sleep are augmented in women with preeclampsia. Am J Hypertens 2001;14:1090–5.

78. Edwards N, Blyton DM, Hennessy A, et al. Severity of sleep-disordered breathing improves following parturition. Sleep 2005;28:737–41.

79. Archer GW Jr, Marx GF. Arterial oxygen tension during apnoea in parturient women. Br J Anaesth 1974;46:358–60.

80. Cheun JK, Choi KT. Arterial oxygen desaturation rate following obstructive apnea in parturients. J Korean Med Sci 1992;7:6–10.

81. D'Ambrosio C, Bowman T, Mohsenin V. Quality of life in patients with obstructive sleep apnea: effect of nasal continuous positive airway pressure a prospective study. Chest 1999;115:123–9.

82. Gay P, Weaver T, Loube D, et al. Evaluation of positive airway pressure treatment for sleep related breathing disorders in adults. Sleep 2006 29:381–401.

83. Giles TL, Lasserson TJ, Smith BJ, et al. Continuous positive airways pressure for obstructive sleep apnoea in adults. Cochrane Database Syst Rev 2006;3:CD001106.

84. Patel SR, White DP, Malhotra A, et al. Continuous positive airway pressure therapy for treating sleepiness in a diverse population with obstructive sleep apnea: results of a meta-analysis. Arch Intern Med 2003;163:565–71.

85. Sullivan CE, Issa FG, Berthon-Jones M, et al. Reversal of obstructive sleep apnoea by continuous positive airway pressure applied through the nares. Lancet 1981;1:862–5.

86. Marin JM, Carrizo SJ, Vicente E, et al. Long-term cardiovascular outcomes in men with obstructive sleep apnoea-hypopnoea with or without treatment with continuous positive airway pressure: an observational study. Lancet 2005;365:1046–53.

87. Shah NA, Yaggi HK, Concato J, et al. Obstructive sleep apnea as a risk factor for coronary events or cardiovascular death. Sleep Breath 2010;14:131–6.

88. Yaggi HK, Concato J, Kernan WN, et al. Obstructive sleep apnea as a risk factor for stroke and death. N Engl J Med 2005;353:2034–41.

89. Bahammam A, Delaive K, Ronald J, et al. Health care utilization in males with obstructive sleep apnea syndrome two years after diagnosis and treatment. Sleep 1999;22:740–7.

90. Kapur VK, Alfonso-Cristancho R. Just a good deal or truly a steal? Medical cost savings and the impact on the cost-effectiveness of treating sleep apnea. Sleep 2009;32:135–6.

91. Centers for Medicare & Medicaid Services (CMS), Department of Health and Human Services. Continuous positive airway pressure (CPAP) therapy for obstructive sleep apnea (OSA). 2005. Available at http://www.cms.gov/Transmittals/downloads/R35NCD pdf. Accessed July 30, 2010.

92. Edwards N, Blyton DM, Kirjavainen T, et al. Nasal continuous positive airway pressure reduces sleep-induced blood pressure increments in preeclampsia. Am J Respir Crit Care Med 2000; 162:252–7.

93. Tuomilehto H, Peltonen M, Partinen M, et al. Sleep duration, lifestyle intervention, and incidence of type 2 diabetes in impaired glucose tolerance: the Finnish Diabetes Prevention study. Diabetes Care 2009;32:1965–71.

94. Bourjeily G. Sleep disorders in pregnancy. Obstet Med 2009;2:100–6.

95. Blyton DM, Sullivan CE, Edwards N. Reduced nocturnal cardiac output associated with preeclampsia is minimized with the use of nocturnal nasal CPAP. Sleep 2004;27:79–84.

96. Mehta A, Qian J, Petocz P, et al. A randomized, controlled study of a mandibular advancement splint for obstructive sleep apnea. Am J Respir Crit Care Med 2001;163:1457–61.

97. Ayrim A, Keskin EA, Ozol D, et al. Influence of self-reported snoring and witnessed sleep apnea on gestational hypertension and fetal outcome in pregnancy. Arch Gynecol Obstet 2009. [Epub ahead of print].

Index

Note: Page numbers of article titles are in **boldface** type.

A

Abdomen, diagnostic/therapeutic radiation of, in women of reproductive age, 40

Acute renal failure, in critically ill obstetric patients, management principles, 58–59

Addiction, tobacco, among offspring of women who smoke during pregnancy, 81

Airway(s)
    pregnancy effects on, 61–63
    upper, pregnancy effects on, 1–2

Airway resistance/conductance, pregnancy effects on, 4–5

Anesthesia/anesthetics, during labor and delivery, pulmonary hypertension management during, 170

Antibiotic(s)
    during pregnancy, in women with cystic fibrosis, 114
    for bacterial/atypical pathogen pneumonia, during pregnancy, 125–126

Anticytoplasmic antibody–associated granulomatosis necrotizing systemic vasculitis, ILDs in pregnancy and, 137

Antimicrobial agents. See *Antibiotic(s)*.

Antithrombic agents, in pulmonary hypertension management during pregnancy, 171–172

Anxiety, asthma in pregnancy and, 102

Arthritis, rheumatoid, ILDs in pregnancy and, 134–135

Aspiration, bacterial/atypical pathogen pneumonia in pregnancy and, 126

Asthma, during pregnancy, **93–110**
    anxiety and, 102
    changes related to, 93–94
        congenital malformations, 99
        long-term changes into childhood, 100
        maternal and infant, 95–100
        mechanisms for, 95
        medical intervention during labor and delivery, 97
        poor neonatal outcomes, 97–98
    depression and, 102
    exacerbations of, risk factors for, 94–95
    management of
        approaches to, 104–105
        barriers to, 100–102
        exacerbations treatment, 103–104
        medications in, 100–101
        safety level of treatments, 102–103
    neonatal complications related to, 100
    perinatal mortality effects of, 98–99
    prevalence of, 93
    smoking with, 101–102

Attention-deficit disorder/hyperactivity, smoking during pregnancy and, 80

B

Bacterial/atypical pathogen pneumonia, in pregnancy, 124–126
    antimicrobial therapy in, 125–126
    aspiration prevention in, 126
    clinical findings in, 124
    diagnostic testing in, 125
    severity of, 124–125
    supportive care in, 126

Behavior, smoking during pregnancy and, 79–81

Behavior modification, in sleep-disordered breathing management during pregnancy, 185

Birth, preterm, sleep-disordered breathing in pregnancy and, 180

Blood, fetal, PO_2 of, 15–16

Blood volume, pregnancy effects on, 8

Breathing, sleep-disordered, in pregnancy, **175–189.** See also *Sleep-disordered breathing, in pregnancy.*

Bronchiolitis, respiratory, ILDs related to, in pregnancy, 140

Bronchoscopic procedures, during pregnancy
    indications for, 64
    risks associated with, 67

C

Cardiac output, pregnancy effects on, 8

Cardiomyopathy(ies), peripartum, in critically ill obstetric patients, management principles, 57

Cardiopulmonary resuscitation, in pregnancy, 57

Cardiovascular system
    dysfunction of, in critically ill obstetric patients, 56–58
        cardiopulmonary resuscitation in pregnancy, 57
        hypertensive crisis, 57
        management principles, 56–58
            shock, 56–57
        perimortem cesarean delivery, 57–58
        peripartum cardiomyopathy, 57

Clin Chest Med 32 (2011) 191–197
doi:10.1016/S0272-5231(11)00009-8
0272-5231/11/$ – see front matter © 2011 Elsevier Inc. All rights reserved.

chestmed.theclinics.com

Cardiovascular (*continued*)
    labor and delivery effects on, 9–10
    pregnancy effects on, 7–8
Cesarean delivery, perimortem, in critically ill
    patients, 57–58
Chest radiography, in VTE assessment in
    pregnancy, 150
Chest wall, pregnancy effects on, 2
Childhood, long-term changes into, maternal
    asthma resulting in, 100
Choriocarcinoma, in pregnancy, 141
Churg-Strauss syndrome, ILDs in pregnancy and,
    137–138
Closing volume, pregnancy effects on, 5
Cognition, smoking during pregnancy and, 79–81
Compression ultrasonography, in VTE assessment
    in pregnancy, 151–152
Conception
    delayed, smoking during pregnancy and, 78
    iatrogenic ILDs effects on, 133–134
Conception counseling, pulmonary
    hypertension–related, 169
Congenital malformations, asthma during
    pregnancy and, 99
Connective tissue diseases, ILDs in pregnancy
    and, 134–137
Contrast media, in VTE assessment in pregnancy,
    151
Counseling
    conception, pulmonary hypertension–related, 169
    for smoking cessation during pregnancy, 86
Critical illness, in obstetric patients, management
    principles, **53–60.** See also specific illness and
    Obstetric patients, critically ill.
Cryptogenic organizing pneumonia,
    in pregnancy, 140
Cystic fibrosis
    described, 111
    fertility effects of, 111–113
        in men, 111
        in women, 112–113
    pregnancy in, **111–120**
        birth outcomes, 117
        diabetes mellitus and, 116–117
        following lung transplantation, 118
        genetic screening for, 113
        maternal lung function effects of, 115–116
        medication use during pregnancy, 113–115
        mortality data, 115–116
        nutrition and, 116–117
        obstetric and postpartum considerations,
            117–118

D

Deep venous thrombosis (DVT), in pregnancy,
    147–148

Depression, asthma in pregnancy and, 102
Dermatomyositis, ILDs in pregnancy and, 136–137
Diabetes, gestational, sleep-disordered breathing
    in pregnancy and, 177, 180
Diabetes mellitus, cystic fibrosis in pregnancy
    and, 116–117
Diffusing capacity
    in high-altitude pregnancy, 23
    pregnancy effects on, 5
Drug(s), during pregnancy
    in pulmonary procedures, 65–67
    lung disease related to, 140
DVT. See *Deep venous thrombosis (DVT).*

E

Edema, pulmonary, in pregnancy, 141–142
Embryo, radiation risks to, 37–39
Eosinophilic pneumonias, in pregnancy, 140
Exercise physiology, in pregnancy, 8–9

F

Fat soluble vitamins, during pregnancy in women
    with cystic fibrosis, 114
Fertility, cystic fibrosis effects on, 111–113
Fetal blood, PO_2 of, 15–16
Fetal heart rate response, sleep-disordered
    breathing in pregnancy and, 181
Fetus(es)
    high altitude effects on, highland ancestry and,
        26–28
    oxygenation of, **15–19**
        maternal ventilation and, 17–18
        sleep-disordered breathing in pregnancy effects
        on, 180–181
Fluoroscopy, during pregnancy, 68
Fungal pneumonia, in pregnancy, 129–130

G

Gas exchange, pregnancy effects on, 5–7
Genetic(s), cystic fibrosis in pregnancy related to,
    screening for, 113
Gestational age, small for, smoking during
    pregnancy and, 78–79
Gestational diabetes, sleep-disordered breathing
    in pregnancy and, 177, 180
Gestational hypertensive disorders, sleep-disordered
    breathing in pregnancy and, 176–177
Granulomatosis necrotizing systemic vasculitis,
    anticytoplasmic antibody–associated, ILDs in
    pregnancy and, 137
Growth restriction, sleep-disordered breathing in
    pregnancy and, 180–181

H

Hematologic considerations, in high-altitude pregnancy, 23
Heparin(s), in peripartum pulmonary embolism management, 153–155
High altitude, during pregnancy, **21–31**
    fetal growth effects of, highland ancestry and, 26–28
    influence of, 22–23
    maternal arterial oxygenation determinants related to, 23–26
    oxygen transport related to, 26
    physiologic compensations related to, 23–26
High-altitude hypoxia, challenge of, 21–22
HIV infection, pneumonia complicating, in pregnancy, 130
Hypertension
    pulmonary. See Pulmonary hypertension.
    pulmonary arterial. See Pulmonary arterial hypertension (PAH).
Hypertensive crisis, in critically ill obstetric patients, management principles of, 57
Hypoxia, high-altitude, challenge of, 21–22

I

Idiopathic interstitial pneumonias, in pregnancy, 140
Idiopathic pulmonary fibrosis, in pregnancy, 140
ILDs. See Infiltrative lung diseases (ILDs).
Infertility, smoking during pregnancy and, 78
Infiltrative lung diseases (ILDs)
    iatrogenic, and conception, 133–134
    in pregnancy, **133–146**
        choriocarcinoma, 141
        connective tissue disease–associated, 134–137
            dermatomyositis, 136–137
            polymyositis, 136–137
            rheumatoid arthritis, 134–135
            SLE, 135–136
            systemic sclerosis, 136
        drug-induced lung disease, 140
        eosinophilic pneumonias, 140
        idiopathic interstitial pneumonias, 140
        LAM, 139–140
        pulmonary alveolar lipoproteinosis, 140–141
        pulmonary edema, 141–142
        pulmonary LCH, 141
        pulmonary lymphangitic carcinomatosis, 141
        pulmonary vasculitis, 137–138
        sarcoidosis, 138–139
    respiratory bronchiolitis–associated, in pregnancy, 140
Influenza virus, in pregnancy, 127–128
Interstitial pneumonia, idiopathic, in pregnancy, 140

Interventional chest procedures, during pregnancy, **61–74.** See also Pregnancy, interventional chest procedures during.
Ionizing radiation, exposure to, by pregnant women, reproductive and developmental risks of, 34

L

Labor and delivery
    cardiovascular physiology in, 9–10
    medical intervention during, asthma during pregnancy and, 97
    pulmonary embolism during, management of, 156
    pulmonary hypertension management during, 170
    respiratory physiology in, 9
Lactation, pharmacotherapy during, **43–52**
LAM. See Lymphangioleiomomatosis (LAM).
Langerhans cell histiocytosis (LCH), pulmonary, in pregnancy, 141
LCH. See Langerhans cell histiocytosis (LCH).
Lipoproteinosis, pulmonary alveolar, in pregnancy, 140–141
Low birth weight, smoking during pregnancy and, 78–79
Lung disease(s)
    drug-induced, in pregnancy, 140
    during pregnancy, symptoms of, 63
Lung function
    maternal, cystic fibrosis in pregnancy and, 115–116
    pregnancy effects on, 2–5, 61–63
    smoking during pregnancy effects on, 82
Lung transplantation, cystic fibrosis–related, pregnancy following, 118
Lymphangioleiomomatosis (LAM), in pregnancy, 139–140

M

Magnetic resonance imaging (MRI), in VTE assessment in pregnancy, 152
Maternal arterial oxygenation, determinants of, in high-altitude pregnancy, 23–26
Maternal ventilation, **15–19**
    in fetal oxygenation, 17–18
MDCT–PA. See Multidetector computed tomography–pulmonary angiography (MDCT–PA).
Microscopic polyangiitis, ILDs in pregnancy and, 138
MRI. See Magnetic resonance imaging (MRI).
Mucolytic(s), during pregnancy, in women with cystic fibrosis, 114
Multidetector computed tomography–pulmonary angiography (MDCT–PA), in VTE assessment in pregnancy, 150

N

Neonate(s), asthma during pregnancy effects on, 100
Neurotransmitter(s), nicotine effects on, 79–80
Nicotine, neurotransmitters effects of, 79–80
Nutrition, cystic fibrosis in pregnancy and, 116–117

O

Obstetric patients, critically ill, management
    principles, **53–60.** See also Pregnancy, critical
    illness in; *specific conditions/disorders, e.g.,*
    Cardiovascular system, dysfunction of, in critically
    ill obstetric patients.
    acute renal failure, 58–59
    cardiovascular dysfunction, 56–58
    critically ill parturients, 54–56
    during pregnancy, 53–54
    respiratory failure, 58–59
Obstructive sleep apnea (OSA)–specific therapy, in
    sleep-disordered breathing management, in
    pregnancy, 185
OSA. See *Obstructive sleep apnea (OSA).*
Oxygen transport, in high-altitude pregnancy, 26

P

PAH. See *Pulmonary arterial hypertension (PAH).*
Pancreatic enzyme replacement therapy, during
    pregnancy, in women with cystic fibrosis, 114
Parturient(s), critically ill, management principles,
    54–56
    airway, 54–55
    breathing, 55
    circulation, 55
    maternal and fetal evaluation, 55–56
Perimortem cesarean delivery, in critically ill patients,
    57–58
Perinatal mortality, asthma during pregnancy and,
    98–99
Peripartum cardiomyopathy, in critically ill obstetric
    patients, management principles, 57
Peripartum pulmonary embolism, **147–164**
    diagnosis of, approach to, 153
    management of, 153–159
        duration of therapy in, 156
        heparins in, 153–155
        thrombolysis therapy in, 155–156
    prevention of, 156–159
Pharmacotherapy
    during lactation, **43–52**
        key principles in, 46–51
    during pregnancy, **43–52**
        for smoking cessation, 86–87
        key principles in, 43–46
        pulmonary medications, 48–50
Pleural disease, during pregnancy, 69–71

Pneumonia(s). See also specific types.
    in pregnancy, **121–132.** See also specific types.
        bacterial/atypical pathogen pneumonia,
            124–126
        causes of, 122–124
        cryptogenic organizing, 140
        described, 121–122
        eosinophilic, 140
        fungal, 129–130
        HIV infection complicated by, 130
        idiopathic interstitial, 140
        varicella, 128–129
        viral, 127–129
Pneumothorax, during pregnancy, 71
PO$_2$ of fetal blood, 15–16
Polyangiitis, microscopic, ILDs in pregnancy and, 13
Polymyositis, ILDs in pregnancy and, 136–137
Polysomnography, in sleep-disordered breathing
    assessment, in pregnancy, 181–184
Postpartum
    cardiovascular physiology, 9–10
    respiratory physiology, 9
Pregnancy. See also *Labor and delivery.*
    airway changes during, 61–63
    asthma during, **93–110.** See also *Asthma, during*
        pregnancy.
    bronchoscopic procedures during
        indications for, 64
        risks associated with, 67
    cardiovascular changes during, 7–8
    chest wall changes during, 2
    critical illness in
        management principles
            cardiopulmonary resuscitation, 57
            perimortem cesarean delivery, 57–58
        obstetric vs. nonobstetric disorders, 54
        parturient, 54–56
        prevalence of, 53
        prognosis of, 53–54
    critically illness in, 53–54
    diagnostic radiological studies/radiation therapy
        during, reproductive risks associated with
        carcinogenic effects, 40
        case report, 39
        described, 33–34
        embryonic risks, 37–39
        evaluation of, 34–37
        importance of determining pregnancy status,
            41
        patient evaluation, 39–40
        pulmonologist's role in, **33–42**
        scheduling of examination, 40–41
    exercise physiology in, 8–9
    gas exchange during, 5–7
    hemodynamic effects of, 63
    high altitude during, **21–31.** See also *High altitude*
        during pregnancy.

ILDs in, **133–146.** See also *Infiltrative lung diseases (ILDs), in pregnancy.*

in cystic fibrosis, **111–120.** See also *Cystic fibrosis, pregnancy in.*

influenza virus during, 127–128

interventional chest procedures during, **61–74**

   bronchoscopic procedures

      indications for, 64

      risks associated with, 67

   described, 61

   diagnostic tools in, 67–68

   fluoroscopy, 68

   medications in, 65–67

   pleural disease–related, 69–71

   pneumothorax, 71

   pulmonary procedures, 64–65

   special issues related to, 67–69

   therapeutic tools, 69

lung disease during, symptoms of, 63

lung function during, 2–5, 61–63

   airway resistance/conductance, 4–5

   spirometry, 4

   static, 2–4

muscle function during, 2

pharmacotherapy during, **43–52.** See also *Pharmacotherapy, during pregnancy.*

pneumonia complicating, **121–132.** See also *Pneumonia(s), in pregnancy.*

pulmonary hypertension and, **165–174.** See also *Pulmonary hypertension, pregnancy and.*

pulmonary response to, 63

respiratory mechanics in, 133

respiratory physiology in, **1–13,** 133

   closing volume, 5

   diffusing capacity, 5

sleep-disordered breathing in, **175–189.** See also *Sleep-disordered breathing, in pregnancy.*

smoking cessation during, **75–91.** See also *Smoking cessation, during pregnancy.*

smoking during, **75–91.** See also *Smoking, during pregnancy.*

upper airway changes in, 1–2

ventilation during, 5–7

VTE in, **147–164.** See also *Venous thromboembolism (VTE).*

Pregnant women, ionizing radiation exposure during, reproductive and developmental risks of exposures of, 34

Preterm birth, sleep-disordered breathing in pregnancy and, 180

Pulmonary alveolar lipoproteinosis, in pregnancy, 140–141

Pulmonary arterial hypertension (PAH). See also *Pulmonary hypertension.*

   classification of, 166

   described, 165

Pulmonary edema, in pregnancy, 141–142

Pulmonary embolism, peripartum, **147–164.** See also *Peripartum pulmonary embolism.*

Pulmonary hypertension

   classification of, 166

   conception counseling related to, 169

   described, 165

   pregnancy and, **165–174**

      classification of, 166

      described, 168–169

      diagnosis and screening for, 166–167

      management of, 169–172

         antithrombic therapy in, 171–172

         during delivery and anesthesia, 170

         medical therapy in, 170–171

         monitoring in, 170

      mortality data, 167–168

      outcomes related to, 167–168

      physiology of, 165–166

Pulmonary lymphangitic carcinomatosis, in pregnancy, 141

Pulmonary procedures, during pregnancy, 64–65

Pulmonary system, pregnancy effects on, 63

Pulmonary vascular system, pregnancy effects on, 8–9

Pulmonary vasculitis, ILDs in pregnancy and, 137–138

R

Race, as factor in VTE, 147

Radiation exposure

   carcinogenic effects, 40

   in VTE assessment in pregnancy, 151

   ionizing radiation, by pregnant women, reproductive and developmental risks of, 34

Radiation therapy, in pregnant women, pulmonologist's role in, **33–42.** See also *Pregnant women, diagnostic risk of diagnostic radiological studies/radiation therapy in, pulmonologist's role in.*

Radiography, chest, in VTE assessment in pregnancy, 150

Radiological studies, in pregnant women. See also *Pregnant women, diagnostic radiological studies/radiation therapy in, reproductive risks associated with.*

   pulmonologist's role in, **33–42**

Renal failure, acute, in critically ill obstetric patients, management principles, 58–59

Reproductive age, women of

   diagnostic/therapeutic abdomen radiation in, 40

   smoking among, 75

Respiratory bronchiolitis, ILDs related to, in pregnancy, 140

Respiratory failure, in critically ill obstetric patients, management principles, 58–59

Respiratory function
  in high-altitude pregnancy, 23, 26
  pregnancy effects on, 2
Respiratory illness, smoking during pregnancy
    and, 82
Respiratory physiology
  postpartum, 9
  pregnancy effects on, **1–13,** 133
Respiratory system
  labor and delivery effects on, 9
  pregnancy effects on, **1–13.** See also *Pregnancy.*
Resuscitation, cardiopulmonary, in pregnancy, 57
Rheumatoid arthritis, ILDs in pregnancy and,
    134–135

S

Sarcoidosis, in pregnancy, 138–139
Shock, in critically ill obstetric patients, management
    principles, 56–57
SIDS. See *Sudden infant death syndrome (SIDS).*
SLE. See *Systemic lupus erythematosus (SLE).*
Sleep-disordered breathing, in pregnancy, **175–189**
  delivery mode effects of, 180
  diagnosis of, 181–184
  epidemiology of, 176
  factors predisposing to, 175–176
  factors protecting against, 176
  fetal outcomes of, 180–181
  gestational diabetes due to, 177, 180
  gestational hypertensive disorders due to,
    176–177
  maternal outcomes of, 176–180
  screening for, 185–186
  treatment of, 184–185
    behavior modification in, 185
    indications for, 184–185
    OSA–specific therapy in, 185
Small for gestational age, smoking during pregnancy
    and, 78–79
Smoking
  among women of reproductive age, 75
  during pregnancy, **75–91**
    adverse effects of
      attention-deficit disorder/hyperactivity, 80
      behavior-related, 79–81
      cognitive impairments, 79–81
      delayed conception, 78
      infertility, 78
      low birth weight, 78–79
      maternal, fetal, and offspring, 77–82
      overweight child, 81
      respiratory illness and lung function, 82
      SIDS, 79
      small for gestational age, 78–79
      tobacco addiction among offspring, 81

complications related to, 78
epidemiology of, 75–77
factors associated with, 76–77
in women with asthma, 101–102
international trends in, 76
US trends in, 75–76
Smoking cessation, during pregnancy, 77, 82–87
  approach to, 86
  counseling related to, 86
  epidemiology of, 75–77
  pharmacologic therapies in, 86–87
  self-help materials for, 86
  timing of, 83, 86
Spirometry, pregnancy effects on, 4
Sudden infant death syndrome (SIDS), smoking
    during pregnancy and, 79
Sulfonylurea(s), during pregnancy, in women with
    cystic fibrosis, 114
Systemic lupus erythematosus (SLE), ILDs in
    pregnancy and, 135–136
Systemic sclerosis, ILDs in pregnancy and, 136

T

Thiazolidinedione(s), during pregnancy, in women
    with cystic fibrosis, 114–115
Thromboembolism, venous, **147–164.** See also
    Venous thromboembolism (VTE).
Thrombolysis therapy, in peripartum pulmonary
    embolism management, 155–156
Transplacental exchange, venous equilibration
    model of, 16–17
Transplantation(s), lung, cystic fibrosis–related,
    pregnancy following, 118

U

Ultrasonography, compression, in VTE assessment
    in pregnancy, 151–152
Upper airways, pregnancy effects on, 1–2

V

Varicella pneumonia, in pregnancy, 128–129
Vascular system, pulmonary, pregnancy effects on,
    8–9
Vasculitis, pulmonary, ILDs in pregnancy and,
    137–138
Venous equilibration model of transplacental
    exchange, 16–17
Venous thromboembolism (VTE)
  described, 147
  epidemiology of, 147–148
  in pregnancy, **147–164**
    clinical presentation of, 149

diagnosis of, 149–152
   DVT, 147–148
   pathophysiology of, 148
   prognosis of, 152–153
   risk factors for, 148–149
  incidence of, 147
  mortality data, 147
  race as factor in, 147
Venous thrombosis, deep. See *Deep venous thrombosis (DVT)*.
Ventilation
  in high-altitude pregnancy, 23
  maternal, **15–19**
   in fetal oxygenation, 17–18
  pregnancy effects on, 5–7

Ventilation perfusion scan, in VTE assessment in pregnancy, 150
Viral pneumonia, in pregnancy, 126
Vitamin(s), fat soluble, during pregnancy in women with cystic fibrosis, 114
VTE. See *Venous thromboembolism (VTE)*.

W

Women
  cystic fibrosis in, fertility effects of, 112–113
  of reproductive age
   diagnostic/therapeutic abdominal radiation in, 40
   smoking among, 75

Moving?

Make sure your subscription moves with you!

To notify us of your new address, find your **Clinics Account Number** (located on your mailing label above your name), and contact customer service at:

Email: **journalscustomerservice-usa@elsevier.com**

800-654-2452 (subscribers in the U.S. & Canada)
314-447-8871 (subscribers outside of the U.S. & Canada)

Fax number: **314-447-8029**

Elsevier Health Sciences Division
Subscription Customer Service
3251 Riverport Lane
Maryland Heights, MO 63043

*To ensure uninterrupted delivery of your subscription, please notify us at least 4 weeks in advance of move.